THROMBOLYTIC THERAPY FOR STROKE

Thrombolytic Therapy for Stroke

Edited by

Patrick D. Lyden, MD

UCSD Stroke Center
San Diego, CA

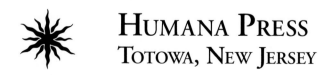

Humana Press
Totowa, New Jersey

© 2001 Humana Press Inc.
999 Riverview Drive, Suite 208
Totowa, New Jersey 07512

For additional copies, pricing for bulk purchases, and/or information about other Humana titles, contact Humana at the above address or at any of the following numbers: Tel.: 973-256-1699; Fax: 973-256-8341; E-mail: humana@humanapr.com

This publication is printed on acid-free paper. ∞
ANSI Z39.48-1984 (American Standards Institute) Permanence of Paper for Printed Library Materials.

Cover design by Patricia F. Cleary.

Printed in the United States of America.   10 9 8 7 6 5 4 3 2 1

Library of Congress Cataloging-in-Publication Data

Thrombolytic therapy for stroke/edited by Patrick D. Lyden.
     p. cm.
    Includes bibliographical references and index.
    ISBN 0-89603-746-0 (alk. paper)
    1. Cerebrovascular disease—Chemotherapy. 2. Thrombolytic therapy I. Lyden, Patrick D.
    [DNLM: 1. Cerebrovascular Accident—drug therapy. 2. Thrombolytic therapy. WL
355 T5307 2001]
RC388.5.T477 2001
616.8'1—dc21
DNLM/DLC
for Library of Congress   00-044910
                                           CIP

This book is dedicated to our families, who daily cope with the vagaries, inconveniences, and turmoil surrounding our involvement in a Stroke Team. It is also dedicated to the patients who volunteered to participate in the placebo-controlled trials of thrombolytic stroke therapy: a more courageous and selfless group act, on such a scale, may not be seen again in medical research.

PREFACE

Thrombolytic Therapy for Stroke is intended for physicians who will be treating patients in the first few hours after stroke: neurologists, neurosurgeons, emergency medicine physicians, internists, and radiologists. In some areas, family medicine general practice physicians may provide the majority of acute stroke care. We will provide the reader with all the data necessary to understand the utility and limitations of thrombolytic therapy. By reading the protocols, and working through the case tutorials, the reader will become sufficiently familiar with the indications and contraindications of thrombolytic therapy to begin evaluating potential patients. Although nothing can replace direct instruction by more experienced physicians, we hope that by imparting our accumulated knowledge we may guide those physicians who cannot attend a "hands-on" workshop, or who, having heard the appropriate lectures, feel the need for further guidance.

We will review the scientific rationale for thrombolysis: first, most ischemic stroke is caused by thrombo-emboli; second, a portion of brain, the penumbra, remains salvageable for a few hours after vascular occlusion; and third, promptly delivered thrombolysis can remove the offending occlusion and restore cerebral blood flow to the penumbra in time to salvage brain and neurologic function. Then we will review the preclinical development of thrombolytics for stroke patients and the early pilot trials. Next, we will present the pivotal clinical trials that demonstrated the efficacy and safety of thrombolysis. Then we will describe the treatment protocol for treating patients: field triage and management, Emergency Department therapy, brain imaging, clinical decision making and patient selection, drug administration, post thrombolysis management and treatment of complications. In the final section of the book, we will demonstrate the use of the protocol using a series of real patient case histories.

Since most medical books are "out of date" when published, we do not include extensive literature on topics that are controversial or in development. Rather, we have assembled the essential papers and protocols that are well accepted and will stand the test of time. We intend this guide to be useful as a starting point, and as a ready reference for the clinician encountering a novel or unusual case.

We recognize that thrombolytic therapy was viewed with some skepticism until recently. In 1999 and early 2000, however, the tide seemed to turn in favor of thrombolysis, despite its risks. One of the prominent early critics, Dr. Lou Caplan, graciously agreed to summarize his arguments against thrombolytic stroke therapy as a chapter in this book (Chapter 13). Together with a rebuttal, this point–counterpoint leads off Section 3. We think the reader will benefit from hearing both sides of the debate. Dr. Caplan points out, however, he is no longer opposed to thrombolytic therapy, having personally treated several patients. He does continue to suggest that patients undergo vascular imaging prior to treatment. On this, and on all other issues raised in this book, we have tried to present multiple viewpoints, supported by data, to allow the reader to decide independently.

   We are hopeful that you will find *Thrombolytic Therapy for Stroke* useful and entertaining. It is brief, because time is precious, and our message is simple. We look forward to a future in which more stroke victims enjoy the benefits of thrombolytic stroke therapy, and are returned to a productive, independent life.

Patrick D. Lyden, MD

ACKNOWLEDGMENTS

Editing a multiauthored book is a harrowing and gratifying experience, one that would be impossible without the able and noble efforts of others. I am grateful to the authors for diligently writing and revising their work. Without the expert and tireless assistance of Alyssa Chardi and Tony Di Lullo, I could never have begun, let alone finished this work. My special thanks go to Dr. Steven Levine, for graciously contributing several case tutorials, and to Dr. Justin Zivin, for years of mentoring. The nurses on staff at the UCSD Stroke Center, phenomenally dedicated to stroke research and patient care, include Nancy Kelly, Janet Werner, and Teri McClean, all of whom helped collect cases for the tutorial section. I most especially recognize my colleague in managing our thrombolytic trials, Karen Rapp, a nurse and clinical researcher of the highest caliber, motivation, and compassion. Finally, my deepest gratitude goes to my colleague, partner, and companion, Dr. Cristy Jackson, sine qua non at work and at home, and our children Jessica, Hannah, and Hillary.

CONTENTS

Dedication v

Preface vii

Acknowledgments ix

Contributors xiii

PART I BACKGROUND AND BASIC INVESTIGATIONS

1 Mechanisms of Thrombolysis 3
   Gregory J. del Zoppo and Naohisa Hosomi
2 Pathogenesis of Cervico-cranial Artery Occlusion 29
   Louis R. Caplan
3 The Ischemic Penumbra and Neuronal Salvage 43
   Patrick D. Lyden

PART II SCIENTIFIC RATIONALE AND CLINICAL TRIALS

4 Pre-Clinical Testing of Thrombolytic Therapy
   for Stroke 65
   Anne M. Guyot and Steven R. Levine
5 Combination of Thrombolytic Therapy with
   Neuroprotectants 75
   James C. Grotta
6 Early Studies of Thrombolytic Therapy for Stroke 91
   Anne M. Guyot, Luchi Quinones, and Steven R. Levine
7 Phase 2 Experience with Intravenous Thrombolytic
   Therapy for Acute Ischemic Stroke 129
   E. Clarke Haley, Jr.
8 Intravenous Thrombolytic Therapy for Acute
   Ischemic Stroke: *Results of Large, Randomized
   Clinical Trials* 141
   Rashmi U. Kothari and Joseph P. Broderick
9 Further Analysis of NINDS Study: *Long-Term Outcome,
   Subgroups, and Cost Effectiveness* 153
   Susan C. Fagan, Thomas Kwiatkowski, and Patrick D. Lyden

10 Intra-Arterial Thrombolysis in Acute
    Ischemic Stroke 175
    Anthony J. Furlan, Randall Higashida, Irene Katzan,
    and Alex Abou-Chebl
11 Combinations of Intravenous and Intra-Arterial
    Thrombolysis 197
    Joseph P. Broderick and Rashmi Kothari

PART III USING THROMBOLYSIS FOR ACUTE STROKE

12 The Case for Thrombolytic Therapy in Stroke Patients 211
    Patrick D. Lyden
13 The Case Against the Present Guidelines for Stroke Thrombolysis:
    The Present Recommendations for Clinical Use Should
    Be Modified 223
    Louis R. Caplan
14 How to Run a Code Stroke 237
    Christopher Lewandowski
15 Interpretation of CT Scans for Acute Stroke 255
    Rüdiger von Kummer
16 Identifying and Overcoming Obstacles to Acute
    Stroke Treatment with rt-PA:
    Establishing Hospital and EMS Protocols 283
    Karen S. Rapp and Patti Bratina
17 The NINDS t-PA for Acute Stroke Protocol 297
    John R. Marler and Patrick D. Lyden
18 Research Directions and the Future of Stroke Therapy 309
    Patrick D. Lyden

PART IV: ILLUSTRATIVE CASES

Illustrative Cases 313
Index 399

CONTRIBUTORS

ALEX ABOU-CHEBL, MD • *Department of Neurology, Cleveland Clinic, Cleveland, OH*

PATTI BRATINA, RN, BSN • *Department of Neurology, University of Texas-Houston Medical School, Houston, TX*

JOSEPH P. BRODERICK, MD • *Department of Neurology, University of Cincinnati, Cincinnati, OH*

LOUIS R. CAPLAN, MD • *Neurology Department, Beth Israel Deaconess Medical Center, Boston, MA*

GREGORY DEL ZOPPO, MD • *Molecular and Experimental Medicine, The Scripps Research Institute, La Jolla, CA*

SUSAN C. FAGAN, PHARMD • *Clinical Pharmacy Program, The Medical College of Georgia, Augusta, GA*

ANTHONY J. FURLAN, MD • *Head Section of Adult Neurology, Cleveland Clinic, Cerebrovascular Center, Cleveland, OH*

JAMES C. GROTTA, MD • *Department of Neurology, University of Texas-Houston Medical School, Houston, TX*

ANNE M. GUYOT, MD • *Department of Neurology, Wayne State University, School of Medicine, University Health Center, Detroit, MI*

E. CLARKE HALEY, JR., MD • *Department of Neurology, University of Virginia Health System, Charlottesville, VA*

RANDALL HIGASHIDA, MD • *UCSF-Radiology, University of California, San Francisco, CA*

NAOHISA HOSOMI, MD, PHD • *The Scripps Research Institute, Molecular and Experimental Medicine, La Jolla, CA*

IRENE KATZAN, MD • *Department of Neurology, Cleveland Clinic, Cleveland, OH*

RASHMI U. KOTHARI, MD • *Borgess Research Institute, Michigan State University, Kalamazoo Center for Medical Studies, Kalamazoo, MI*

THOMAS KWIATKOWSKI, MD • *Department of Emergency Medicine, Long Island Jewish Medical Center, New Hyde Park, NY*

STEVEN R. LEVINE, MD • *Wayne State University, School of Medicine, University Health Center, Detroit, MI*

CHRISTOPHER LEWANDOWSKI, MD • *Department of Emergency Medicine, Henry Ford Hospital, Detroit, MI*

PATRICK D. LYDEN, MD • *UCSD Stroke Center, San Diego, CA*

JOHN R. MARLER, MD • *NINDS–Neurodegeneration, Neuroscience Center, Rockville, MD*

LUCHI QUINONES, MD • *Wayne State University, School of Medicine, University Health Center, Detroit, MI*

KAREN S. RAPP, RN, BSN • *UCSD Stroke Center, San Diego, CA*

RÜDIGER VON KUMMER, MD • *Department of Neuroradiology, University of Technology, Dresden, Germany*

JUSTIN A. ZIVIN, MD • *Department of Neurosciences, University of California, San Diego, La Jolla, CA*

I BACKGROUND AND BASIC INVESTIGATIONS

1   Mechanisms of Thrombolysis

Gregory J. del Zoppo, MD and Naohisa Hosomi, MD, PhD

CONTENTS

INTRODUCTION
THROMBUS FORMATION
FIBRINOLYSIS
PLASMINOGEN ACTIVATORS
REGULATION OF ENDOGENOUS FIBRINOLYSIS
CONSEQUENCES OF THERAPEUTIC PLASMINOGEN ACTIVATION
LIMITATIONS TO THE CLINICAL USE OF FIBRINOLYTIC AGENTS
PLASMINOGEN ACTIVATORS IN CEREBRAL TISSUE
PLASMINOGEN ACTIVATORS
    IN EXPERIMENTAL CEREBRAL ISCHEMIA
REFERENCES

INTRODUCTION

The pharmacologic use of plasminogen activators has been associated with symptomatic improvement in patients with coronary artery thrombosis, peripheral arterial occlusions, and thrombosis of the venous system. Based upon prospective angiographic studies and planned programs *(1–5)*, thrombolysis has attained a place in the acute treatment of ischemic stroke *(6–8)* under limited circumstances. Currently, recombinant tissue plasminogen activator (rt-PA) is licensed in the United States and several other countries for the treatment of ischemic stroke within 3 h of onset *(6)*.

The development of agents that promote fibrinolysis by *exogenous* application stems from observations beginning in the 19th century *(9)* of the liquefaction of clotted blood and spontaneous dissolution of fibrin thrombi. Enquiry into the mechanisms of streptococcal fibrinolysis *(10)* was paralleled by a growing

From: *Thrombolytic Therapy for Stroke*
Edited by: P. D. Lyden © Humana Press Inc., Totowa, NJ

understanding of plasma proteolytic digestion of fibrin *(11)*. Streptokinase was first employed to dissolve closed space (intrapleural) fibrin clots *(12)*, but purified preparations were required for lysis of intravascular thrombi *(13)*. Development of plasminogen activators for therapeutic vascular thrombus lysis has progressed in concert with insights into the mechanisms of thrombus formation and degradation.

The growth, dissolution, and migration of a thrombus depends upon the relative contributions of platelet activation, coagulation system activation, and fibrinolysis. These processes are inextricably connected. Clinically, excess vascular fibrin or excess fibrin degradation may contribute to thrombosis or hemorrhage, respectively. Plasminogen activators have been exploited clinically to dissolve significant (symptomatic) thrombi; however, all substances that promote plasmin formation retain the potential to increase the risk of hemorrhage.

THROMBUS FORMATION

Thrombosis and thrombus growth involve the processes of endothelial injury, platelet adherence and aggregation, and thrombin generation. The relative contributions of these processes to the thrombus composition depend upon other factors including the degree of vascular injury, shear stress, and the presence of antithrombotic agents.

Thrombin is the central player in clot formation, acting as a link between platelet activation and coagulation. Thrombin cleaves fibrinogen, which contributes fibrin to the clot matrix. The growing fibrin matrix forms the scaffolding for the thrombus *(14)*. Inter-fibrin strand crosslinking is accomplished by factor XIII, a transglutaminase bound to fibrinogen, which is itself activated by thrombin and contributes to thrombus stabilization *(15)*. Thrombin mediates fibrin polymerization through the cleavage of the NH_2-terminal fragments of the Aα and Bβ chains of fibrinogen *(16,17)*. This leads to the generation of fibrin I and fibrin II monomers, and the release of fibrinopeptide A (FPA) and fibrinopeptide B (FPB), respectively.

Thrombin-mediated fibrin formation occurs simultaneously with platelet activation by several mechanisms. Thrombin is locally generated by both extrinsic and intrinsic pathways of coagulation in a process involving platelet membrane receptors and phospholipid *(18)*. Additionally, platelets promote activation of the early stages of intrinsic coagulation by a process that involves the factor XI receptor and high-molecular-weight kininogen (HMWK) *(19)*. Also, factors V and VIII interact with specific platelet membrane phospholipids (receptors) to facilitate the activation of factor X to Xa and the conversion of prothrombin to thrombin on the platelet surface *(20)*. Platelet-bound thrombin-modified factor V (factor Va) serves as a high affinity platelet receptor for factor Xa *(21)*. Consequently, the rate of thrombin generation is significantly accelerated by a potent positive feedback mechanism, which leads to further fibrin network formation.

This process also leads to the conversion of plasminogen to plasmin and the activation of endogenous fibrinolysis. Thrombin provides one direct connection between thrombus formation and plasmin generation through localized generation of plasminogen activators from endothelial cells. Active thrombin has been shown in vitro and in vivo to markedly stimulate tissue plasminogen activator (t-PA) release from endothelial stores (22–24). In one experiment, infusion of factor Xa and phospholipid into nonhuman primates resulted in a pronounced increase in circulating t-PA activity (25), suggesting that significant vascular stores of this plasminogen activator may be released by active components of coagulation. Other vascular and cellular stimuli may also augment PA release, thereby pushing the balance toward thrombus lysis.

The relative platelet-fibrin composition of a specific thrombus is dependent upon regional blood flow or shear stress. At arterial flow rates thrombi are predominantly platelet rich, whereas at lower shear rates characteristic of venous flow, activation of coagulation seems to predominate. It has been suggested that the efficacy of pharmacologic thrombus lysis is dependent upon 1) the relative fibrin content and 2) the degree of fibrin crosslinking (26,27). The latter may reflect thrombus age.

Thrombus development requires abrogation of the constitutive antithrombotic characteristics of the endothelial cell (28). Alternatively, thrombus formation may occur following lodgment of a thrombus in a downstream vascular bed. In addition to both endothelial cell-derived antithrombotic characteristics and circulating anticoagulants (i.e., activated protein C, protein S), thrombus growth is limited by the *endogenous* thrombus lytic system. One effect of fibrinolysis is to continually remodel the thrombus. This results from the preferential conversion of plasminogen to plasmin on the thrombus surface where fibrin binds t-PA in proximity to its substrate plasminogen, thereby accelerating local plasmin formation. In concert with local shear stress, these processes may lead to the further embolization into downstream cerebral vasculature (29). However, little is known about the *endogenous* generation and secretion of PAs within the cerebral vessels (30). *Exogenous* application of pharmacologic doses of PAs accelerate conversion of thrombus bound plasminogen to plasmin, and prevent thrombus formation as discussed below.

FIBRINOLYSIS

Plasmin formation is central to thrombus dissolution. The *endogenous* fibrinolytic system is comprised of plasminogen, plasminogen activators, and inhibitors of fibrinolysis. Fibrin (and fibrinogen) degradation requires plasmin generation. Plasminogen, its activators, and the inhibitors of the fibrinolytic components contribute to the balance between hemorrhage and thrombosis (Tables 1 and 2).

Table 1
Plasminogen Activators

Plasminogen activators	M_R (kDa)	Chains	Plasma concentration (mg dl^{-1})	$t_{1/2}$	Substrates
Endogenous					
plasminogen	92	2	20	2.2 d	(Fibrin)
t-PA	68(59)	1→2	5×10^{-4}	5–8 min	Fibrin/plasminogen
scu-PA	54(46)	1→2	2–20×10^{-4}	8 min	Fibrin/plasmin(ogen)
u-PA	54(46)	2	8×10^{-4}	9–12 min	Plasminogen
Exogenous					
streptokinase	47	1	0	41 and 30 min	Plasminogen, fibrin(ogen)
APSAC	131	complex	0	70–90 min	Fibrin(ogen)
staphylokinase	16.5		0		Plasminogen

Table 2
Plasminogen Activator Inhibitors

Inhibitor	M_R (kDa)	Chains	Plasma concentration (mg dL^{-1})	$t_{1/2}$	Substrates
Plasmin Inhibitors					
α_2-antiplasmin	65	1	7	3.3 min	Plasmin
α_2-macroglobulin	740	4	250		Plasmin (excess)
Plasminogen Activator Inhibitors					
PAI-1	48–52	1	5×10^{-2}	7 min	t-PA, u-PA
PAI-2	47,70	1	$<5 \times 10^{-4}$	24 h	t-PA, u-PA
PAI-3	50				u-PA, t-PA

Plasmin formation occurs 1) in the plasma, where it can cleave circulating fibrinogen and fibrin, and 2) on reactive surfaces (e.g., thrombi or cells). The fibrin matrix offers a setting for plasminogen activation, whereas various cell types, including polymorphonuclear (PMN) leukocytes, platelets, and endothelial cells, express receptors for plasminogen binding *(31)*. Specific cellular receptors concentrate plasminogen and specific activators (e.g., urokinase plasminogen activator [u-PA]), which thereby enhance local plasmin production. Similar receptors on tumor cells are also involved with the dissolution of basement membranes and the metastatic process. Plasmin can also mediate the proteolytic cleavage of matrix ligands, which comprise basement membranes and vascular basal lamina.

Plasminogen

The naturally circulating plasminogen activators, single-chain t-PA and single-chain urokinase plasminogen activator (scu-PA), catalyze plasmin formation from plasminogen *(32–35)*. Plasmin, generated in the circulation, degrades circulating fibrinogen and the fibrin lattice of thrombi into soluble products *(36)*.

Plasmin is derived from the zymogen, plasminogen, a single-chain 92 kDa glycosylated serine protease *(37,38)*. Plasminogen (Fig. 1) is present in two forms: glu-plasminogen, which has an NH_2-terminal glutamic acid, and lys-plasminogen, lacking an 8 kDa peptide, which has an NH_2-terminal lysine. Plasmin cleavage of the NH_2-terminal fragment converts glu-plasminogen to lys-plasminogen *(39,40)*. Glu-plasminogen has a plasma clearance $t_{1/2}$ of approx 2.2 d, while lys-plasminogen has a $t_{1/2}$ of 0.8 d *(13)*. Both t-PA and u-PA catalyze the conversion of glu-plasminogen to lys-plasmin through either of two intermediates, glu-plasmin or lys-plasminogen *(41)*. Structurally, plasminogen contains five kringles, two of which (K_1 and K_5) mediate the binding of plasminogen to fibrin through characteristic lysine binding sites *(37,42,43)*, and a protease domain (Fig. 1). The lysine-binding sites also mediate the binding of plasminogen to $α_2$-antiplasmin, thrombospondin, components of the vascular extracellular matrix (ECM), and histidine rich glycoprotein *(38)*. $α_2$-antiplasmin prevents binding of plasminogen to fibrin by this mechanism *(41)*. Partial degradation of the fibrin network enhances the binding of glu-plasminogen to fibrin, promoting further local fibrinolysis.

Plasminogen Activation

The activation of plasminogen is 1) tied to thrombus formation by coagulation system activation ("intrinsic activation") or 2) augmented by the secretion of physiological plasminogen activators ("extrinsic activation"). It has been suggested that kallikrein, factor XIa, and factor XIIa in the presence of HMWK may directly activate plasminogen in the "intrinsic activation" method *(44,45)*. Sev-

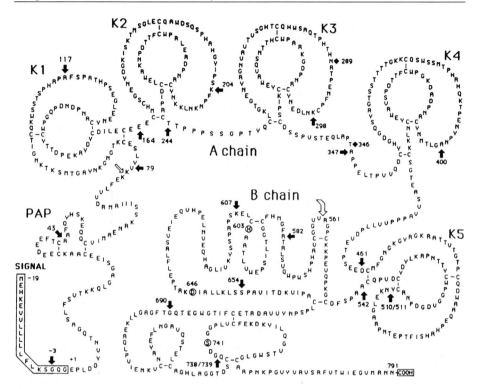

Fig. 1. The secondary structure of plasminogen. The molecule contains five kringle structures (K_1-K_5) in the A chain. Glycosylation sites are located at asn[289] and thr[346] (diamonds).

eral lines of evidence suggest that scu-PA may be an activator of plasminogen *(46–48)*. This pathway appears to be less important than the extrinsic pathway for physiologic fibrinolysis *(13)*. The primary contributor to "extrinsic activation" appears to be t-PA, which is secreted from the endothelium and other cellular sources. Thrombin generated by either intrinsic or extrinsic coagulation stimulates t-PA secretion from endothelial stores *(22,49,50)*.

Several serine proteases can mediate the conversion of plasminogen to plasmin by cleaving the arg[560]-val[561] bond *(38,51,52)*. Serine proteases have common structural features including an NH_2-terminal "A" chain with substrate binding affinity, a COOH-terminal "B" chain with the active site, and intrachain disulfide bridges. Plasminogen-cleaving serine proteases include the coagulation proteins factor IX, factor X, prothrombin (factor II), protein C, chymotrypsin and trypsin, various elastases (of leukocyte origin), the plasminogen activators u-PA and t-PA, and plasmin itself *(38)*. t-PA activates plasminogen in accordance with models described by Collen and colleagues *(53,54)*. In the circulation, plasmin binds rapidly to the inhibitor α_2-antiplasmin and is thereby inactivated. Within the thrombus, plasminogen is protected from α_2-antiplasmin. Plasminogen activation by t-PA is markedly enhanced by the presence of fibrin through the ternary complex t-PA/fibrin/plasminogen *(54,55)*. Activation of thrombus-bound plasminogen also protects plasmin from the inhibitors α_2-antiplasmin and α_2-macroglobulin *(38)*. Here, the lysine-binding sites and catalytic site of plasmin are occupied by fibrin, thereby blocking its interaction with α_2-antiplasmin *(53,54)*. Furthermore, fibrin and fibrin-bound plasminogen render t-PA relatively inaccessible to inhibition by other circulating plasma inhibitors *(56)*.

Thrombus Dissolution

Fibrinolysis occurs predominantly within the thrombus and at its surface *(57–60)*. Thrombus lysis is augmented by contributions from local blood flow. During thrombus consolidation, plasminogen bound to fibrin and to platelets allows local release of plasmin 61. In the circulation, plasmin cleaves the fibrinogen Aα chain appendage, and generates fragment X (DED), Aα fragments, and Bβ 1-42. Further cleavage of fragment X leads to the generation of fragments DE, D, and E. In contrast, degradation of the fibrin network generates YY/DXD, YD/DY, and the unique DD/E (fragment X = DED and fragment Y = DE) *(36,57,62)*. Incorporation of some of these products into forming thrombus destabilizes the fibrin network. Crosslinkage of DD with fragment E is vulnerable to further cleavage allowing the generation of D-dimer fragments. The measurement of D-dimer levels may have clinical utility. The presence of D-dimers in plasma reflects the breakdown of fibrin-containing thrombi by plasmin. The absence of circulating D-dimer indicates the absence of massive thrombosis *(63)*. Ordinarily, in the setting of focal cerebral ischemia the thrombus load is small and the meaning of D-dimer elevations is uncertain. However, the alteration in circulating fibrinogen and the generation of breakdown products of fibrin(ogen) limits the protection from hemorrhage.

PLASMINOGEN ACTIVATORS

All fibrinolytic agents in current use are obligate plasminogen activators (Table 1). t-PA, scu-PA, and u-PA are considered *endogenous* plasminogen activators because they are involved in physiological fibrinolysis. t-PA and scu-PA have relative fibrin and thrombus specificity *(35,63)*. Recombinant t-PA, scu-PA, and u-PA as well as streptokinase (SK), acylated plasminogen streptokinase activator complex (APSAC), staphylokinase, plasminogen activators of vampire bat origin, and other novel agents have all been used clinically as *exogenous* plasminogen activators. Their conversion of plasminogen to plasmin in the circulation involves different mechanisms than those of the *endogenous* agents *(58–60)*.

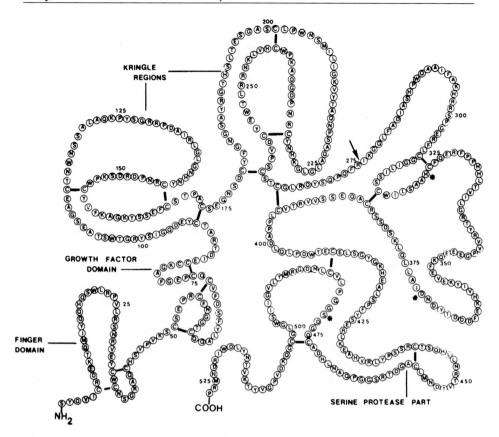

Fig. 2. The secondary structure of t-PA. The active site is formed by residues his[322], asp[371], and ser[478] (asterisks). Conversion of single chain t-PA to two chain t-PA by plasmin occurs at the arg[275]-isoleu[276] bond (arrow). Adapted and reproduced with permission of the publisher *(109)*, from the original source *(69)*.

Endogenous Plasminogen Activators

Tissue-type Plasminogen Activator

t-PA is a 70 kDa single-chain glycosylated serine protease *(51,64)* (Fig. 2). It has four distinct domains, which include a finger (F-) domain, a growth factor (E-) domain, two kringle regions (K$_1$ and K$_2$), and a serine protease domain *(65)*. The finger domain residues 4–50 and the K$_2$ domain *(35,64,66)* are responsible for fibrin affinity. The growth factor domain (residues 50–87) is homologous with epidermal growth factor (EDF), and the COOH-terminal serine protease domain contains the active site for plasminogen cleavage. The two kringle domains are homologous to the kringle regions of plasminogen.

The single-chain form is converted to the two-chain form by plasmin cleavage of the arg[275]-isoleu[276] bond. Both single-chain and two-chain species are enzymatically active and have relatively fibrin-selective properties. The catalytic efficiency of single-chain and two-chain t-PA for conversion of plasminogen to plasmin in vitro is stimulated to similar activity in the presence of fibrin *(64,67)*. Infusion studies in humans indicate that both single-chain and two-chain species have circulating plasma $t_{1/2}$s of 3–8 min *(35)*, although the biologic $t_{1/2}$s are longer. t-PA is considered to be fibrin-dependent because of its favorable binding constant for fibrin-bound plasminogen and its activation of plasminogen in association with fibrin *(35,65)*. Significant inactivation of circulating factors V and VIII does not occur with infused recombinant t-PA (rt-PA), and an anticoagulant state is generally not produced *(35)*. However, if sufficiently high doserates are employed, clinically measurable fibrinogenolysis and plasminogen consumption may be produced.

t-PA may be secreted from cultured endothelial cells following stimulation by thrombin *(49,50,68)*, activated protein C (APC) *(69)*, histamine *(49)*, phorbol myristate esterase, and other mediators *(70–74)*. However, the location of storage pools of t-PA in vivo remain unclear. In patients, release or synthesis of t-PA may be enhanced by various stimuli, some of which probably release endothelial stores in vivo *(75–77)*. Physical exercise and certain vasoactive substances produce measurable increases in circulating t-PA levels. Desmopressin acetate (DDAVP) may produce a three- to fourfold increase in t-PA antigen levels within 60 min of parenteral infusion. Heparin and heparan sulfate have been associated with significant increases in t-PA activity, whereas synthetic anabolic steroids potentiate fibrinolytic activity modestly. t-PA is cleared by the liver *(78)*. t-PA and u-PA have been reported to be secreted by endothelial cells, neurons, astrocytes, and microglia in vivo or in vitro *(30,79–86)*. The reasons for this broad cell expression are uncertain.

Urokinase Plasminogen Activator

Single-chain urokinase plasminogen activator (scu-PA or pro-UK) is a 54 kDa glycoprotein synthesized by endothelial and renal cells, and certain malignant cells (Fig. 3) *(31)*. This single-chain proenzyme of u-PA is unusual in possessing fibrin-selective plasmin-generating activity *(87,88)*. It has also been synthesized by recombinant techniques for use as an *exogenous* agent *(35,89)*.

The relationship of scu-PA to u-PA is complex: Cleavage or removal of lys[158] from scu-PA by plasmin produces high-molecular-weight (54 kDa) two-chain u-PA linked by the disulfide bridge at cys[148] and cys[279]. This consists of an A-chain (157 residues) and a glycosylated B-chain (253 residues). Further cleavages at lys[135] and arg[156] produce the low-molecular-weight (31 kDa) u-PA *(64)*. Both high- and low-molecular-weight species are enzymatically active.

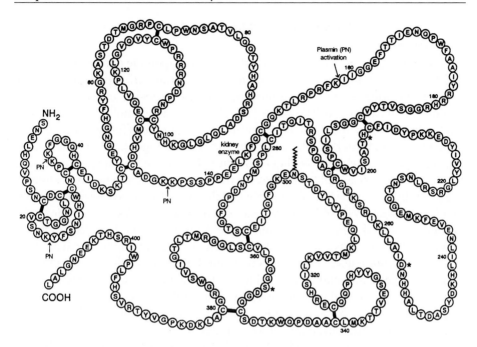

Fig. 3. The secondary structure of scu-PA (54 kDa). The active site is formed by residues his[204], asp[255], and ser[356] (asterisks). Activation by plasmin takes place at the 158–159 bond (arrow). The zig-zag line represents the glycosylation site. With the kind permission of A. Sasahara.

High-molecular-weight urokinase 54 kDa (u-PA) activates plasminogen to plasmin directly by first-order kinetics *(58,90)*. The two forms of u-PA exhibit measurable fibrinolytic and fibrinogenolytic activities in vitro and in vivo *(91,92)*, and have a plasma $t_{1/2}$ of 9–12 min. When infused as *exogenous* therapeutic agents, u-PA leads to consumption of plasminogen and inactivation of factors II (prothrombin), V, and VII. The latter changes constitute the systemic lytic state.

In hemostasis, t-PA and u-PA differ primarily in the domain organization of their noncatalytic regions, which regulate the function of the two plasminogen activators by binding to cofactors in a manner suggesting that they play quite different biological roles. Therefore, although both PAs can generate plasmin by cleavage of plasminogen, t-PA may be primarily involved in the maintenance of hemostasis through the dissolution of fibrin, whereas u-PA may be involved in generating pericellular proteolytic activity in relation to cells expressing u-PAR, needed for degradation of extracellular matrix. The roles of these two PAs in central nervous system function are yet to be fully appreciated (*see* Plasminogen Activators in Cerebral Tissue).

Exogenous Plasminogen Activators

STREPTOKINASE

Streptokinase (SK) is a 47 kDa single-chain polypeptide derived from group C β-hemolytic streptococci *(93)*. It combines stoichiometrically with plasminogen to form [streptokinase-plasminogen] complex, exposing an active site in the complexed plasminogen. The active [SK-plasminogen] complex converts circulating plasminogen directly to plasmin, and itself undergoes further intramolecular activation to form [SK-plasmin]. The [SK-plasminogen], [SK-plasmin], and plasmin species circulate together *(94)*. The [SK-plasmin] complex is not bound by the inhibitor α_2-antiplasmin, leaving this uninhibited form and free circulating plasmin to degrade both fibrinogen and fibrin, and to inactivate prothrombin, and factors V and VIII *(61)*. The kinetics of elimination of SK are complex, with an initial $t_{1/2}$ of 4 min and a second $t_{1/2}$ of 30 min (for the [SK-plasminogen] complex) *(95)*. Because of the bacterial origin of SK, antistreptococcal antibodies formed from antecedent infections neutralize infused SK. The anamnestic response is generally maximal 4–7 d following the initiation of the SK infusion. Neutralization of circulating antistreptococcal antibodies is necessary, and usually requires at least 3.5×10^5 U SK. However, because of the variable presence of anti-SK antibodies, the doses of SK required to achieve a steady-state plasminogen activation must be individualized. Depletion of plasminogen through conversion to plasmin and by as yet poorly understood clearance mechanisms for the [SK-plasminogen] complex can lead to hypoplasminogenemia. Generation of plasmin is then limited at low and at high SK infusion dose-rates because of inadequate plasminogen conversion and depletion of plasminogen, respectively. In the latter case, an increase in SK infusion will not increase fibrinogenolysis.

ANISOYLATED PLASMINOGEN-STREPTOKINASE ACTIVATOR COMPLEX (APSAC)

Anisoylated plasminogen-streptokinase activator complex (e.g., APSAC [Anistreplase]) is an artificial activator construct consisting of plasminogen and SK bound noncovalently. It displays fibrin selectivity by virtue of the fibrin-attachment properties of the plasminogen kringle structures *(35)*. The activity of APSAC depends upon the deacylation rate of the acyl-plasminogen component and the dissociation of SK from the complex. Hydrolytic activation of the acyl-protected active site of plasminogen allows plasmin formation by streptokinase within the complex in the presence of fibrin. The $t_{1/2}$ for deacylation of APSAC in plasma is approx 110 min, providing a $t_{1/2}$ for APSAC of 70 min *(96,97)*. From those observations and based on the terminal $t_{1/2}$ of SK, it is clear that APSAC has a longer circulation time than streptokinase. APSAC has not, despite its fibrin selectivity, found a place in the treatment of vascular thrombosis.

STAPHYLOKINASE

Staphylokinase (STK) is a 16.5 kDa polypeptide derived from certain strains of *Staphylococcus aureus (98–100)*. It combines stoichiometrically (1:1) with plasminogen to form an irreversible complex that activates free plasminogen. The binding of STK to plasmin has been worked out in detail *(100)*. The [STK-plasmin] complex has relative fibrin-specificity, based partly upon the observation that in the absence of fibrin the complex is inhibited by α_2-antiplasmin *(98,101)*. Recombinant STK has been prepared from the known gene nucleotide sequence, and has been tested in the setting of acute myocardial infarction.

PLASMINOGEN ACTIVATORS DERIVED FROM *DESMODUS ROTUNDUS*

Recombinant plasminogen activators identical to those derived from the saliva of the vampire bat *(Desmodus rotundus)* have been prepared that have fibrin-dependent plasminogen activating properties in vitro and in vivo. The α form of *Desmodus* salivary plasminogen activator (DSPA-α) and vampire bat salivary plasminogen activator (Bat-PA) are more fibrin-dependent than t-PA *(102,103)*. "Fluid phase" plasmin is not produced *(104)*. Experimental studies have suggested that rDSPA-α_1 *(105)* and Bat-PA *(106)* may be superior to t-PA in terms of sustained recanalization without fibrinogenolysis. The plasma $t_{1/2}$ of DSPA is significantly longer than that of rt-PA *(102)*. With regard to fibrin selectivity, Bat-PA has a fastidious requirement for fibrin I and fibrin II polymer, which is unlike that of rt-PA *(103,107)*. Both novel PAs have not been vigorously tested for utility in central nervous system (CNS) ischemia.

NOVEL PLASMINOGEN ACTIVATORS

Modifications of the DNA sequences of u-PA and t-PA by point mutations and deletions have provided molecules with altered stability and specificity *(108,109)*. t-PA mutants lacking the K_1 and K_2 kringle domains (fibrin- and lysine-binding regions) exhibits fibrin specificity, normal specific activity, but reduced inhibition by PAI-1 *(66)*. Altered t-PAs containing deletions of F- (and/ or E-) domain and single-site mutations with longer $t_{1/2}$, have been tested in various animal models of coronary artery thrombosis and pulmonary artery thrombosis *(110)*. Several mutant t-PAs with prolonged plasma $t_{1/2}$ have been under study *(108,109)*.

TNK, an rt-PA mutant with delayed clearance and prolonged $t_{1/2}$, has been tested in small animal models *(111,112)*. TNK, in addition, has enhanced fibrin specificity and relative resistance to inhibition by PAI-1 compared to rt-PA *(112)*, which has been shown in modeling to produce superior recanalization. Development of this mutant t-PA has included application as bolus infusion in acute myocardial infusion where safety and coronary artery recanalization have been confirmed *(113–116)*. Application of TNK to clinical ischemic stroke has not yet been formally tested. However, it is unclear in this setting what advantages the delayed clearance will provide *(117)*. Although there is so far no substantial evidence that there is an increased risk of serious hemorrhage with extended PA circulation (given dose adjustments), efficacy relative to cerebrovascular thrombosis may be compromised to reduce the risk of intracerebral hemorrhage.

Other novel plasminogen activator constructs have included single-site mutants and variants of rt-PA and recombinant scu-PA; t-PA/scu-PA and t-PA/u-PA chimerae *(118)*; u-PA/anti-fibrin monoclonal antibodies *(119)*, u-PA/anti-platelet monoclonal antibodies *(120)*, and bifunctional antibody conjugates *(121)*; and scu-PA deletion mutants *(122)*.

REGULATION OF ENDOGENOUS FIBRINOLYSIS

Endogenous fibrinolysis is modulated by several families of inhibitors of plasmin and of plasminogen activators. For streptokinase, APSAC, and staphylokinase, circulating neutralizing antibodies appear.

α_2-antiplasmin is the primary inhibitor of fibrinolysis through direct plasmin inhibition. Excess plasmin is inactivated by covalent binding to α_2-macroglobulin. Thrombospondin interferes with fibrin-associated plasminogen activation by t-PA *(123)*. Inhibitors of the contact activation system and complement (C1 inhibitor) have an indirect effect on fibrinolysis. Histidine-rich glycoprotein (HRG) is a competitive inhibitor of plasminogen. Generally, though, these physiological modulators of plasmin activity are overwhelmed by pharmacological concentrations of PAs, leading to the thrombus lytic effect and fibrinogenolysis (e.g., with SK and u-PA).

Circulating plasmin generated in the plasma during fibrinolysis is bound by α_2-antiplasmin. Two forms of α_2-antiplasmin may be found in the plasma: 1) the native form that binds plasminogen, and 2) a second form that cannot bind plasminogen *(124)*. Ordinarily, α_2-antiplasmin is found in either plasminogen-bound or free circulating forms *(125)*. For fibrin-bound plasmin, as when t-PA activates fibrin-bound plasminogen, both the active site and the usual site of interaction with α_2-antiplasmin are already occupied. This confers some protection for fibrin-bound plasmin from the inhibitor.

Excess free plasmin is bound by α_2-macroglobulin. It is a relatively nonspecific inhibitor of fibrinolysis, inactivating plasmin, kallikrein, t-PA, u-PA, and APSAC *(126)*.

In addition to inhibitors of plasmin, specific plasminogen activator inhibitors directly reduce the activity of t-PA, scu-PA, and u-PA (Table 2). Plasminogen activator inhibitor-1 (PAI-1) specifically inhibits both plasma t-PA and u-PA. PAI-1 is derived from both endothelial cell and platelet compartments *(127–129)*. Several lines of evidence indicate that K_2 of t-PA is responsible for the interaction between t-PA and PAI-1 and that this interaction is altered by the presence of fibrin *(130)*. PAI-1 is also an acute phase reactant *(131)*. "Shut down" of the fibrinolytic system following surgery is partially attributable to an increase in PAI-1 *(132)*, and deep venous thrombosis, septicemia, and type II diabetes mellitus are associated with elevated plasma PAI-1 levels. The potential risk of thrombosis then reflects the relative concentration of circulating PAI-1 and of t-PA.

PAI-2 is derived from placental tissue, granulocytes, monocytes/macrophages, and histiocytes *(133,134)*. The kinetics of PA inhibition by PAI-2 differs from that of PAI-1. PAI-2, which is found in a 70 kDa high-molecular-weight form and a 47 kDa low-molecular-weight form, has a lower K_i for u-PA and two-chain t-PA. This inhibitor probably plays little role in the physiologic antagonism of t-PA, and is most important in the uteroplacental circulation *(135)*.

PAI-3 is a serine protease inhibitor of u-PA, t-PA, and APC found in plasma and urine *(136,137)*.

CONSEQUENCES OF THERAPEUTIC PLASMINOGEN ACTIVATION

Pharmacologic concentrations (doses) of plasminogen activators can have significant effects upon hemostasis. u-PA, SK, and occasionally t-PA produce systemic fibrinogen degradation, with a fall in fibrinogen concentration. Rapid generation of plasmin in the circulation produces both a reduction in circulating plasminogen and α_2-antiplasmin. Inactivation of factors V and VIII may contribute to the "systemic lytic state" or "anticoagulant state" associated with the plasminogen activators u-PA and SK *(138)*. The systemic lytic state is marked by a decrease or depletion of circulating plasminogen, fibrinogen, and factors V and VIII with reciprocal generation of fragments of fibrin(ogen). The fragments interfere with fibrin multimerization and contribute to thrombus destabilization, whereas the circulating fragments, hypofibrinogenemia, and factor depletion produce a transient anticoagulant state that may limit thrombus extension as well as thrombus formation. For SK infusions, a severe hypoplasminogenemia may result, which makes dose adjustment particularly difficult. The clinical consequences of u-PA or SK infusion include a progressive decrease or depletion of measurable circulating plasminogen and fibrinogen, with prolongation of the activated partial thromboplastin time (aPTT) secondary to significant fibrinogen reduction and/or inactivation of factors V and VIII.

Certain plasminogen activators may also affect platelet function. Clinical studies of rt-PA in acute myocardial infarction (MI) have demonstrated prolongation of standardized template bleeding times *(139)*. rt-PA infusion in experimental systems has been shown to produce prolonged hemorrhage or increased erythrocyte extravasation *(140,141)*. t-PA is known to cause disaggregation of human platelets, inhibitable by α_2-antiplasmin, through selective proteolysis of intraplatelet fibrin *(142)*. Lys-and glu-plasminogen can potentiate the disaggregation effect of rt-PA on platelets *(143)*. It is likely that the risk of intracerebral hemorrhage that attends PA infusion involves disruption of sustained platelet aggregation and dissolution of fibrin being formed at the site of vascular injury.

LIMITATIONS TO THE CLINICAL USE
OF FIBRINOLYTIC AGENTS

The clinical setting in which plasminogen activators are used is an important and relevant variable in risk reduction. Intracerebral hemorrhage is a known feature of plasminogen activator exposure. The use of fibrinolytic agents in pharmacologic doses in clearly defined thrombotic disorders should conform to criteria established by an NIH Consensus Conference *(144)*, which attempt to limit the risk of hemorrhagic events. An abbreviated summary of strict contraindications to the use of fibrinolytic agents includes a history of previous intracranial hemorrhage; septic embolism; malignant hypertension or sustained diastolic or systolic blood pressure in excess of 180/110; conditions consistent with ongoing parenchymal hemorrhage (e.g., gastrointestinal source); pregnancy or parturition; history of recent trauma or surgery; and known hemorrhagic diatheses. These contraindications apply for the use of rt-PA in select ischemic stroke patients <3 h from symptom onset *(6)*, as well as other approved indications for the use of pharmacologic rt-PA, u-PA, or SK.

PLASMINOGEN ACTIVATORS IN CEREBRAL TISSUE

Although current clinical interests focus on the use of plasminogen activators as therapeutic agents for vascular reperfusion, cerebral tissue also expresses *endogenous* plasminogen activators. Various roles for specific PAs have been suggested. For instance, PA activity has been associated with development, vascular remodeling, cell migration, and tumor development and vascular invasion in the central nervous system. In normal cerebral tissue, t-PA antigen is associated with microvessels of a size similar to those of the vasa vasorum of the aorta *(30)*. Expression of plasminogen activator activity has been reported in nonischemic tissues of mouse, spontaneously hypertensive rats (>nonhypertensive counterparts), and primates *(145,146)*.

Resident nonvascular cells of the central nervous system have been reported to variously express t-PA, u-PA, or PAI-1. t-PA and u-PA have been reported to be secreted by endothelial cells, neurons, astrocytes, and microglia in vivo or in vitro *(79–86)*.

Plasminogen activators may be involved in cell migration, development, vascular remodeling, and neuron viability in the central nervous system. u-PA mRNA is expressed in neurons and oligodendrocytes during process outgrowth in rodent brain *(147)*. t-PA is expressed by neurons in many brain regions, but extracellular proteolysis seems confined to specific discrete brain regions *(148)*. Recent studies suggesting that t-PA may mediate hippocampal neurodegeneration during excitotoxicity or following focal cerebral ischemia *(149)*, have opened a discussion that PAs may play roles in cellular viability outside the fibrinolytic system.

However, at this writing, conflicting evidence of increasing injury by t-PA has been balanced against credible reports of no effect or reductions in infarct volume in rodent focal cerebral ischemia models *(149,150) (see below)*.

PLASMINOGEN ACTIVATORS IN EXPERIMENTAL CEREBRAL ISCHEMIA

Demonstration of improved clinical (behavioral and/or neurological) outcomes has been confined to rodent models of focal cerebral ischemia exposed to PAs (mostly rt-PA) very early following thromboembolism *(151–153)*. Significant improvement in clinical outcome over untreated controls accompanied early infusion of rt-PA in a rabbit multiple thromboembolism model *(151)*. More recent work, coupling PA exposure with putative inhibitors of PMN leukocyte adhesion have supported this impression, although differences among rt-PA cohorts were observed in various experimental sets *(154,155)*. In a rt-PA dose-rate study in the nonhuman primate, no significant difference in clinical outcome, according to a motor-weighted semiquantitated neurologic outcome score relative to controls was observed *(156,157)*.

Nonetheless, the overall experience is consistent with the view that direct intervention with PAs early after ischemia/infarction is not associated with a significant increase in intracerebral hemorrhage, and may result in rapid thrombus lysis, function recovery, and decreased mortality in certain small animal stroke thromboembolism models. Infusion of rt-PA as late as 3 h after MCA occlusion and reperfusion, did not enhance outcome in the nonhuman primate, but hemorrhagic infarction was not increased *(158)*. In contradistinction, although a set of uncontrolled and placebo-controlled studies of rt-PAs in acute ischemic stroke have demonstrated no substantial increase in the frequency of parenchymatous hematoma formation, all recent clinical placebo-controlled tests of PAs in acute focal cerebral ischemia have demonstrated significant increases in the frequency of symptomatic intracerebral hemorrhage over control *(6–8)*. In all cases hemorrhage contributed to morbidity and mortality.

REFERENCES

1. del Zoppo GJ, Ferbert A, Otis S, Brückmann H, Hacke W, Zyroff J, Harker LA, Zeumer H. Local intra-arterial fibrinolytic therapy in acute carotid territory stroke: A pilot study. *Stroke* 1988;19:307–313.
2. Mori E, Tabuchi M, Yoshida T, Yamadori A. Intracarotid urokinase with thromboembolic occlusion of the middle cerebral artery. *Stroke* 1988;19:802–812.
3. del Zoppo GJ, Poeck K, Pessin MS, Wolpert SM, Furlan AJ, Ferbert A. Recombinant tissue plasminogen activator in acute thrombotic and embolic stroke. *Ann Neurol* 1992;32:78–86.
4. Mori E, Yoneda Y, Tabuchi M, Yoshida T, Ohkawa S, Ohsumi Y. Intravenous recombinant tissue plasminogen activator in acute carotid artery territory stroke. *Neurology* 1992;42:976–982.

5. Yamaguchi T, Hayakawa T, Kikuchi H. Intravenous tissue plasminogen activator amelio-rates the outcome of hyperacute embolic stroke. *Cerebrovasc Dis* 1993;3:269–272.

6. The National Institutes of Neurological Disorders and Stroke rt-PA Stroke Study Group. Tissue plasminogen activator for acute ischemic stroke. *N Engl J Med* 1995;333:1581–1587.

7. Hacke W, Kaste M, Fieschi C, Toni D, Lesaffre E, von Kummer R, for the ECASS Study Group. Intravenous thrombolysis with recombinant tissue plasminogen activator for acute hemispheric stroke. The European Cooperative Acute Stroke Study (ECASS). *JAMA* 1995;274:1017–1025.

8. Hacke W, Kaste M, Fieschi C, von Kummer R, Davalos A, Meier D, for the Second Euro-pean-Australasian acute Stroke Study Investigators. Randomised double-blind placebo-controlled trial of thrombolytic therapy with intravenous alteplase in acute ischaemic stroke (ECASS II). *The Lancet* 1998;352:1245–1251.

9. Sherry S. The history and development of thrombolytic therapy. In: *Thrombolytic Therapy for Peripheral Vascular Disease*, Comerota AJ, ed. J. B. Lippincott Co: Philadelphia. 1995; pp. 67–86.

10. Kaplan MH. Nature and role of the lytic factor in hemolytic streptococcal fibrinolysis. *Proc Soc Exp Biol Med* 1944;57:40–43.

11. Christensen LR, MacLeod CM. A proteolytic enzyme of serum: Characterization, activa-tion, and reaction with inhibitors. *J Gen Physiol* 1945;28:559–583.

12. Tillett WS, Sherry S. The effect in patients of streptokinase fibrinolysis (streptokinase) and streptococcal deoxyribonuclease on fibrinous, purulent and sanguineous pleural exudations. *J Clin Invest* 1949;28:173–190.

13. Johnson AJ, Tillett WS. Lysis in rabbits of intravascular blood clots by the streptococcal fibrinolytic system (streptokinase). *J Exp Med* 1952;95:449–464.

14. Hermans J, McDonagh J. Fibrin: Structure and interactions. *Semin Thromb Hemost* 1982;8:11–24.

15. Davie EW, Fujikawa K, Kisiel W. The coagulation cascade: Initiation, maintenance, and regulation. *Biochemistry* 1991;30:10,363–10,370.

16. Nossel HL. Relative proteolysis of fibrin B-beta chain by thrombin and plasmin as a deter-minant of thrombosis. *Nature* 1981;291:754–762.

17. Alkjaersig N, Fletcher AP. Catabolism and excretion of fibrinopeptide A. *Blood* 1982;60: 148–156.

18. Majerus PW, Miletich JP, Kane WP, Hoffmann SL, Stanford N, Jackson CM. The formation of thrombin on platelet surface. In: *The Regulation of Coagulation*, Mann KG, Taylor FB, eds. Elsevier/North Holland: New York. 1980; pp. 215–215.

19. Kaplan AP. Initiation of the intrinsic coagulation and fibrinolytic pathways of man: The role of surfaces, Hageman factor, prekallikrein, high molecular weight kininogen, and factor XI. *Prog Hemost Thromb* 1978;4:127–175.

20. Nesheim ME, Hibbard LS, Tracy PB, Bloom JW, Myrmel KH, Mann KA: Participation of factor Va in prothrombinase. In: *The Regulation of Coagulation*, Mann KG, Tayler FB, eds. Elsevier/North Holland: New York. 1980; pp. 145–159.

21. Miletich JP, Jackson CM, Majerus PW. Properties of the factor Xa binding site on human platelets. *J Biol Chem* 1978;253:6908–6916.

22. Levin EG, Marzec U, Anderson J, Harker LA. Thrombin stimulates tissue plasminogen activator release from cultured human endothelial cells. *J Clin Invest* 1984;74:1988–1995.

23. Van Hinsbergh VWM. Regulation of the synthesis and secretion of plasminogen activators by endothelial cells. *Haemostasis* 1988;18:307–327.

24. Liesi P, Kirkwood T, Vaheri A. Fibronectin is expressed by astrocytes cultured from embry-onic and early postnatal rat brain. *Exp Cell Res* 1986;163:175–185.

25. Giles AR, Nosheim ME, Herring SW, Hoogendoorn H, Stump DC, Heldebrant CM. The fibrinolytic potential of the normal primate following the generation of thrombin in vivo. *Thromb Haemost* 1990;63:476–481.

26. Schwartz ML, Pizzo SV, Hill RL, McKee PA. Human factor XIII from plasma and platelets. Molecular weight, subunit structures, proteolytic activation and cross-linking of fibrinogen and fibrin. *J Biol Chem* 1973;248:1395–1407.

27. Gaffney PJ, Whittaker AN. Fibrin cross-links and lysis rates. *Thromb Res* 1979;14:85–94.

28. Nawroth PP, Stern DM. Endothelial cells as active participants in procoagulant reactions. In: *Vascular Endothelium in Hemostasis and Thrombosis*, Gimbrone MA, ed. Churchill-Livingstone: Edinburgh. 1986; pp. 14–39.

29. Collen D, de Maeyer L. Molecular biology of human plasminogen. I. Physiocochemical properties and microheterogeneity. *Thromb Diath Haemorhag* 1975;34:396–402.

30. Levin EG, del Zoppo GJ. Localization of tissue plasminogen activator in the endothelium of a limited number of vessels. *Am J Pathol* 1994;144:855–861.

31. Plow EF, Felez J, Miles LA. Cellular regulation of fibrinolysis. *Thromb Haemost* 1991;66:132–136.

32. Bachmann F, Kruithof IEKO. Tissue plasminogen activator: Chemical and physiological aspects. *Semin Thromb Hemost* 1984;10:6–17.

33. Aoki N, Harpel PC. Inhibitors of the fibrinolytic enzyme system. *Semin Thromb Hemost* 1984;10:24–41.

34. Collen D, Lijnen HR. New approaches to thrombolytic therapy. *Arteriosclerosis* 1984;4:579–585.

35. Verstraete M, Collen D. Thrombolytic therapy in the eighties. *Blood* 1986;67:1529–1541.

36. Gaffrey PJ, Lane DA, Kakkar VV, Brahser M. Characterization of a soluble D-dimer-E complex in cross-linked fibrin digests. *Thromb Res* 1975;7:89–99.

37. Forsgren M, Raden B, Israelsson M, Larsson K, Heden LO. Molecular cloning and characterization of a full-length cDNA clone for human plasminogen. *FEBS Lett* 1987;213:254–260.

38. Bachmann F. Molecular aspects of plasminogen, plasminogen activators and plasmin. In: *Haemostasis and Thrombosis*, Bloom AL, Forbes CD, Thomas DP, Tuddneham EGD, eds. Churchill Livingstone: Edinburgh. 1994; pp. 575–613.

39. Wallen P, Wiman B. Characterization of human plasminogen. II. Separation and partial characterization of different molecular forms of human plasminogen. *Biochim Biophys Acta* 1973;257:122–134.

40. Holvoet P, Lijnen HR, Collen D. A monoclonal antibody specific for lys-plasminogen. Application to the study of the activation pathways of plasminogen *in vivo*. *J Biol Chem* 1985;260:12,106–12,111.

41. Thorsen S, Mullertz S, Svenson E, Kok P. Sequence of formation of molecular forms of plasminogen and plasminogen-inhibitor complexes in plasma activated by urokinase or tissue-type plasminogen activator. *Biochem J* 1984;223:179–187.

42. Peterson LC, Serenson E. Effect of plasminogen and tissue-type plasminogen activator on fibrin gel structure. *Fibrinolysis* 1990;5:51–59.

43. Tran-Thong C, Kruithof EKO, Atkinson J, Bachmann F. High-affinity binding sites for human glu-plasminogen unveiled by limited plasmic degradation of human fibrin. *Eur J Biochem* 1986;160:559–604.

44. Miles LA, Greengard JS, Griffin JH. A comparison of the abilities of plasma kallikrein, Beta-Factor XIIa, Factor XIa and urokinase to activate plasminogen. *Thromb Res* 1983;29:407–417.

45. Kluft C, Dooijewaard G, Emeis JJ. Role of the contact system in fibrinolysis. *Semin Thromb Hemost* 1987;13:50–68.

46. Wun TC, Ossowski L, Reich E. A proenzyme of human urokinase. *J Biol Chem* 1982;257:7262–7276.

47. Wun TC, Schleuning E, Reich E. Isolation and characterization of urokinase from human plasma. *J Biol Chem* 1982;257:3276–3287.

48. Ichinose A, Fujikawa K, Suyama T. The activation of pro-urokinase by plasma kallikrein and its inactivation by thrombin. *J Biol Chem* 1986;261:3486–3489.

49. Hanss M, Collen D. Secretion of tissue-type plasminogen activator and plasminogen activator inhibitor by cultured human endothelial cells: Modulation by thrombin endotoxin and histamine. *J Lab Clin Med* 1987;109:97–104.

50. Levin EG, Stern DM, Nawrath PP, Marlar RA, Fair DS, Fenton II JW, Harker LA. Specificity of the thrombin-induced release of tissue plasminogen activator from cultured human endothelial cells. *Thromb Haemost* 1986;56:115–119.

51. Robbins KC, Summaria L, Hsieh B, Shah RJ. The peptide chains of human plasmin. *J Biochem* 1967;242:2333–2342.

52. Robbins KC. The plasminogen-plasmin system. In: *Thrombolytic Therapy for Peripheral Vascular Disease*, Comerota AJ, ed. J. B. Lippincott: Philadelphia. 1995; pp. 41–65.

53. Wiman B, Collen D. Molecular mechanism of physiological fibrinolysis. *Nature* 1979;272:549–550.

54. Collen D. On the regulation and control of fibrinolysis. *Thromb Haemost* 1980;43:77–89.

55. Hoylaerts M, Rijken DC, Lijnen HR, Collen D. Kinetics of the activation of plasminogen by human tissue plasminogen activator. Role of fibrin. *J Biol Chem* 1982;257:2912–2919.

56. Wun T-C, Capugno A. Initiation and regulation of fibrinolysis in human plasma at the plasminogen activator level. *Blood* 1987;69:1354–1362.

57. Bloom AL, Thomas DP. *Haemostasis and Thrombosis*. Edinburgh, Churchill-Livingstone, 1987.

58. Kakkar VV, Scully MF. Thrombolytic therapy. *Br Med Bull* 1978;34:191–199.

59. Sharma GVRK, Cella G, Parish AF, Sasahara AA. Drug therapy: Thrombolytic therapy. *N Engl J Med* 1982;306:1268–1276.

60. Verstraete M. Biochemical and clinical aspects of thrombolysis. *Semin Hematol* 1978;15:35–54.

61. Castellino FJ. Biochemistry of human plasminogen. *Semin Thromb Hemost* 1984;10:18–23.

62. Yasaka M, Yamaguchi T, Miyashita T, Tsuchiya T. Regression of intracardiac thrombus after embolic stroke. *Stroke* 1990;21:1540–1544.

63. Bounameaux H, de Moerloose P, Perrier A, Reber G. Plasma measurement of D-dimer as diagnostic aid in suspected venous thromboembolism: An overview. *Thromb Haemost* 1994;71:1–6.

64. Rijken DC. Structure/function relationships of t-PA. In: *Tissue Type Plasminogen Activator (t-PA): Physiological and Clinical Aspects Vol. 1*, Kluft C, ed. CRC Press: Boca Raton. 1988; pp. 101–122.

65. Pennica D, Holmes WE, Kohr WJ, Harkins RN, Vehar GA, Ward CA. Cloning and expression of human tissue-type plasminogen activator cDNA in *E coli*. *Nature* 1983;301:214–221.

66. Ehrlich HJ, Bang NW, Little SP, Jaskunas SR, Weigel BJ, Mattler LE, Harms CS. Biological properties of a kringleless tissue plasminogen activator (t-PA) mutant. *Fibrinolysis* 1987;1:75–81.

67. Ranby M, Bergsdorf N, Norrman B, Svenson E, Wallen P. Tissue plasminogen activator kinetics. In: *Progress in Fibrinolysis Vol. VI*, Davison JF, Bachmann F, Bouvier CA, Kruithof EKO, eds. Churchill-Livingstone: New York. 1982; pp. 182–182.

68. Gelehrter TD, Sznycer-Laszuk R. Thrombin induction of plasminogen activator-inhibitor in cultured human endothelial cells. *J Clin Invest* 1986;77:165–169.

69. Sakata Y, Curriden S, Lawrence D, et al. Activated protein C stimulates the fibrinolytic activity of cultured endothelial cells and decreases antiactivator activity. *Proc Natl Acad Sci USA* 1985;82:1121–1125.

70. Moscatelli D. Urokinase-type and tissue-type plasminogen activators have different distributions in cultured bovine capillary endothelial cells. *J Cell Biochem* 1986;30:19–29.

71. Bulens F, Nelles L, Van den Panhuyzen N, Collen D. Stimulation by retinoids of tissue-type plasminogen activator secretion in cultured human endothelial cells: Relations of structure to effect. *J Cardiovasc Pharmacol* 1992;19:508–514.
72. Thompson EA, Nelles L, Collen D. Effect of retinoic acid on the synthesis of tissue-type plasminogen activator and plasminogen activator inhibitor-I in human endothelial cells. *Eur J Biochem* 1991;201:627–632.
73. Saksela O, Moscatelli D, Rifkin DB. The opposing effects of basic fibroblast growth factor and transforming growth factor beta on the regulation of plasminogen activator activity in capillary endothelial cells and decreases antiactivator activity. *J Cell Biol* 1987;105:957–963.
74. Levin EG, Marotti KR, Santell L. Protein kinase C and the stimulation of tissue plasminogen activator release from human endothelial cells. Dependence on the elevation of messenger RNA. *J Biol Chem* 1989;264:16,030–16,036.
75. Smith D, Gilbert M, Owen WG. Tissue plasminogen activator release *in vivo* in response to vasoactive agents. *Blood* 1985;66:835–839.
76. Brommer EJP. Clinical relevance of t-PA levels of fibrinolytic assays. In: *Tissue-Type Plasminogen Activator (t-PA): Physiological and Clinical Aspects Part 2*, Kluft C, ed. CRC Press: Boca Raton. 1988; pp. 89–89.
77. Agnelli G. The pharmacological basis of thrombmolytic therapy. In: *Thrombolysis Yearbook 1995*, Agnelli G, ed. Excerpta Medica: Amsterdam. 1995; pp. 31–61.
78. Verstraete M, Bounameaux H, de Cock F, Van de Loerf F, Collen D. Pharmacokinetics and systemic fibrinogenolytic effects of recombinant human tissue-type plasminogen activator (rt-PA) in humans. *J Pharmacol Exp Ther* 1986;235:506–512.
79. Krystosek A, Seeds NW. Normal and malignant cells, including neurons, deposit plasminogen activator on growth substrata. *Exp Cell Res* 1986;166:31–46.
80. Pittman RN. Release of plasminogen activator and a calcium-dependent metalloprotease from cultured sympathetic and sensory neurons. *Dev Biol* 1985;110:91–101.
81. Vincent VA, Lowik CW, Verheijen JH, de Bart AC, Tilders FJ, Van Dam AM. Role of astrocyte-derived tissue-type plasminogen activator in the regulation of endotoxin-stimulated nitric oxide production by microglial cells. *GLIA* 1998;22:130–137.
82. Toshniwal PK, Firestone SL, Barlow GH, Tiku ML. Characterization of astrocyte plasminogen activator. *J Neurol Sci* 1987;80:277–287.
83. Tsirka SE, Rogove AD, Bugge TH, Degen JL, Strickland S. An extracellular proteolytic cascade promotes neuronal degeneration in the mouse hippocampus. *J Neurosci* 1997;17: 543–552.
84. Masos T, Miskin R. Localization of urokinase-type plasminogen activator mRNA in the adult mouse brain. *Brain Res Mol Brain Res* 1996;35:139–148.
85. Tranque P, Naftolin F, Robbins R. Differential regulation of astrocyte plasminogen activators by insulin-like growth factor-I and epidermal growth factor. *Endocrinology* 1994;134: 2606–2613.
86. Nakajima K, Tsuzaki N, Shimojo M, Hamanoue M, Kohsaka S. Microglia isolated from rat brain secrete a urokinase-type plasminogen activator. *Brain Res* 1992;577:285–292.
87. Lijnen HR, Zamarron C, Blaber M, Winkler ME, Collen D. Activation of plasminogen by pro-urokinase. I. Mechanism. *J Biol Chem* 1986;261:1253–1258.
88. Peterson LC, Lund LR, Nielsen LS, Dano K, Shriver L. One-chain urokinase-type plasminogen activator from human sarcoma cells is a proenzyme with little or no intrinsic activity. *J Biol Chem* 1988;263:11,189–11,195.
89. Gunzler WA, Steffens GJ, Otting F, Buse G, Flohe L. Structural relationship between human high and low molecular mass urokinase. *Hoppe Seylers Z Physiol Chem* 1982;563:133–141.
90. White FW, Barlow GH, Mozen MM. The isolation and characterization of plasminogen activators (urokinase) from human urine. *Biochemistry* 1966;5:2160–2169.

91. Fletcher AP, Alkjaersig N, Sherry S, Genton E, Hirsh J, Bachmann F. The development of urokinase as a thrombolytic agent. Maintenance of a sustained thrombolytic state in man by its intravenous infusion. *J Lab Clin Med* 1965;65:713–731.
92. Stump DC, Mann KH. Mechanisms of thrombus formation and lysis. *Ann Emerg Med* 1988;17:1138–1147.
93. Davies MC, Englert ME, De Rezo EC. Interaction of streptokinase and human plasminogen observed in the ultracentrifuge under a variety of experimental conditions. *J Biol Chem* 1964;239(8):2651–2656.
94. Reddy KN, Marcus B. Mechanisms of activation of human plasminogen by streptokinase. *J Biol Chem* 1972;246:1683–1691.
95. Fletcher AP, Alkjaersig N, Sherry S. The clearance of heterologous proteins from the circulation of normal and immunized man. *J Clin Invest* 1958;37(9):1306–1315.
96. Standing R, Fears R, Ferres H. The protective effect of acylation on the stability of APSAC (Eminase) in human plasma. *Fibrinolysis* 1988;2:157.
97. Ferres H. Preclinical pharmacological evaluation of Eminase (APSAC). *Drugs* 1987; 33(Suppl 3):33–50.
98. Lignen HR, de Cock F, Matsuo O, Collen D. Comparative fibrinolytic and fibrinogenolytic properties of staphylokinase and streptokinase in plasma of different species in vitro. *Fibrinolysis* 1992;6:33–37.
99. Collen D. Staphlyokinase: a potent, uniquely fibrin-selective thrombolytic agent. *Nature Medicine* 1998;4(3):279–282.
100. Jespers L, Vanwetswinkel S, Lijnen HR, Van Herzeele N, Van Hoef B, Demarsin E, et al. Structural and functional basis of plasminogen activation by staphylokinase. *Thromb Haemost* 1999;81(4):479–484.
101. Lijnen HR, Van Hoef B, Matsuo O, Collen D. On the molecular, interactions between plasminogen- staphylokinase, α_2-antiplasmin and fibrin. *Biochim Biophys Acta* 1992;1118: 144–148.
102. Witt W, Maass B, Baldus B, Hildebrand M, Donner P, Schleuning WD. Coronary thrombosis with Desmodus salivary plasminogen activator in dogs. Fast and persistent recanalization by intravenous bolus administration. *Circulation* 1994;90:421–426.
103. Bergum PW, Gardell SJ. Vampire bat salivary plasminogen activator exhibits a strict and fastidious requirement for polymeric fibrin as its cofactor, unlike human tissue-type plasminogen activator. A kinetic analysis. *J Biol Chem* 1992;267:17,726–17,731.
104. Hare TR, Gardell SJ. Vampire bat salivary plasminogen activator promotes robust lysis of plasma clots in a plasma milieu without causing fluid phase plasminogen activation. *Thromb Haemost* 1992;68:165–169.
105. Witt W, Baldus B, Bringmann P, Cashion L, Donner P, Schleuning WD. Thrombolytic properties of Desmodus rotundus (vampire bat) salivary plasminogen activator in experimental pulmonary embolism in rats. *Blood* 1992;79:1213–1217.
106. Mellot MJ, Stabilito II, Holahan MA, Cuca GC, Wang S, Li P, Barrett JS, Lynch JJ, Gardell SJ. Vampire bat salivary plasminogen activator promotes rapid and sustained reperfusion without concomitant systemic plasminogen activation in a canine model of arterial thrombosis. *Arterioscler Thromb* 1992;12:212–221.
107. Gardell SJ, Ramjit DR, Stabilito II, Fujita T, Lynch JJ, Cuca GC, et al. Effective thrombolysis without marked plasminemia after bolus intravenous administration of vampire bat salivary plasminogen activator in rabbits. *Circulation* 1991;84:244–253.
108. Lijnen HR, Collen D: Development of new fibrinolytic agents. In: *Haemostasis and Thrombosis*, Bloom AL, Forbes CD, Thomas DP, Tuddenham EGD, eds. Churchill-Livingstone: Edinburgh. 1994; pp. 625–637.
109. Van de Werf F. New thrombolytic strategies. *Aust N Z J Med* 1993;23:763–765.

110. Barnathan ES, Kuo A, Van der Keyl H, McCrae KR, Larsen GR, Cines DB. Tissue-type plasminogen activator binding to human endothelial cells. *J Biol Chem* 1988;263: 7792–7799.
111. Smalling RW. Pharmacological and clinical impact of the unique molecular structure of a new plasminogen activator. *Eur Heart J* 1997;18(F):F11–F16.
112. Benedict CR, Refino CJ, Keyt BA, Pakala R, Paoni NF, Thomas GR, Bennett WF. New variant of human tissue plasminogen activator (TPA) with enhanced efficacy and lower incidence of bleeding compared with recombinant human TPA. *Circulation* 1995;92(10): 3032–3040.
113. Cannon CP, McCabe CH, Gibson CM, Ghali M, Sequeira RF, McKendall GR, et al. TNK-tissue plasminogen activator in acute myocardial infarction. Results of the Thrombolysis in Myocardial Infarction (TIMI) 10A dose-ranging trial. *Circulation* 1997;95(2):351–356.
114. Cannon CP, Gibson CM, McCabe CH, Adgey AA, Schweiger MJ, Sequeira RF, et al. TNK-tissue plasminogen activator compared with front-loaded alteplase in acute myocardial infarction: results of the TIMI 10B trial. Thrombolysis in Myocardial Infarction (TIMI) 10B Investigators. *Circulation* 1998;98(25):2805–2814.
115. Van de Werf F, Cannon CP, Luyten A, Houbracken K, McCabe CH, Berioli S, et al. Safety assessment of single-bolus administration of TNK tissue-plasminogen activator in acute myocardial infarction: the ASSENT-1 trial. The ASSENT-1 Investigators. *Am Heart J* 1999;137(5):786–791.
116. Gibson CM, Cannon CP, Murphy SA, Adgey AA, Schweiger MJ, Sequeira RF, Grollier G, Fox NL, Berioli S, Weaver WD, Van de Werf F, Braunwald E. Weight-adjusted dosing of TNK-tissue plasminogen activator and its relation to angiographic outcomes in the thrombolysis in myocardial infarction 10B trial. TIMI 10B Investigators. *Am J Cardiol* 1999;84(9):976–980.
117. Modi NB, Eppler S, Breed J, Cannon CP, Braunwald E, Love TW. Pharmacokinetics of a slower clearing tissue plasminogen activator variant, TNK-tPA, in patients with acute myocardial infarction. *Thromb Haemost* 1998;79(1):134–139.
118. Pierard L, Jacobs P, Gheysen D, Hoylaerts M, André B, Topisirovic L, et al. Mutant and chimeric recombinant plasminogen activators. *J Biol Chem* 1987;262:11,771–11,778.
119. Runge MS, Bode C, Matsueda GR, Haber E. Antibody-enhanced thrombolysis: Targeting of tissue plasminogen activator *in vivo. Proc Natl Acad Sci USA* 1987;84:7659–7662.
120. Bode C, Meinhardt G, Runge MS, et al. Platelet-targeted fibrinolysis enhances clot lysis and inhibits platelet aggregation. *Circulation* 1991;84:805–813.
121. Jones RD, Donaldson IM, Parkin PJ. Impairment and recovery of ipsilateral sensory-motor function following unilateral cerebral infarction. *Brain* 1989;112:113–132.
122. Kasper W, Meinertz T, Hohnloser S, Engler H, Hasler C, Rossler W, et al. Coronary thrombolysis in man with prourokinase: Improved efficacy with low dose urokinase. *Klin Wochenschr* 1988;66:109–114.
123. Bachmann F. Fibrinolysis. In: *Thrombosis and Haemostasis*, Verstraete M, Vermylen J, Lijnen HR, Arnout J, eds. Leuven, ISTH/University of Leuven Press: 1987; pp. 227–265.
124. Kluft C, Los N. Demonstration of two forms of α_2-antiplasmin in plasma by modified crossed immunoelectrophoresis. *Thromb Res* 1981;21:65–71.
125. Winman B, Nilsson T, Cedergren B. Studies on a form of α_2-antiplasmin in plasma which does not interact with the lysine-binding sites in plasminogen. *Thromb Res* 1982; 28:193–200.
126. Aoki N, Harpel P. Inhibitors of the fibrinolytic enzyme system. *Semin Hemostat Thromb* 1984;10:24–39.
127. Philips M, Juul AG, Thorsen S. Human endothelial cells produce a plasminogen activator inhibitor and a tissue-type plasminogen activator-inhibitor complex. *Biochim Biophys Acta* 1984;802:99–110.

128. Loskutoff DJ, van Mourik JA, Erickson LA, Lawrence DA. Detection of an unusually stable fibrinolytic inhibitor produced by bovine endothelial cells. *Proc Natl Acad Sci USA* 1983;80:2956–2960.

129. Thorsen S, Philips M, Selmer J, Lecander I, Astedt B. Kinetics of inhibition of tissue-type and urokinase-type plasminogen activator by plasminogen-activator inhibitor type 1 and type 2. *Eur J Biochem* 1988;175:33–39.

130. Wilhelm OG, Jaskunas SR, Vlahos CJ, Bang NU. Functional properties of the recombinant kringle-2 domain of tissue plasminogen activator produced in Escherichia coli. *J Biol Chem* 1990;265:14,606–14,611.

131. Juhan-Vague I, Moerman B, de Cock F, Aillaud MF, Collen D. Plasma levels of a specific inhibitor of tissue-type plasminogen activator (and urokinase) in normal and pathological conditions. *Thromb Res* 1984;33:523–530.

132. Kluft C, Verheihen J-H, Jie AFH, Rijken DC, Preston FE, Sue-Ling HM, et al. The postoperative fibrinolytic shutdown: A rapidly reverting acute-phase pattern for the fast-acting inhibitor of tissue-type plasminogen activator after trauma. *Scand J Clin Lab Invest* 1985;45:605–610.

133. Schleuning W-D, Medcalf RL, Hession C, Rothenbühler R, Shaw A, Kruithof EKO. Plasminogen activator inhibitor 2: Regulation of gene transcription during phorbol ester-mediated differentiation of U- 937 human histiocytic lymphoma cells. *Mol Cell Biol* 1987;7: 4564–4567.

134. Kruithof EKO, Tran-Thang C, Gudinchet A, Hauert J, Nicoloso G, Genton C, et al. Fibrinolysis in pregnancy: A study of plasminogen activator inhibitors. *Blood* 1987;69:460–466.

135. Bonnar J, Daly L, Sheppard BL. Changes in the fibrinolytic system during pregnancy. *Semin Thromb Hemost* 1990;16:221–229.

136. Stump D, Thienpoint M, Collén D. Purification and characterization of a novel inhibitor of urokinase from human urine: Quantitation and preliminary characterization in plasma. *J Biol Chem* 1986;261:12759–12766.

137. Heeb MJ, Espana F, Geiger M, Collen D, Stump D, Griffin JH. Immunological identity of heparin-dependent plasma and urinary protein C inhibitor and plasminogen activator inhibitor-3. *J Biol Chem* 1987;262:15813–15816.

138. Marder VJ, Sherry S. Thrombolytic therapy. Current status. *N Engl J Med* 1988;388: 1512–1520.

139. Gimple LW, Gold HK, Leinbach RC, Coller BS, Werner W, Yasuda T, et al. Correlation between template bleeding times and spontaneous bleeding during treatment of acute myocardial infarction with recombinant tissue plasminogen activator. *Circulation* 1989;80:581–588.

140. Agnelli G, Buchanan MR, Fernandez F, Boneu B, Van Ryn J, Hirsh J, Collén D. A comparison of the thrombolytic and hemorrhagic effects of tissue-type plasminogen activator and streptokinase in rabbits. *Circulation* 1985;72:178–182.

141. Marder VJ, Shortell CK, Fitzpatrick PG, Kim C, Oxley D. An animal model of fibrinolytic bleeding based on the rebleed phenomenon: Application to a study of vulnerability of hemostatic plugs of different age. *Thromb Res* 1992;67(1):31–40.

142. Loscalzo J, Vaughan DB. Tissue plasminogen activator promotes platelet disaggregation in plasma. *J Clin Invest* 1987;79:1749–1755.

143. Chen LY, Muhta JL. Lys- and glu-plasminogen potentiate the inhibitory effect of recombinant tissue plasminogen activator on human platelet aggregation. *Thromb Res* 1994;74:555–563.

144. NIH Consensus Conference. Thrombolytic therapy in treatment. *Br Med J* 1980;280: 1585–1587.

145. Danglet G, Vinson D, Chapeville F. Qualitative and quantitative distribution of plasminogen activators in organs from healthy adult mice. *FEBS Lett* 1986;194:96–100.

146. Matsuo O, Okada K, Fukao H, Suzuki A, Ueshima S. Cerebral plasminogen activator activity in spontaneously hypertensive stroke-prone rats. *Stroke* 1992;23:995–999.
147. Dent MA, Sumi Y, Morris RJ, Seeley PJ. Urokinase-type plasminogen activator expression by neurons and oligodendrocytes during process outgrowth in developing rat brain. *Eur J Neurosci* 1993;5:633–647.
148. Sappino A-P, Madani R, Huarte J, Belin D, Kiss JZ, Wohlwend A, Vassalli J-D. Extracellular proteolysis in the adult murine brain. *J Clin Invest* 1993;92:679–685.
149. Wang YF, Tsirka SE, Strickland S, Stieg PE, Soriano SG, Lipton SA. Tissue plasminogen activator (t-PA) increases neuronal damage after focal cerebral ischemia in wild-type and t-PA-deficient mice. *Nature Medicine* 1998;4:228–231.
150. del Zoppo GJ. t-PA: A neuron buster, too? (Editorial). *Nature Medicine* 1998;4:148–150.
151. Zivin JA, Fisher M, DeGirolami U, Hemenway CC, Stashak JA. Tissue plasminogen activator reduced neurological damage after cerebral embolism. *Science* 1985;230:1289–1292.
152. Overgaard K, Sereghy T, Boysen G, Pedersen H, Diemer NH. Reduction of infarct volume by thrombolysis with rt-PA in an embolic rat stroke model. *Scand J Clin Lab Invest* 1993;53:383–393.
153. Hamann GF, del Zoppo GJ. Leukocyte involvement in vasomotor reactivity of the cerebral vasculature. *Stroke* 1994;25:2117–2119.
154. Kunkel EJ, Jung U, Bullard DC, Norman KE, Wolitzky BA, Vestweber D, Beaudet AL, Ley K. Absence of trauma-induced leukocyte rolling in mice deficient in both P-selectin and intercellular adhesion molecule 1. *J Exp Med* 1996;183:57–65.
155. Bowes MP, Rothlein R, Fagan SC, Zivin JA. Monoclonal antibodies preventing leukocyte activation reduce experimental neurologic injury and enhance efficacy of thrombolytic therapy. *Neurology* 1995;45:815–819.
156. Spetzler RF, Selman WR, Weinstein P, Townsend J, Mehdoric M, Telks D, et al. Chronic reversible cerebral ischemia: Evaluation of a new baboon model. *J Neurosurg* 1980;7:257–261.
157. del Zoppo GJ, Copeland BR, Anderchek K, Hacke W, Koziol JA. Hemorrhagic transformation following tissue plasminogen activator in experimental cerebral infarction. *Stroke* 1990;21:596–601.
158. del Zoppo GJ, Copeland BR, Hacke W, Dietrich JE, Harker LA. Intracerebral hemorrhage following rt-PA infusion in a primate stroke model. *Stroke* 1988;19:134–134.

2 Pathogenesis of Cervico-cranial Artery Occlusion

Louis R. Caplan, MD

CONTENTS

INTRODUCTION
BRAIN EMBOLISM
IN SITU ARTERIAL DISORDERS—THROMBOSIS
REFERENCES

INTRODUCTION

Brain ischemia is caused by a heterogeneous array of different vascular disorders. The general categories of vascular disorders most often used are embolism, "thrombosis" (referring to a local *in situ* process that narrows and often occludes an artery or vein), and systemic hypoperfusion. Systemic disorders that lead to brain ischemia include cardiac disorders (cardiac arrest, arrythmias, low cardiac output), conditions that cause hypovolemia and lack of adequate oxygen-carrying blood (blood loss, severe anemia, shock, carbon monoxide poisoning, hypotension), and acute pulmonary conditions (pulmonary embolism). Since patients with systemic disorders are not candidates for thrombolysis and there ordinarily is no associated intracranial vascular occlusions, this large category will not be discussed herein. I will focus entirely on embolic and "thrombotic" disorders.

BRAIN EMBOLISM

Embolism has been variously defined and categorized. Although some use this category only to include cardiac-origin embolism, I urge a more general approach. An embolus refers to a particle that originates in one place and moves to another site: a traveling particle rather than one that stays at the place it

From: *Thrombolytic Therapy for Stroke*
Edited by: P. D. Lyden © Humana Press Inc., Totowa, NJ

originated ("thrombus"). Embolism is the process of particle migration within the vascular bed.

There are three main descriptors of embolism: the *donor site* that is the source of the embolus; the *material* that makes up the embolus; and the *recipient site* where the embolus rests or remains. All are important determinants when considering treatment *(1–3)*.

Donor Sources

The donor sites for embolic material are the heart, aorta, and extracranial and intracranial arteries. Emboli originating from the heart are usually called cardiogenic, whereas emboli originating within the aorta or proximal arteries are called intra-arterial but are sometimes referred to as local emboli.

Some emboli arise in the venous system and simply pass through the heart to reach the brain and other systemic arteries. These emboli traverse communications between the right heart-pulmonary system and the left heart-systemic circulation. The most common of such communications are intraatrial septal defects and patent foramen ovales. Occasionally incriminated are ventricular septal defects and pulmonary arteriovenous malformations. These emboli are often referred to as *paradoxical emboli*. Studies now show that paradoxical embolism is much more common than previously recognized.

A variety of different cardiac disorders can provide the source for embolism. I have listed the most common categories in Table 1. In all published series, arrythmias such as atrial fibrillation and coronary artery disease related conditions are the most common sources followed by valve disorders. Table 2 enumerates the most frequent cardiac sources in the Stroke Data Bank *(1,4,5)* and that studies' categorization of high and medium risk heart conditions with respect to their importance in serving as sources of emboli. Table 3 lists the most frequent potential cardiac sources of embolism in the Lausanne Stroke Registry *(1,6,7)*.

The aorta is now recognized as a very important source of emboli to the brain, especially during and after cardiac surgery *(8–10)*. Clamping of an atheromatous aortic arch often leads to release of particles into the brain and systemic arteries. Atherosclerosis is often severe in the aorta and the plaques often are located in the ascending aorta and the arch proximal to the origins of the carotid and brachiocephalic arteries *(11)*. Protuberant mobile large plaques are most often associated with brain embolism.

Arterial sources of embolism are also quite varied. Emboli arise from a variety of different disorders and from a variety of different sites. Although atherosclerosis is by far the most common condition that leads to intra-arterial embolism, other vascular diseases can also serve as donor sources. Trauma and dissections of arteries leads to local thrombus formation and embolism. Occasionally inflammatory diseases of the brachiocephalic branches of the aortic arch such as temporal arteritis and Takayasu's disease are sources of intra-arterial embolism.

Table 1
Most Frequent Cardiac Disorders Associated with Brain Embolism

Arrythmias
   atrial fibrillation
   sick-sinus syndrome (brady-tachy syndrome)
Valve diseases
   rheumatic mitral and aortic valve disease
   calcific aortic and mitral valve disease
   prosthetic valves
   bacterial endocarditis
   nonbacterial thrombotic endocarditis (marantic endocarditis) (commonest causes:
      lupus erythematosis, cancer, antiphospholipid antibody syndrome)
   myxomatous valve degeneration (mitral valve prolapse)
   mitral annulus calcification
   ? valve strands
Myocardial disorders
   myocardial infarction
   hypokinetic regions
   myocardial aneurysms
   myocarditis
   cardiomyopathies
Septal lesions
   patent foramen ovale
   atrial septal defects
   ventricular septal defects
   atrial septal aneurysms
Cardiac chamber lesions
   cardiac tumors (myxomas, rhabdomyomas, fibrouelastomas)
   ball thrombi
   "spontaneous echo contrast"

Thrombi sometimes form within arterial aneurysms, saccular, dissecting, and fusiform dolichoectatic aneurysms, and can then break off and embolize to distal branch arteries. Fibromuscular dysplasia (FMD) is an important but relatively uncommon vascular disease that affects the pharyngeal and occasionally the intracranial portions of the carotid and vertebral arteries, which can also occasionally serve as a source of distal intra-arterial embolism. Thrombi can, on occasion, form within large arteries in the absence of important arterial disease in patients with cancer and other causes of hypercoagulability (12). These luminal thrombi then embolize to intracranial arteries causing strokes.

Table 2
Patients in the NIH Stroke Data Bank with Selected Cardiac Characteristics
in High and Medium Cardiac Risk Groups (Modified from *[5]* with Permission)

Cardiac risk categories	High Risk; n = 250	Medium Risk; n = 166
High-risk categories		
Valve surgery	15	
A fib, A flutter, sick sinus with valve disease	28	
A fib, A flutter, sick sinus but no valve disease	**162**	
Ventricular aneurysm*	5	
Mural thrombus*	12	
Cardiomyopathy or left ventricle hypokinesis*	7	
Akinetic region*	**52**	
Medium-risk categories		
Myocardial infarct within 6 mo	25	18
Valve disease without A fib,Aflutter, sick sinus	31	19
Congestive heart failure	**92**	**95**
Decreased left ventricle function*	0	3
Hypokinetic segment*	0	12
Mitral valve prolapse (by history or echocardiogram)	5	13
Mitral annulus calcification*	14	**46**

*By echocardiography some patients had more than one characteristic.

I will discuss some of these conditions further when I consider *in situ* arterial "thrombosis" below.

Embolic Material

The actual "stuff" that embolizes is of great importance *(1–3)*. As far as is known, thrombolytic drugs lyse red erythrocyte thrombi. Of course, fresh soft red thromboemboli are more easily lysed than old organized fibrotic thromboemboli. There are a variety of different particles that can embolize from cardiac and arterial sources. These are listed in Table 4.

Recipient Sites and Resultant Infarct Patterns

About 80% of emboli that arise from the heart go into the anterior (carotid artery) circulation, equally divided between the left and right sides. The remaining 20% of emboli go into the posterior (vertebrobasilar) circulation, a rate roughly equal to the proportion of the blood supply that goes into the vertebrobasilar arteries. The recipient artery destination depends on the size and nature of the particles. Calcific particles from heart valves or mitral annular calcifications are less mobile and adapt less well to the shape of their recipient artery resting places than red (erythrocyte-fibrin) and white (platelet-fibrin)

Table 3
Potential Cardiac Sources of Embolism in the Lausanne Stroke Registry
(Modified from *[7]* with Permission)

Cardiac abnormalities	n patients (%)
Isolated myocardial abnormalities	84 (27.5%)
Focal left ventricle akinesia without thrombus	**61 (20%)**
Focal left ventricle akinesia with thrombus	7 (2.3%)
Global ventricular hypokinesia	7 (2.3%)
Patent foramen ovale	6 (2%)
Left atrial myxoma	2 (0.7%)
Left ventricle thrombus	1 (0.3%)
Isolated valve abnormalities	71 (23.3%)
Mitral valve prolapse	**51 (16.7%)**
Mitral stenosis or insufficiency	10 (3.3%)
Prosthetic mitral or aortic valve	10 (3.3%)
Isolated arrythmia	**127 (41.6%)**
Atrial fibrillation	118 (38.7%)
Sick sinus syndrome	9 (2.9%)
Arrythmias + myocardial abnormalities	12 (3.9%)
Atrial fibrillation + Focal left ventricular akinesia without thrombus	6 (2%)
Atrial fibrillation+ Focal left ventricular akinesia with thrombus	1 (0.3%)
Atrial fibrillation + Global hypokinesia	3 (1%)
Atrial fibrillation + Left ventricular thrombus	2 (0.7%)
Arrythmias + valve abnormalities	11 (3.6%)
Atrial fibrillation + Mitral valve prolapse	6 (2%)
+ mitral stenosis	2 (0.7%)
+ prosthetic valve	3 (1%)

thrombi. The circulating blood stream seems to be able to somehow bypass obstructing cholesterol crystal emboli, especially in the retinal arteries.

Within the anterior and posterior circulations, there are predilection sites for the destination of embolic particles. Large emboli entering a common carotid artery may become lodged in the common or internal carotid artery, especially if atheromatous plaques had already narrowed the lumens of these vessels. If the emboli were able to pass through the carotid arteries in the neck, the next common lodging place is the intracranial bifurcation of the internal carotid arteries (ICAs) into the anterior cerebral (ACA) and middle cerebral (MCA) arteries. Bifurcations are common resting places for emboli. Emboli that pass through the carotid intracranial bifurcations most often go into the MCAs and their branches. Gacs et al. *(13)* showed that balloon emboli placed in the circulation nearly always followed the same pathway and ended up in the MCAs and their branches. Embolism in experimental animals produced by the introduction of silicone

Table 4
Embolic Materials

Cardiac origin	Arterial
red: erythrocyte-fibrin clots	red: erythrocyte-fibrin clots
white: platelet-fibrin clots	white: platelet-fibrin clots
calcific particles	calcific particles
bacteria	cholesterol crystals
fibrous strands	parts of plaques
myxomatous tumors	
prosthetic valve parts	

cylinders or spheres, elastic cylinders, and autologous blood clots, also showed a very high incidence of MCA territory localization *(14)*. Emboli often pass into the superior and inferior divisions of the MCA and the cortical branches of these divisions. The superior division supplies the cortex and white matter above the sylvian fissure including the frontal and superior parietal lobes. The inferior division supplies the area below the sylvian fissure including the temporal and inferior parietal lobes. The ACA supplies the paramedian frontal lobe. Emboli seldom go into the penetrating artery (lenticulostriate arteries) branches of the MCAs or the penetrators from the ACAs because these vessels originate at about a 90 degree angle from the parent arteries.

Embolism into the MCAs causes a variety of different patterns of infarction *(1,15)*. Blockage of the mainstem MCA before the lenticulostriate branches can cause a large infarct that encompasses the entire MCA territory including the deep basal ganglia and internal capsule as well as the cerebral cortex and subcortical white matter of both the suprasylvian and infrasylvian MCA territories. In some patients an embolus has blocked the intracranial carotid artery causing infarction of the ACA territory as well as the entire MCA territory. In young patients when the mainstem MCA is blocked, the rapid development of collateral circulation over the convexity of the brain, often leads to sparing of the superficial territory of the MCA. The lenticulostriate branches are blocked by the clot in the mainstem MCA and collateral circulation to the deep MCA territory is poor. The resultant infarct is limited to the basal ganglia and surrounding cerebral white matter and is usually referred to as a striatocapsular infarct. Passage of an embolus into the superior division of the MCA leads to a cortical/subcortical infarct in the region of the suprasylvian convexity, and embolism to the inferior division leads to an infarct limited to the temporal and inferior parietal lobes below the sylvian fissure. When an embolus rests first in the mainstem MCA and then travels to one of the divisional branches, infarction involves the deep terri-

Table 5
Location and Distribution of Infarcts in the Lausanne Stroke Registry
in Patients with Potential Cardiac Sources of Embolism [7]

Anterior circulation	213 (70%)
Global MCA	33 (11%)
Superior division MCA	60 (20%)
Inferior division MCA	54 (18%)
Deep subcortical	56 (18%)
Anterior Cerebral Artery (ACA)	9 (3%)
ACA and MCA together	1 (0.3%)
Posterior circulation	69 (23%)
Brainstem	18 (6%)
Thalamus (deep PCA)	12 (4%)
Superficial PCA	21 (7%)
Superficial and deep PCA	3 (1%)
Cerebellum	10 (3%)

tory and cortex above or below the sylvian fissure. Small emboli block cortical branches and cause small cortical/subcortical infarcts involving one or several gyri. Occasionally emboli block the anterior cerebral artery or its distal branches. This causes an infarct in the paramedian area of one frontal lobe.

Emboli that enter the posterior circulation can block the vertebral arteries in the neck or intracranially. Emboli that pass through the intracranial vertebral arteries (ICVAs) will usually be able to pass through the proximal and middle portions of the basilar artery, which are wider than the ICVAs. The basilar artery becomes narrower as it courses craniad. Emboli often block the distal basilar artery bifurcation ("top of the basilar") or one of its branches (16–18). The main branches of the basilar artery bifurcation are penetrating arteries to the medial portions of the thalami and midbrain, the superior cerebellar artery, which supplies the upper surface of the cerebellum, and the posterior cerebral arteries (PCAs), which supply the lateral portions of the thalami and the temporal and occipital lobe territories of the posterior cerebral arteries. The most frequent brain areas infarcted are the posterior inferior portion of the cerebellum in the territory of the posterior inferior cerebellar artery (PICA) branch of the ICVA; the superior surface of the cerebellum in the territory of the superior cerebellar artery; the thalamic and hemispheral territories of the PCAs. The clinical and imaging findings in patients with these lesions are described in detail elsewhere (16).

Table 5 notes the most frequent locations of brain infarction in the Lausanne Stroke Registry in patients with potential cardiac sources of embolism (7).

When emboli arise from arteries, the emboli can, of course, only go into more distal portions of that artery. Emboli that originate in the internal carotid artery usually go into the MCA and its branches but occasionally may go into the anterior cerebral, and anterior choroidal arteries and their branches. Occasional emboli go into penetrating artery branches. Within the posterior circulation, emboli that originate from the vertebral arteries in the neck go to the ipsilateral intracranial vertebral artery and its PICA branch and more distally into the basilar artery and any of the branches on either side of the basilar artery and the SCAs and PCAs.

IN SITU ARTERIAL DISORDERS—THROMBOSIS

Atherosclerosis of Large Arteries

Atherosclerosis is by far the most common condition leading to stenosis and occlusion of large extracranial and intracranial arteries. The initial arterial lesion is a fatty streak that develops in the intima and then enlarges into a raised atherosclerotic plaque. Plaques contain a mixture of lipid, smooth muscle, fibrous and collagen tissues, and inflammatory cells *(19,20)*. Plaques can enlarge quickly when hemorrhages occur within the plaques. When a critical plaque size and reduction in the lumen are reached, the atherosclerotic process accelerates. Reduced luminal area and the bulk of the protruding plaque alter the physical and mechanical properties of blood flow and create regions of local turbulence and stasis. Platelets adhere to the irregular surfaces of plaques. Secretion of chemical mediators within platelets and within the underlying vascular endothelium causes aggregation and further adherence of platelets to the endothelium. A "white clot" composed of platelets and fibrin develops and, at first, is rather loosely adherent to the vascular wall. Plaques often interrupt the endothelium and ulcerate. Breaches in the endothelium allow cracks and fissures to form allowing contact of the constituents of the plaque with the luminal contents. The coagulation cascade is activated by this contact and a "red thrombus" composed of erythrocytes and fibrin forms within the lumen. Platelet secretion can also activate the serine proteases that form the body's coagulation system and also promote red clot formation. When thrombi first form, they are poorly organized and only loosely adherent. Often they then propagate and embolize. Within a period of one to two weeks, thrombi organize and become more adherent and fragments are less likely to break off and embolize *(15)*.

There are important sex and racial differences in the distribution of arteriosclerotic occlusive lesions *(21–24)*. In white men, the predominant cerebrovascular occlusive lesions are in the carotid and vertebral arteries in the neck *(15,21,25–27)*. Blacks, individuals of Asian origin, and women, more often have occlusive lesions in the large intracranial arteries and their main branches, and less often have severe occlusive vascular lesions in the neck. White men who have carotid artery disease also have a high frequency of coexisting coronary artery and occlusive lower limb artery disease, as well as hypertension, hypercholesterolemia, and smoking. After menopause, the frequency of extracranial occlusive disease increases in women.

Within the anterior circulation, the most frequent and most important occlusive lesion in white men is within the ICA in the neck. Atherosclerotic lesions usually begin within the common carotid artery (CCA) along the posterior wall of that vessel opposite the flow-divider between the ICA and the external carotid artery (ECA) *(19,20)*. Atherosclerotic plaques grow in diameter and often spread rostrally within the CCA, and the proximal ICA and ECAs. The next most common atherosclerotic lesions in white men are found within the intracranial ICA in the proximal intracranial portion of the artery, the carotid siphon, and within the proximal portions of the MCAs. These lesions all produce symptoms by causing hypoperfusion of supplied brain territories and/or by embolism of fragments of clots that form upon the vascular endothelium of plaques or of particles of the plaques themselves. Women, blacks, and Asians often develop occlusive lesions within the MCAs and their branches *(21–24)*. ICA siphon and neck lesions are less often found. Blacks, Asians, and women who develop occlusive neck lesions usually smoke and have important coexisting atherosclerotic risk factors such as hypertension and hypercholesterolemia.

Within the posterior circulation, the commonest occlusive lesion among white men is at the origins of the vertebral arteries in the neck and within the adjacent subclavian artery. The next most common lesion is within the basilar artery. White men with occlusive extracranial vertebral artery (ECVA) disease also have a high frequency of coexisting carotid artery disease *(16,26,27)*, as well as hypertension and hypercholesterolemia. Intracranial lesions are also very common both in white men and in women, blacks, and Asians. The predominant lesions are within the ICVAs. Atherosclerotic lesions within the ICVAs are often bilateral. Atherosclerotic lesions involving the posterior cerebral arteries are more common in women, blacks, and Asians *(16)*.

Arterial Dissections

Arterial dissections are probably the second most common disease that leads to thrombi forming within arteries. Dissections are often related to mechanical injury. When there is an obvious direct injury, the dissections are usually called traumatic but even so-called "spontaneous" dissections usually involve some mechanical perturbation of the arterial wall. Stretching or tearing within the arterial media causes formation of an intramural hematoma. Blood within the media dissects longitudinally along the vessel wall. Expansion of the arterial wall compromises the lumen. The expanding intramural hematoma can tear through the intima and inject fresh red congealed hematoma containing thrombus-like material into the arterial lumen. This material is, at first, not adherent to the endothelium and often embolizes. The intimal tear and the underlying medial hematoma cause some irritation of the endothelium, which, in turn, causes activation of platelets and the coagulation cascade promoting the formation of a thrombus *in situ* within the lumen. Compromise of the lumen by the expanding intramural lesion alters blood flow within the lumen, which also promotes thrombus formation. Thus, thrombus can form *in situ* within the dissected artery or reach the lumen by introduction of the intramural contents. In either case, the acute lumenal thrombus is poorly organized and nonadherent and readily embolizes distally *(15,16)*.

Arterial dissections most often involve the pharyngeal portions of the extracranial carotid and vertebral arteries *(15,16,28–30)*. The pharyngeal portions of the neck arteries are relatively mobile, whereas the origins of the arteries and their penetrations into the cranial cavity are relatively anchored and much less mobile. Tearing most often occurs in portions of arteries that are flexible and stretch with motion. Within the ECVAs, the most common site of dissection is the most distal portion of the artery, which emerges from the intervertebral foramina and courses around the atlas to penetrate the dura mater and enter the foramen magnum *(16,29,30)*. Dissections also occur in the mobile part of the proximal portion of the ECVAs above the origin of the arteries from the subclavian arteries but before the arteries enter the vertebral column at the intervertebral foramen of the sixth or fifth cervical vertebrae. Intracranial dissections are much less common than extracranial dissections. In the anterior circulation, dissections most often affect the intracranial ICA and extend into the middle and anterior cerebral arteries. Within the posterior circulation the commonest site is the intracranial vertebral artery *(30,31)*. Dissections within the ICVAs often spread into the basilar artery. Occasionally the basilar artery is the primary site of dissection *(16)*.

Other Large Artery Diseases

Other vascular conditions cause large artery occlusions at a much lower frequency than atherosclerosis and arterial dissections. *Fibromuscular dysplasia (FMD)* is a heterogeneous condition characterized mostly by abnormalities in the smooth muscle and connective tissue within the arterial media *(15,16)*. The lesions can occur in the pharyngeal carotid artery and in the vertebral arteries within the vertebral column. Occasionally the lesions involve the intracranial large arteries. Thrombi can develop in regions of narrowing of arteries related to FMD. Various types of arteritis can on rare occasions cause arterial occlusions. The most important such disorder is arteritis related to the Herpes zoster-varicella virus *(32)*. The virus can spread from the trigeminal ganglion to the middle cerebral artery and cause endothelial lesions that promote thrombus formation. Although other forms of arteritis are frequently mentioned as part of obligatory differential diagnoses, they are extremely rare causes of brain infarction and are not often complicated by thrombosis of sizable intracranial arteries. *Migraine* can be accompanied by arterial vasoconstriction. Narrowing of intracranial arteries, especially the PCA, and perturbation of the endothelium can promote thrombus formation (16,33).

Hypercoagulable States (34,35)

Occasionally occlusion of extracranial arteries is caused by hypercoagulability. There may also be an underlying endothelial lesion, e.g., a plaque within the carotid or vertebral arteries. Polycythemia, thrombocytosis, hereditary and acquired deficiencies of coagulation factors (antithrombin III, protein C, protein S, and activated Factor V Leiden), cancer, increased serum levels of fibrinogen, deficiencies of fibrinolytic factors all can cause or contribute to hypercoagulability. Cancer, especially mucinous adenocarcinomas, and inflammatory diseases such as Crohn's disease and ulcerative colitis, can also lead to increased coagulability. Acute and chronic infections induce an increase in acute phase reactants that increase coagulability.

In hypercoagulable patients, thrombi can form anywhere. Thrombi can form in regions of endothelial abnormalities. Often there are multiple small intracranial thrombi.

Penetrating Artery Disease

The arteries that penetrate into the deeper regions of the brain are susceptible to somewhat different disease processes than the superficial branches of the same intracranial arteries. These vessels supply the basal ganglia, caudate nuclei, thalami, pons, and portions of the midbrain and medulla as well as regions of the internal capsules, corona radiata, and centrum semiovale. The small, penetrating artery branches mostly arise at nearly right angles from the anterior, middle, and posterior cerebral arteries and the basilar artery. The predominant conditions that affect these penetrating arteries are lipohyalinosis (36–38) and intracranial atheromatous branch disease (39–41).

Lipohyalinotic arteries have walls thickened by the deposition of hyaline material and lipids. This process can lead to the narrowing of arterial lumens with subsequent brain infarction in tissue supplied by the compromised penetrating artery (36–38). Atheromas can also develop within the parent arteries and block or extend into the orifices of the penetrating branches (39–41). Microatheromas can also form within the proximal portion of the branches. Pathological studies are scant and it is not well-known how often microthrombi form in these penetrating arteries. Microdissections have been discovered at necropsy within the proximal portions of relatively large penetrating arteries (40).

REFERENCES

1. Caplan LR. Brain embolism. In: Practical Clinical Neurocardiology, Caplan LR, Chimowitz M, Hurst JW, eds. Marcel Dekker: New York. 2000, pp. 35–185.

2. Caplan LR. Brain embolism, revisited. *Neurology* 1993;43:1281–1287.

3. Caplan LR. Of birds, and nests and brain emboli. *Rev Neurol* (Paris) 1991;147:265–273.

4. Foulkes MA, Wolf PA, Price TR, Mohr JP, Hier DB. The Stroke Data Bank: Design, methods, and baseline characteristics. *Stroke* 1988;19:547–554.

5. Kittner SJ, Sharkness CM, Price TR, et al. Infarcts with a cardiac source of embolism in the NINCDS Stroke Data Bank: historical features. *Neurology* 1990;40:281–284.

6. Bogousslavsky J, van Melle G, Regli F. The Lausanne Stroke Registry: Analysis of 1000 consecutive patients with first stroke. *Stroke* 1988;19:1083–1092.

7. Bogousslavsky J, Cachin C, Regli F, et al. Cardiac sources of embolism and cerebral infarction. Clinical consequences and vascular concomitants. *Neurology* 1991;41:855–859.

8. Amarenco P, Duyckaerts C, Tzourio C, et al. The prevalence of ulcerated plaques in the aortic arch in patients with stroke. *N Engl J Med* 1992;326:221–225.

9. Amarenco P, Cohen A, Baudrimont M, Bousser M-G. Transesophageal echocardiographic detection of aortic arch disease in patients with cerebral infarction. *Stroke* 1992;23:1005–1009.

10. The French Study of Aortic Plaques in Stroke Group. Atherosclerotic disease of the aortic arch as a risk factor for recurrent ischemic stroke. *N Engl J Med* 1996;334:1216–1221.

11. Tobler HG, Edwards JE. Frequency and location of atherosclerotic plaques in the ascending aorta. *J Thor Cardiovasc Surg* 1988;96:304–306.

12. Caplan LR, Stein R, Patel D, et al. Intraluminal clot of the carotid artery detected radiographically. *Neurology* 1984;34:1175–1181.

13. Gacs G, Merer FT, Bodosi M. Balloon catheter as a model of cerebral emboli in humans. *Stroke* 1982;13:39–42.

14. Helgason C. Cardioembolic stroke topography and pathogenesis. *Cerebrovasc Brain Metab Rev* 1992;4:28–58.

15. Caplan LR. Caplan's Stroke, a clinical approach, 3rd ed. Butterworth-Heinemann: Boston. 2000.

16. Caplan LR. Posterior circulation disease. In: *Clinical findings, diagnosis, and management.* Blackwell Science: Boston. 1996.

17. Caplan LR. Top of the basilar syndrome: selected clinical aspects. *Neurology* 1980;30:72–79.

18. Caplan LR, Tettenborn B. Vertebrobasilar occlusive disease: review of selected aspects. 2. Posterior circulation embolism. *Cerebrovasc Dis* 1992;2:320–326.

19. Hennerici M, Sitzer G, Weger H-D. Carotid artery plaques. Basel, Karger, 1987.

20. Fisher CM, Ojemann RG. A clinico-pathologic study of carotid endarterectomy plaques. *Rev Neurol (Paris)* 1986;142:573–589.

21. Caplan JR, Gorelick PB, Hier DB. Race, sex, and occlusive cerebrovascular disease: a review. *Stroke* 1986;17:648–655.

22. Gorelick PB, Caplan LR, Hier DB, et al. Racial differences in the distribution of anterior circulation occlusive disease. *Neurology* 1984;34:54–59.

23. Gorelick PB, Caplan LR, Hier DB, Langenberg P, Pessin MS, Biller J, Kornack D. Racial differences in the distribution of posterior circulation occlusive disease. *Stroke* 1985;16:785–790.

24. Feldmann E, Daneault N, Kwan E, Ho KJ, Pessin MS, Langenberg P, Caplan LR. Chinese-White differences in the distribution of occlusive cerebrovascular disease. *Neurology* 1990;40:1541–1545.

25. Fisher CM, Gore I, Okabe N, White PD. Atherosclerosis of the carotid and vertebral arteries-extracranial and intracranial. *J Neuropathol Exp Neurol* 1965;24:455–476.

26. Hutchinson EC, Yates PO. Carotico-vertebral stenosis. *Lancet* 1957;1:2–8.

27. Hutchinson EC, Yates PO. The cervical portion of the vertebral artery. A clinicopathological study. *Brain* 1956;79:319–331.

28. Fisher CM, Ojemann R, Roberson G. Spontaneous dissection of cervicocerebral arteries. *Can J Neuro Sci* 1978;5:9–19.

29. Caplan LR, Zarins C, Hemmatti M. Spontaneous dissection of the extracranial vertebral artery. *Stroke* 1985;16:1030–1038.

30. Caplan LR, Tettenborn B. Vertebrobasilar occlusive disease:review of selected aspects. 1. Spontaneous dissection of extracranial and intracranial posterior circulation arteries. *Cerebrovasc Dis* 1992;2:256–265.
31. Caplan LR, Baquis G, Pessin MS, et al. Dissection of the intracranial vertebral artery. *Neurology* 1988;38:868–877.
32. Hilt DC, Buchholz D, Krumholz A, et al. Herpes zoster opthalmicus and delayed contralateral hemiparesis caused by cerebral angiitis: diagnosis and management approaches. *Ann Neurol* 1983;14:543–553.
33. Caplan LR. Migraine and vertebrobasilar ischemia. *Neurology* 1991;41:55–61.
34. Markus HS, Hambley H. Neurology and the blood: Haematological abnormalities in ischaemic stroke. *J Neurol Neurosurg Psychiatry* 1998;64:150–159.
35. Feinberg WM. Coagulation in Brain ischemia. In: *Basic concepts and clinical relevance*, Caplan LR, ed. Springer-Verlag: London. 1995; pp. 85–96.
36. Fisher CM. The arterial lesions underlying lacunes. *Acta Neuropathol* 1969;12:1–15.
37. Fisher CM. Cerebral miliary aneurysms in hypertension. *Am J Pathol* 1972;66:313–324.
38. Rosenblum WJ. Miliary aneurysms and "fibrinoid" degeneration of cerebral blood vessels. *Hum Pathol* 1977;8:133–139.
39. Fisher CM, Caplan LR. Basilar artery branch occlusion: a cause of pontine infarction. *Neurology* 1971;21:900–905.
40. Fisher CM. Bilateral occlusion of basilar artery branches. *J Neurol Neurosurg Psychiatry* 1977;40:1182–1189.
41. Caplan LR. Intracranial branch atheromatous disease: a neglected, understudied, and underused concept. *Neurology* 1989;39:1246–1250.

3

The Ischemic Penumbra and Neuronal Salvage

Patrick D. Lyden, MD

CONTENTS

INTRODUCTION
THE ISCHEMIC PENUMBRA
EXCITOTOXICITY AND NEUROINHIBITORY THERAPY
APOPTOSIS AND NECROSIS
THE ROLE OF GRANUOLCYTES
COMBINATORIAL NEUROPROTECTION
HEMORRHAGIC INFARCTION AND INTRACRANIAL HEMORRHAGE
REFERENCES

INTRODUCTION

The majority of focal cerebral ischemic events result from arterial occlusion due to embolism or *in situ* thrombosis. This interruption in blood flow, if severe and prolonged, leads to cerebral infarction. Brain infarction results from a disruption in blood flow causing a reduction in oxygen and glucose supplied to the tissue. Glucose and oxygen deprivation causes a metabolic shift toward the production of lactic acidic. Coincident with this impairment of the Na^+/Ca^{2+} exchange pump, excessive glutamate release causes an unregulated amount of calcium to enter the cells. Intracellular calcium increases trigger a variety of processes that result in the breakdown of membranes and nucleic acids. In addition, the release of free radicals, the breakdown of the blood-brain barrier, and development of the inflammatory response all work together to promote further cellular injury.

For centuries, the brain was believed to tolerate no more than a few minutes of ischemia; brain cell death was considered irreversible. In the 1980s, a series

From: *Thrombolytic Therapy for Stroke*
Edited by: P. D. Lyden © Humana Press Inc., Totowa, NJ

of investigations proved that only a portion of the brain tissue is irreparably damaged so quickly after focal ischemia. The surrounding region may remain viable for several hours. This concept has been referred to as the "ischemic penumbra" *(1–6)*. Restoration of blood flow to this area within a certain period of time may salvage the "viable" cells and diminish the degree of neurological deficits. One way to reestablish blood flow is by dissolution of the thrombus. This concept led to thoughts about thrombolysis as a possible treatment for stroke.

The clinician contemplating the use of thrombolysis is acknowledging de facto the existence of a penumbra that cannot be measured or documented. Using somewhat circular logic, the successful thrombolytic trials support the notion that some portion of ischemic brain remains salvageable for hours after symptom onset. Limited direct evidence suggests that salvageable brain cells may reside in penumbral zones. It is critical to understand the genesis of the penumbra concept prior to cerebral thrombolysis.

THE ISCHEMIC PENUMBRA

After vascular occlusion, there is a heterogeneous depression of cerebral blood flow (CBF) in the territory of the occluded artery. The *penumbra* is identified as the brain region receiving regional CBF (rCBF) between two critical values *(2,5)*. The first, higher, critical value is associated with neuronal paralysis: brain areas receiving rCBF less than 18–20 mL/100g/min do not function. The second, lower, critical value is associated with cell death: brain areas receiving less than 8–10 mL/100 mg/min do not survive, and this area becomes the *core* of the infarction *(2)*. Neurons in the penumbra are sometimes identified as "idling" to suggest that they are salvageable, although the mechanism of such a phenomenon is unknown. The time course of cell death in the core is rapid whereas cells in the penumbra may survive up to several hours *(7)*.

Soon after the original description of the penumbra, it was recognized that cells do not survive forever, idling in the penumbra *(8,9)*. Thus, it became clear that the penumbra involved two different parameters: blood flow and time. In baboons, for example, cells in a zone of blood that is receiving 20cc/100g/min will survive for a few hours, but cells receiving 12cc/100g/min may only survive for 2 h. This idea suggests that over time the "core" of the infarct enlarges, eventually subsuming the penumbra, giving rise to the clinical dictum that "time is brain." In other words, an increasing fraction of brain loses blood flow below the critical threshold for neuronal survival.

In rats, temporary occlusion of the middle cerebral artery longer than 30 min results in varying degrees of infarction *(10)*. Reperfusion after occlusion will result in some diminution of the infarct, compared to permanent occlusion, up to 120 min. After 2 h, however, reperfusion does not alter infarction volume. Around the infarction, there is a variable amount of neuronal loss *(11)*. Degenerating neurons can be detected within about 3 mm of the infarction border for up to 3 wk after stroke. After that, no further cell loss can be seen using routine stains. In cats, a similar phenomenon has been documented *(12)*. There was a close correlation between rCBF and neuron density around the infarction: the farther away from the edge of the cyst, the greater the blood flow and density of neurons. In humans, it is difficult to document a similar loss of neurons within a few millimeters of areas of complete infarction, or cyst formation *(11)*. These data are consistent with the interpretation that over the long term, there is no survival of penumbral tissue. If reperfusion begins early, however, penumbral tissue may survive; otherwise, the marginal tissue is eventually included in the cyst formed by the core of the infarct.

Baron and colleagues have obtained elegant data using positron emission tomography (PET) scanning to explore the penumbra concept. They showed that over time after stroke an area of excessive oxygen extraction, perhaps reflecting the core, does in fact enlarge *(13)*. Unfortunately, for us designing therapy, the temporal evolution of the penumbra was highly variable. In some patients, a penumbra could be identified as late as 16 h after stroke onset, but in others there was no penumbra by 5 h. In another similar study, possibly viable tissue could be identified in the penumbra for up to 48 hours in some patients *(14)*. Mosely and colleagues at Stanford conducted similar sorts of experiments using magnetic resonance imaging (MRI) of water diffusion, a possible marker of the core, and blood perfusion, a possible marker of the penumbra. In such studies, some patients do indeed exhibit patterns that indicate a core smaller than the penumbra. In untreated patients, the ultimate size of the infarction is comparable to the size of the "penumbra" suggesting that the core did enlarge to subsume the penumbra. In some patients who underwent recanalization, the ultimate infarct was smaller, only the size of the core, suggesting that thrombolysis in fact prevented enlargement of the core. The MRI conceptualization of the penumbra was also documented in rats by Fisher and colleagues *(15)*. After one hour occlusion, a core diffusion-weight image abnormality was surrounded by a larger area of low flow. After 2 h of occlusion, the core and penumbra were identical and the outcome was much poorer.

Until very recently, our concept of the penumbra simply included two zones, one surrounding the other, as shown in Fig. 1. There are a number of problems with the simple penumbra concept. Despite the interesting data obtained by some groups, the vast majority of patients with focal ischemia do not exhibit such consistent patterns. Many more patients who respond to thrombolysis with a gratifying recovery do NOT show a pattern on PET or MRI consistent with a presumed core and a larger penumbra. It is increasingly clear that the penumbra concept should be expanded to include more complicated flow patterns. For example, in Fig. 2 we illustrate a possible scenario in which a central core is surrounded by patches of penumbral flow, some of which include additional

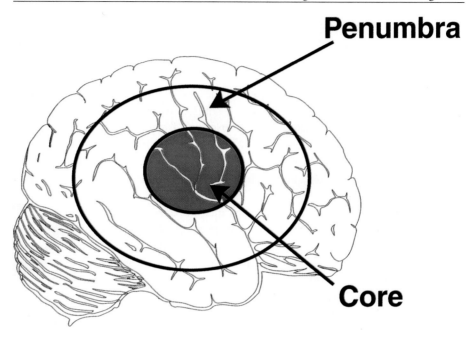

Fig. 1. Traditional concept that the infarct core is surrounded by an enveloping penumbra.

zones of very low, or core, flow. It is quite likely that variable areas of brain receive penumbral levels of flow and that the distribution of these areas in the brain is determined by variable degrees of collateralization from other blood vessels. Such collaterals generally connect in the pia between end-branches of the larger arteries. There is some limited pathological data to support this concept of "islands" of penumbral flow near to areas of complete infarction *(16)*.

No matter what the spatial pattern of blood flow changes, it is clear that cells in penumbral regions do not survive indefinitely. The exact duration of survival is unknown, and is likely different under differing circumstances. Cells in zones receiving 10 to 20cc/100g/min likely survive for hours, but the number of hours is not known. Many factors may reduce the time such marginally perfused cells might survive. For example, it is known that hyperthermia of 1 or 2°C will accelerate cell death *(17)*. Elevations of serum glucose also accelerate cell death *(18)*. Such marginal levels of blood flow do not support neuronal survival indefinitely, but could be sufficient to deliver neuroprotectants into the ischemic zone. Therefore, pending recanalization and restoration of blood flow, a number of therapies could be directed at idling neurons in the penumbra. Such neuroprotectants might salvage brain by preserving neurons until blood flow is restored. The possible mechanisms of neuroprotection include interrupting ischemic

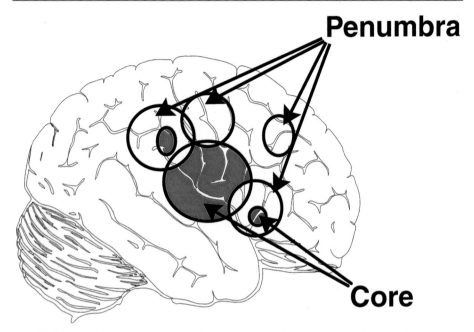

Fig. 2. Alternative concept that regions corresponding to core and penumbra may be heterogeneous.

excitotoxicity, blocking apoptosis, and blocking the inflammatory response that follows ischemia.

EXCITOTOXICITY AND NEUROINHIBITORY THERAPY

The elucidation of the excitotoxic cell death mechanism advanced stroke neurology considerably. An understanding of the biochemical events outlined below spawned a plethora of therapeutic trials. As of this writing (2000) no agent has yet proven successful in humans, despite considerable excitement from laboratory studies. Future successful neuroprotection depends upon further delineation of the steps in the ischemic cascade, and identifying candidate points for intervention.

The Ischemic Cascade and the Role of Intracellular Calcium

The sudden deprivation of oxygen and glucose sets into motion a set of events called the ischemic cascade. The use of the term cascade implies that ischemia proceeds in an orderly manner from the beginning of the cascade to the end. Alternatively, it is becoming clear that the several steps in the cascade occur simultaneously, rather than sequentially and in addition there appear to be multiple feed-forward, feed-back, and amplification steps (e.g., *19–21*). A simple sketch of some of these phenomena is presented as Fig. 3.

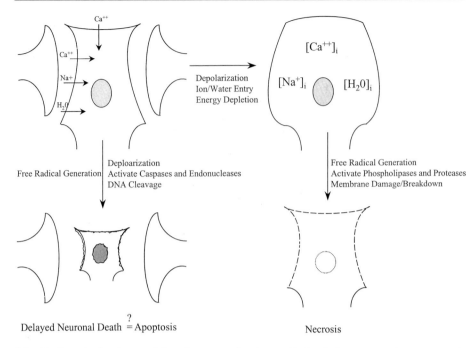

Fig. 3. Depolarization and ion flux may lead to cell death by apoptosis or necrosis pathways.

Glutamate exposure is associated with cell death and degeneration in cell culture *(22–24)* (reviewed in *25*) and glutamate receptor antagonists protect cultured cells from exposure to glutamate, hypoglycemia, and hypoxia *(26,27)*. At least three glutamate receptor subtypes are identified based on ligand binding studies: *N*-methyl-D-aspartate (NMDA), α-amino-3-hydroxy-5-methyl-4-isoxazoleproionate (AMPA)-kainate, and metabotropic *(28)*. Of these subtypes, the NMDA receptor appears to be critical in mediating the effects of ischemia, although interest in AMPA/kainate receptors continues, especially in studies of global ischemia *(27,29)* and the role of the metabotropic receptor subtype remains unclear *(30)*.

Depolarization of the post-synaptic cell occurs in response to application of glutamate, and appears to be a necessary step in the sequence of events leading to cell death *(23,24)*. During excitation of the postsynaptic membrane, there is an influx of sodium, chloride, calcium, and water into the cell *(27,31,32)*. Inflow of ions and water leads to edema, and if severe or prolonged, such edema may lead to cell lysis and death *(32)*. Glutamate does not cause edema or lysis of mature neurons in culture unless sodium and/or chloride are present in the culture medium *(32)*. Inflow of calcium may lead to delayed neuronal death through unknown mechanisms after comparatively brief exposure to ischemia or excitotoxins *(31,33)*. There is some evidence, albeit preliminary and often contradictory, that this delayed cell death may be mediated through apoptotic mechanisms *(34,35)*. This effect persists in culture if sodium is not present in the medium but is blocked by Mg^{2+} or by removing calcium from the medium *(24,32)*.

During ischemia, intracellular calcium concentrations increase through mechanisms other than the ligand-gated channels described above. Some calcium channels are voltage gated, and depolarization to a membrane voltage that opens some of these channels may be a critical determinant of calcium influx *(24,31)*. However, since calcium appears to enter the cell through the NMDA receptor itself, ligand-gated influx appears to continue even in voltage clamped cells *(24,36)*. Nevertheless, it seems reasonable to suspect that prevention of glutamate-stimulated depolarization ought to prevent some of the early cellular edema due to sodium, chloride, and water movement, and some of the calcium flow that leads to delayed toxicity. In support of this expectation, it was observed that hyperpolarization reduced or blocked calcium inflow into neurons *(37)* and reduced the probability of discharge *(38)*. Other routes of influx include the release of calcium from intracytoplasmic stores *(39)* (mediated in part via metabotropic receptors linked to protein kinase C) and loss of adenosine triphosphate (ATP) dependent calcium extrusion mechanisms *(40)*. Also, with membrane damage there is influx of calcium down an electrochemical gradient *(41)*.

There is now a growing consensus that the increase in intracellular calcium sets into motion a variety of events that lead to cell death, most especially the activation of cytosolic phospolipases, and proteases *(19,42)*. Proteases may play a central role in activating programmed cell death; phospholipases may be critically involved in further excitotoxin release, and the generation of reactive oxygen species; as a direct result of early glutamate mediated increases in intracellular calcium, a vicious cycle is created that causes spread of the core zone of infarction *(19)*.

Several direct glutamate antagonists (MK-801, CGS-19755, and dextrophan) and indirect agents that bind at the NMDA glycine site (ACEA1021, felbamate, GV150526a) appear to protect brain during focal ischemia *(43–51)*. The direct agents resemble dissociative anesthetics such as ketamine and phencyclidine and humans experience significant side effects during treatment with NMDA antagonists that ended development efforts for these agents. Therefore, others have chosen to pursue an alternative strategy for brain protection during cerebral ischemia: to use agents that block the effect of excitotoxins without causing such severe side effects. We chose gamma-aminobutyric acid (GABA) agonists for this purpose. The events discussed below are sketched in Fig. 4.

In mammalian brain, GABA is considered the principal inhibitory neurotransmitter *(52)*. Inhibitory neurotransmitters increase chloride conductance, lower the resting membrane potential of the neuron, and reduce the probability that glutamate stimulation leads to action potential *(38,52,53)*. GABA mediates its

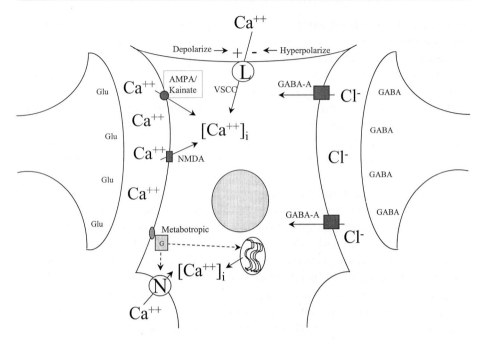

Fig. 4. GABA receptor activation leads to a hyperpolarizing influx of chloride that blocks voltage-gated calcium influx via the L-type voltage-sensitive calcium channel (VSCC). There may also be inhibition of the *N*-type calcium channel.

effects through two receptor subtypes, A and B. The GABA-A receptor is a ligand-gated chloride channel found throughout the brain that mediates a fast inhibitory response *(54,55)*. The GABA-B receptor appears to participate in presynaptic release of several neurotransmitters and postsynaptically to mediate the late inhibitory postsynaptic potential *(56)*. When GABA or a suitable analog occupies the postsynaptic GABA-A receptor, the resting membrane potential may not increase and voltage-gated calcium channels are prevented from opening *(37,38,57)*. Also, GABA-A agonists reduce the cerebral metabolic rate for glucose at doses that do not cause sedation or impair respiration or cardiac function *(58,59)*. GABA-A receptors are found on cerebral blood vessels and cause dilation of cerebral, but not extracranial, vessels. This effect is blocked by competitive antagonists of the GABA receptor *(60)*. GABA-B agonists reduce the presynaptic release of glutamate and ought to be neuroprotective via a presynaptic mechanism. Despite this rationale, and the preliminary work presented below, there may be conditions under which GABA is neurotoxic *(61,62)*.

A new strategy for utilizing GABAergic mechanisms emerged with the development of GABA modulators. Some steroid molecules have nongenomic actions on cells that appear to be mediated via binding sites on membrane-bound iono-phores *(63,64)* (for review *see 65,66*). Of particular relevance to our work are the 5-reduced, 3α-hydroxylated pregnane steroids, which appear to be potent modu-lators of chloride flux through the GABA-A ion channel *(67)*. On the other hand, other neurosteroids, such as pregnenolone sulfate, may have GABA-antagonist actions, and some have agonist or antagonist properties at the NMDA receptor. Pregnenolone and allopregnenolone are potent sedatives and anticonvulsants *(68)*. We are unaware of any studies of neurosteroids in ischemia.

APOPTOSIS AND NECROSIS

Despite the obvious difference in blood flow between the core and the pen-umbra, the mechanisms of cell death in the two regions are not fully known. *Necrosis* is obviously one mechanism for cell death in both the penumbra and the core. During necrosis the cell initially swells, then shrinks and can be observed as a small, pyknotic form on sections *(69)*. Finally, microglia and macrophages remove the debris of the dead cell. If necrosis includes the adja-cent glia and structural matrix, a cyst is formed and the process is termed *pannecrosis*. Recently, *apoptosis*, or programmed cell death, has been observed in ischemic brain *(70)*. In this type of cell death, ischemia is thought to activate "suicide" proteins that are latent in all cells. These proteins are normally expressed during embryogenesis and enable the organism to remove cells that will not be needed during further development. The morphometry of apoptosis is quite different from necrosis, and special techniques are available to study the two forms of cell death *(71)*. The role of apoptotic cell death in the core and in the penumbra is not known. Figure 3 illustrates the factors involved in these two forms of cell death. How cells end up "choosing" one form of death over the other is not known.

The cellular and molecular events leading to cell death have been described in cell culture systems. Relating these findings to living subjects, and to ischemia in particular, is problematic. A thorough review of recent in vitro findings is available and not repeated here *(71–73)*. A few pertinent findings are described.

Injuries such as hypoglycemia, anoxia, and excitotoxin exposure kill cells via necrosis. Necrotic cell death is clearly associated with elevations of intracellular calcium, which has been demonstrated in culture, brain slices, and intact brain. The histopathologic sequence of cellular changes leading to necrosis has been documented *(69,74)*. After focal or global ischemia, swollen, eosinophilic neu-rons appear within 2 to 8 h. Pyknotic, shrunken neurons appear within 24 to 36 h. Phagocytosis of neurons, astrocytes, and surrounding matrix occurs over days. Once the necrotic cell death pathway begins, it probably cannot be interrupted easily. In areas of severe ischemia (core), a cyst is formed after phagocytosis and removal of all brain elements. In surrounding brain (penumbra) some cells are removed and astrocytes may proliferate, leaving a zone of "incomplete" infarction that is depleted of neurons but not cystic. The behavioral consequences of this incomplete infarction are unknown.

Another mechanism of cell death has been proposed *(71)*. Programmed cell death via a series of events that may represent apoptosis can also be simulated in neuronal cell culture. The initial events are shrinkage of the nucleus and cytoplasm, chromatin condensation followed by nuclear fragmentation, and the separation of cell membrane protuberances (blebs). A hallmark is the cleavage of DNA by endonucleases into segments of nonrandom length, which results in "laddering" on DNA isolation gels. Ultimately the cell separates into small, pyknotic bodies that are phagoctytosed by cells resident in the tissue. There is little or no inflammatory infiltrate associated with apoptosis *(71)*. During some phases, it is difficult to distinguish apoptotic from necrotic cells using morphologic criteria *(71)*. There is a suggestion that the morphologic changes may not occur simultaneously with endonuclease cleavage of DNA *(75)*. Following focal cerebral injury, including middle cerebral artery occlusion, apoptotic-like changes can be documented in brain *(70,76–79)*. Specifically, focal ischemia is associated with DNA nicking as documented with labels specific for free DNA strands, nonrandom DNA fragmentation as documented by the "laddering" phenomenon on DNA extraction gels, and ultrastructural findings consistent with apoptosis. It is not clear if apoptotic-like cell death occurs in the core, the penumbra, or both. It is also not clear whether this pathway can be interrupted. Of most concern, it is not clear whether apoptotic-like cell death occurs separately from necrotic death, or whether the two phenomena represent different manifestations of one underlying cell death process *(80)*. It is very clear that necrotic and apoptotic appearing cells can be found in the same regions of brain at the same time *(76)*.

There is some evidence supporting the existence of apoptosis as a separate event in the central nervous system. Deprivation of growth factors (adrenalectomized rats) results in apoptotic-like death of some populations of hippocampal neurons *(81)*. Administration of cycloheximide, an inhibitor of protein synthesis required for apoptotic cell death, blocks the death of spinal cord cells after trauma and hippocampal cells after 2VO forebrain ischemia *(82,83)*. In the spinal cord study, this histopathologic finding was correlated with amelioration of the behavioral sequelae of the trauma, paraparesis *(82)*. These findings suggest that blocking steps related to apoptotic cell death might ameliorate the functional sequelae of ischemia. Candidate treatments have yet to emerge or enter clinical trials.

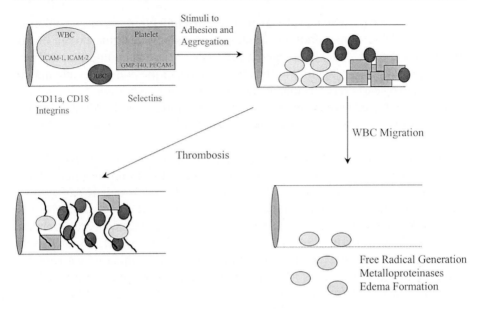

Fig. 5. Following occlusion, granulocytes leave the circulation to enter ischemic brain.

THE ROLE OF GRANULOCYTES

Restoration of arterial blood flow after several hours of occlusion may not result in complete tissue reperfusion, the so-called "no-reflow phenomenon" *(84,85)*. The mechanism is not certain, but may involve endothelial swelling, occlusion of microvessels with platelet-fibrin aggregates, red cell microthrombi, or perivascular swelling. The no-reflow effect does not occur if white blood cells are removed from the circulation *(85)*. Granulocytes may adhere to ischemic endothelium, blocking capillaries and stimulating platelet aggregation and formation of micro-thrombi, as illustrated in Fig. 5. The receptor complex on the granulocyte that mediates adherence is composed of the integrins CD18/CD11 (for review *see* 86). This complex binds to the intercellular adhesion molecule (ICAM) on the endothelial cell.

In addition to mediating the no-reflow phenomenon, granulocytes may have direct toxic effects in the brain. After adhesion, granulocytes migrate into the brain (diapedesis), and can be observed in the peri-ischemic zone within hours of permanent or transient arterial occlusion *(87)*. Once in the brain, granulocytes release phagocytic chemotactic factors as well as cytokines that may promote cellular destruction. Granulocytes also release enzymes that lead to the formation of free radicals, which lead to an increase in hypochlorous acid and chloramines *(88)*. These compounds then activate granulocytic serine proteases and metalloproteinases, which together begin to destroy surrounding tissue. These events proceed independently of the energy status of the brain cells and may be augmented by early reperfusion, the *reperfusion injury syndrome*. Granulocytes have been detected in the penumbra in multiple animal models *(89,90)*. There is very little evidence of reperfusion injury in humans after cerebral thrombolysis, however.

A monoclonal antibody directed against the ICAM receptor effectively blocks granulocyte adherence to endothelial cells, prevents the no-reflow phenomenon and trans-migration into brain *(89,90)*. In animal models anti-ICAM reduces neurologic injury after focal ischemia *(90–92)*. The anti-ICAM-1 antibody (dose of 1 mg/kg given iv 2 h after ischemia onset, plus 0.5 mg/kg 24 h after ischemia onset) has been tested previously in the suture occlusion model in rats *(90)*, where it was effective in reducing infarction volume by 41%. In this study, all animals were subjected to the same 120 min occlusion duration; infarction volume in vehicle treated subjects was 171 ± 38 mm^3 or 17% of cerebrum *(90)*. This was associated with a significant reduction in the numbers of granulocytes found in the cortex ipsilateral to the occlusion.

COMBINATORIAL NEUROPROTECTION

As outlined previously, there are a variety of interacting events proceeding simultaneously during ischemia and it now seems unlikely that a single agent will prove sufficient to salvage most of the ischemic brain in most patients. On the other hand, multiple agents targeted at different receptors or events in the ischemic cascade may cooperatively improve outcome. Attempts have been made to design a combination of neuroprotective agents, with some success, but it is difficult to predict the doses of the two agents to use. Furthermore, the combination may manifest benefit as increased potency compared to the single agents or it may lengthen the treatment delay time window, or both. A study of nimodipine (0.25 microgram/min × 24-hour iv infusion) plus MK-801 (5 mg/kg iv), or both in combination showed that the calcium channel blocker added to efficacy in the rat 4-vessel occlusion model *(93)*. In an MCA occlusion model, the combination (MK-801 2 mg/kg and nimodipine 5 μg/kg/min × 3 min and 1 μg/kg/min for 230 min) resulted in lower levels of intracellular calcium and less histologic damage, compared to MK-801 treatment alone *(94)*. In neither study were higher doses of the single agents used, so no truly synergistic effect could be demonstrated. Zivin et al., found that adding MK-801 to tissue plasminogen activator (t-PA) resulted in a significant increase in ED$_{50}$ for the combination *(95)*. In this study, 1.0 mg/kg MK-801 was given 5 min and t-PA was given 60 min after ischemia. The ED$_{50}$ for the combination was significantly greater than that for t-PA alone. However, the combination was not effective if t-PA was delayed to 90 min. The combination of a free radical scavenger plus MK-801 plus insulin plus diazepam appeared to be more effective than the single drug, but no effort was made to simulate the benefit of the combination by increasing the doses of the single agents *(96)*. Bowes et al. attempted to delay the use of thrombolysis by combining t-PA and anti-ICAM-1 in a rabbit cerebral embolism model *(91)*. When both treatments were given 30 min after ischemia onset, each was effective, as was the combination. After a treatment delay of 90 min, t-PA and the combination were effective, but the ED_{50}'s were the same (no synergistic benefit). After a delay of 180 min, t-PA was not effective when used alone, nor when combined with anti-ICAM given 5 or 175 min after ischemia. In this study, no evidence of treatment interaction could be found, either by examining the potencies of single vs combined treatments, or by examining the maximum effective treatment delay. In a follow-up study, the same group studied longer time intervals *(97)*. In this study, t-PA given 2 h after embolization was not effective, but the combination of anti-ICAM 15 min after and t-PA 2 h after embolization was quite effective. Again, the dose of t-PA alone was not increased to see whether a maximal dose of the single agent was equipotent to the combination. However, this is highly unlikely because the dose of t-PA used, 3 mg/kg, is known to thrombolyse the majority of the injected emboli. Therefore, this study suggests that the use of the two agents conferred a benefit that could not be obtained from higher doses of either agent alone, i.e., synergism.

HEMORRHAGIC INFARCTION
AND INTRACRANIAL HEMORRHAGE (ICH)

Ischemic etiologies account for the majority of stroke cases *(98)*. On the other hand, cerebral hemorrhage accounts for about 12% of all stroke cases, yields a much higher mortality and morbidity than ischemia, may be responsible for a disproportionate share of the neurologic disability attributed to stroke, and responds to no known effective therapy. Recent experience with hyperacute treatment of ischemic stroke suggests that about 40% of all "911" strokes (emergency transport to hospital within 60 min of stroke onset) may be hemorrhagic *(99)*. Thus, of the population that presents early to hospital, a large proportion suffer from an etiology for which there is no known treatment and few clinical trials.

Cerebral hemorrhage can be identified as one of two forms that probably occupy opposite ends of one pathophysiologic continuum *(100)*. Hematoma is a large, homogeneous, solid collection of blood that occupies space, displaces, and destroys surrounding brain. Hemorrhagic infarction, also called transformation, is the leakage of blood cells into adjacent, ischemic brain without displacing or necessarily destroying brain cells.

Spontaneous hematoma probably results from a ruptured blood vessel, rather than from brain ischemia primarily. There is much speculation about the factors that lead to vessel wall rupture, and chronic hypertensive vasculopathy is often noted in such patients *(101)*. Other illnesses that affect the vessel wall are also associated with hematoma, such as diabetes, polyarteritis nodosa, and amyloid angiopathy. There is some evidence that matrix metalloproteinases play a role in the genesis of hematoma, and this observation led to the development of the intracerebral collagenase model of hematoma. The factors that cause the bleeding to start and then stop, and the time course of hemorrhage development are not known. After the hematoma has occurred, however, there are extensive areas of ischemia around the expanding mass.

There is no treatment for hematoma. Removal of the hematoma by aspiration seems to improve neurologic outcome in animals, if the clot is removed soon enough after stroke onset *(102)*. All of the effects of the mass begin to resolve after its removal: intracranial pressure declines toward normal; blood flow increases toward normal; and edema begins to resorb. In humans, however, aspiration or prompt removal of the mass has not been shown to be effective. This is very likely owing to the fact that it is logistically difficult to get patients from the field, through radiology, and into the operating room rapidly *(103,104)*. Therefore, there is a very great need to develop a strategy that protects brain long enough for the patient to undergo removal of the hematoma. Since the subcortical hematoma causes a large area of cortical ischemia *(105)* it seems reasonable to suggest that anti-ischemia therapy directed at protecting the cortex may be successful, even though the hematoma itself is subcortical.

Thrombolytic therapy for acute ischemic stroke produces an increase in the native rate of hemorrhagic transformation. Asymptomatic hemorrhage was noted in about 20% of patients in a recent trial of t-PA for acute stroke and in nearly 40% of patients receiving streptokinase for acute stroke in the Australian and European multicenter stroke trials *(106,107)*. Hematoma with symptomatic deterioration occurred in 6% of the NINDS trial *(108)*. The factors that may promote transformation are poorly understood, although suspects include hypertension, anticoagulation, and timing of reperfusion after stroke onset.

Neuroprotectants could be useful during thrombolysis in a number of ways. As mentioned above, neuroprotectants might preserve neurons in the penumbra longer, pending recanalization. That is, neuroprotection might delay the time at which areas of penumbra become irretrievably damaged. Also, neuroprotectants might limit the incidence of hemorrhagic transformation after ischemia. That is, neuroprotection might prevent hemorrhages that occur because a portion of the ischemic brain dies prior to recanalization. To date there have been no completed studies of thrombolytic plus neuroprotectant combinations, although such studies are underway. For the time being, then, such combinations remain experimental.

REFERENCES

1. Astrup J, Siesjo BK, Symon L. Thresholds in cerebral ischemia: The ischemic penumbra. *Stroke* 1981;12:723–725.
2. Astrup J, Symon L, Branston NM, Lassen NA. Cortical evoked potential and extracellular K+ and H+ at critical levels of brain ischemia. *Stroke* 1977;8:51–57.
3. Garcia JH, Liu K-F, Ye Z-R, Gutierrez JA. Incomplete Infarct and Delayed Neuronal Death After Transient Middle Cerebral Artery Occlusion in Rats. *Stroke* 1997;28:2303–2310.
4. Heiss WD. Experimental evidence of ischemic thresholds and functional recovery. *Stroke* 1992;23:1668–1672.
5. Heiss W-D. Progress in cerebrovascular disease: flow thresholds of functional and morphological damage of brain tissue. *Stroke* 1983;14:329–331.
6. Hossmann K-A. Viability thresholds and the penumbra of focal ischemia. *Ann Neurol* 1994;36:557–565.
7. Kaplan B, Brint S, Tanabe J, Jacewicz M, Wang X-J, Pulsinelli W. Temporal thresholds for neocortical infarction in rats subjected to reversible focal cerebral ischemia. *Stroke* 1991;22:1032–1039.
8. Jones TH, Morawetz RB, Crowell RM, Marcoux FW, FitzGibbon SJ, DeGirolami U, Ojemann RG. Thresholds of focal cerebral ischemia in awake monkeys. *J Neurosurg* 1981;54:773–782.
9. Heiss WD, Rosner G. Functional recovery of cortical neurons as related to degree and duration of ischemia. *Ann Neurol* 1983;14:294–301.
10. Memezawa H, Smith M-L, Siesjo BK. Penumbral tissues salvaged by reperfusion following middle cerebral artery occlusion in rats. *Stroke* 1992;23:552–559
11. Nedergaard M. Neuronal injury in the infarct border: a neuropathological study in the rat. *Acta Neuropathol* 1987;73:267–274.
12. Mies G, Auer LM, Ebhardt G, Traupe H, Heiss W-D. Flow and Neuronal Density in Tissue Surrounding Chronic Infarction. *Stroke* 1983;14:22–27.
13. Baron JC. Mapping the Ischaemic Penumbra with PET: Implications for Acute Stroke Treatment. *Cerebrovasc Dis* 1999;9:193–201.
14. Heiss W-D, Huber M, Fink GR, Herholz K, Pietrzyk U, Wagner R, Weinhard K. Progressive derangement of periinfarct viable tissue in ischemic stroke. *Journal of Cerebral Blood Flow and Metabolism* 1992;12:193–203.
15. Minematsu K, Li L, Sotak CH, Davis MA, Fisher M. Reversible focal ischemic injury demonstrated by diffusion-weighted magnetic resonance imaging in rats. *Stroke* 1992;23:1304–1310.
16. Clark WM, Madden KP, Rothlein R, Zivin JA. Reduction of central nervous system ischemic injury in rabbits using leukocyte adhesion antibody treatment. *Stroke* 1991;22:877–883.
17. Busto R, Dietrich W, Mordecai G. Small differences in intraischemic brain temperature critically determines the extent of neuronal injury. *J Cereb Blood Flow Metab* 1987;7:729–738.
18. Bruno A, Biller J, Adams HP, Clarke WR, Woolson RF, Williams LS, Hansen MD, TOAST Investigators. Acute blood glucose level and outcome from ischemic stroke. *Neurology* 999;52:280–284.
19. Strijbos PJLM, Leach MJ, Garthwaite J. Vicious cycle involving Na+ channels, glutamate release, and NMDA receptors mediates delayed neurodegeneration through nitric oxide formation. *J Neurosci* 1996;16:5004–5013.

20. Pellegrini-Giampietro DE, Cherici G, Alesiani M, Carla V, Moroni F. Excitatory amino acid release and free radical formation may cooperate in the genesis of ischemia-induced neuronal damage. *J Neurosci* 1990;10:1035–1041.
21. Lu YM, Yin HZ, Chiang J, Weiss JH. Ca^{2+}-permeable AMPA/kainate and NMDA channels: High rate of Ca^{2+} influx underlies potent induction of injury. *J Neurosci* 1996;16:5457–5465.
22. Choi DW, Maulucci-Gedde M, Kriegstein AR. Glutamate neurotoxicity in cortical cell culture. *J Neurosci* 1987;7:357–368.
23. Rothman SM. Synaptic activity mediates death of hypoxic neurons. *Science* 1983;220:536–537.
24. Rothman SM, Thurston JH, Hauhart RE. Delayed neurotoxicity of excitatory amino acids in vitro. *Neuroscience* 1987;22:471–480.
25. Rothman SM, Olney JW. Glutamate and the pathophysiology of hypoxic-ischemic brain damage. *Ann Neurol* 1986;19:105–111.
26. Weiss J, Goldberg MP, Choi DW. Ketamine protects cultured neocortical neurons from hypoxic injury. *Brain Res* 1986;380:186–190.
27. Hartley DM, Kurth MC, Bjerkness L, Weiss JH, Choi DW. Glutamate receptor-induced $^{45}Ca^{2+}$ accumulation in cortical cell culture correlates with subsequent neuronal degeneration. *J Neurosci* 1993;13:1993–2000.
28. Nakanishi S. Molecular diversity of glutamate receptors and implications for brain function. *Science* 1992;258:597–603.
29. Carriedo SG, Yin HZ, Weiss JH. Motor neurons are selectively vulnerable to AMPA/kainate receptor-mediated injury *in vitro*. *J Neurosci* 1996;16:4069–4079.
30. Choi S, Lovinger DM. Metabotropic glutamate receptor modulation of voltage-gated Ca^{2+} channels involves multiple receptor subtypes in cortical neurons. *J Neurosci* 1996;16:36–45.
31. Choi DW. Glutamate neurotoxicity in cortical cell culture is calcium-dependent. *Neurosci Lett* 1985;58:293–297.
32. Choi DW. Ionic dependence of glutamate neurotoxicity. *J Neurosci* 1987;7:369–379.
33. Goldberg MP, Choi DW. Combined oxygen and glucose deprivation in cortical cell culture: Calcium-dependent and calcium-independent mechanisms of neuronal injury. *J Neurosci* 1993;13:3510–3524.
34. Bhat RV, DiRocco R, Marcy VR, Flood DG, Zhu Y, Dobrzanski P, Siman R, Scott R, Contreras PC, Miller M. Increased expression of IL-1β converting enzyme in hippocampus after ischemia: Selective localization in microglia. *J Neurosci* 1996;16:4146–4154.
35. Schulz JB, Weller M, Klockgether T. Potassium deprivation-induced apoptosis of cerebellar granule neurons: A sequential requirement for new mRNA and protein synthesis, ICE-like protease activity, and reactive oxygen species. *J Neurosci* 1996;16:4696–4706.
36. MacDermott AB, Mayer ML, Westbrook GL, Smith SJ, Barker JL. NMDA-receptor activation increases cytoplasmic calcium concentration in cultured spinal cord neurones. *Nature (Lond)* 1986;321:519–522.
37. Riveros N, Orrego F. N-Methylaspartate-activated calcium channels in rat brain cortex slices. Effect of calcium channel blockers and of inhibitory and depressant substances. *Neuroscience* 1986;17:541–546.
38. Hirayama T, Ono H, Fukuda H. Effects of excitatory and inhibitory amino acid agonists and antagonists on ventral horn cells in slices of spinal cord isolated from adult rats. *Neuropharmacology* 1990;29:1117–1122.
39. Frandsen A, Schousboe A. Mobilization of dantrolene-sensitive intracellular calcium pools is involved in the cytotoxicity induced by quisqualate and *N*-methyl-D-aspartate but not by 2-amino-3-(3-hydroxy-5-methylisoxazol-4-yl)propionate and kainate in cultured cerebral cortical neurons. *Proc Natl Acad Sci USA* 1992;89:2590–2594.
40. Katchman AN, Hershkowitz N. Early anoxia-induced vesicular glutamate release results from mobilization of calcium from intracellular stores. *J Neurophysiol* 1993;70:1–7.

41. Bickler PE, Hansen BM. Causes of calcium accumulation in rat cortical brain slices during hypoxia and ischemia: Role of ion channels and membrane damage. *Brain Res* 1994;664:269–276.
42. O'Regan MH, Smith-Barbour M, Perkins LM, Phillis JW. A possible role for phospholipases in the release of neurotransmitter amino acids from ischemic rat cerebral cortex. *Neurosci Lett* 1995;185:191–194.
43. Ozyurt E, Graham D, Woodruff G, McCullogh J. Protective effect of the glutamate antagonist MK-801 in focal cerebral ischemia in the cat. *J Cereb Blood Flow Metab* 1988;8:138–143.
44. Yum SW, Faden AI. Comparison of the neuroprotective effects of the N-methyl-D- aspartate antagonist MK-801 and the opiate-receptor antagonist nalmefene in experimental spinal cord ischemia. *Arch Neurol* 1990;47:277–281.
45. Park CK, Nehls DG, Graham DI, Teasdale GM, McCulloch J. The glutamate antagonist MK-801 reduces focal ischemic brain damage in the rat. *Ann Neurol* 1988;24:543–551.
46. Boast CS, Gerhardt B, Pastor G, Lehmann J, Etienne PE, Liebman JM. The N-methyl-D-aspartate antagonist CGS19755 and CPP reduce ischemic brain damage in gerbils. *Brain Res* 1988;442:345–348.
47. George CP, Goldberg MP, Choi DW, Steinberg GK. Dextromethorphan reduces neocortical ischemic neuronal damage in vivo. *Brain Res* 1988;440:375–379.
48. Prince DA, Feeser HR. Dextromethorphan protects against cerebral infarction in a rat model of hypoxia-ischemia. *Neurosci Lett* 1988;85:291–296.
49. Steinberg GK, Saleh J, Kunis D. Delayed treatment with dextromethorphan and dextrophan reduces cerebral damage after transient focal ischemia. *Neurosci Lett* 1988;89:193–197.
50. Newell DW, Barth A, Malouf AT. Glycine site NMDA receptor antagonists provide protection against ischemia-induced neuronal damage in hippocampal slice cultures. *Brain Res* 1995;675:38–44.
51. Tsuchida E, Bullock R. The effect of the glycine site-specific *N*-Methyl-D-Aspartate antagonist ACEA1021 on ischemic brain damage caused by acute subdural hematoma in the rat. *J Neurotrauma* 1995;12:279–288.
52. Roberts E. γ-Aminobutyric acid and nervous system function—a perspective. *Biochem Pharmacol* 1974;23:2637–2649.
53. Bachelard HS. Biochemistry of centrally active amino acids. In: Mandel P, DeFeudis FV, eds. Advances in Biochemical Psychopharmacology. New York: Raven Press, 1981:475–498.
54. Albin RL, Sakurai SY, Makowiec RL, Higgins DS, Young AB, Penney JB. Excitatory amino acid, $GABA_A$, and $GABA_B$ binding sites in human striate cortex. *Cerebral Cortex* 1991;1:499–509.
55. Jansen KLR, Faull RLM, Dragunow M, Leslie RA. Distribution of excitatory and inhibitory amino acid, sigma, monoamine, catecholamine, acetylcholine, opioid, neurotensin, substance P, adenosine and neuropeptide Y receptors in human motor and somatosensory cortex. *Brain Res* 1991;566:225–238.
56. Karlsson G, Olpe H-R. Late inhibitory postsynaptic potentials in rat prefrontal cortex may be mediated by GABA-B receptors. *Experi* 1989;45:157–148.
57. Scharfman HE, Sarvey JM. Responses to γ-aminobutric acid applied cell bodies and dendrites of rat visual cortical neurons. *Brain Res* 1985;358:385–389.
58. Kelly PAT, McCulloch J. Effects of the putative GABAergic agonists, muscimol and THIP, upon local cerebral glucose utilisation. *J Neurochem* 1982;39:613–624.
59. Kelly PAT, McCulloch J. The effects of the GABAergic agonist muscimol upon the relationship between local cerebral blood flow and glucose utilization. *Brain Res* 1983;258:338–342.
60. Edvinsson L, Krause DN. Pharmacological characterization of GABA receptors mediating vasodilation of cerebral arteries in vitro. *Brain Res* 1979;173:89–97.
61. Erdo SL, Michler A, Wolff JR. GABA accelerates excitotoxic cell death in cortical cultures: Protection by blockers of GABA-gated chloride channels. *Brain Res* 1991;542:254–258.

62. van den Pol AN, Obrietan K, Chen G. Excitatory actions of GABA after neuronal trauma. *J Neurosci* 1996;16:4283–4292.

63. Akhondzadeh S, Stone TW. Potentiation by neurosteroids of muscimol/adenosine interactions in rat hippocampus. *Brain Res* 1995;677:311–318.

64. Frye CA. The neurosteroid 3α,5α-THP has antiseizure and possible neuroprotective effects in an animal model of epilepsy. *Brain Res* 1995;696:113–120.

65. Gee KW, McCauley LD, Lan NC. A putative receptor for neurosteroids on the GABA$_A$ receptor complex: The pharmacological properties and therapeutic potential of epalons. *Crit Revs Neurobiology* 1995;9:207–227.

66. Lambert JJ, Belelli D, Hill-Venning C, Peters JA. Neurosteroids and GABA$_A$ receptor function. *Trends Pharmacol Sci* 1995;16:295–303.

67. Devaud LL, Purdy RH, Morrow AL. The Neurosteroid, 3α-hydroxy-5α-pregnan-20-one, protects against bicuculline-induced seizures during ethanol withdrawal in rats. *Alcohol Clin Exp Resp* 1995;19:350–355.

68. Hauser CAE, Wetzel CHR, Rupprecht R, Holsboer F. Allopregnanoline acts as an inhibitory modulator on α$_1$-and α$_6$-containing GABA$_A$ receptors. *Biochem Biophys Res Commun* 1996;219:531–536.

69. Brown AW, Brierley JB. The nature, distribution, and earliest stages of anoxic-ischemic nerve cell damage in the rat brain as defined by the optical microscope. *Br J Exp Pathol* 1968;49:87–106.

70. Linnik MD, Zobrist RH, Hatfield MD. Evidence supporting a role for programmed cell death in focal cerebral ischemia in rats. *Stroke* 1993;24:2002–2009.

71. Wyllie AH, Kerr JFR, Currie AR. Cell Death: The significance of apoptosis. *Int Rev Cytol* 1980;68:251–305.

72. Oppenheim RW. Cell death during development of the nervous system. *Annu Rev Neurosci* 1991;14:453–501.

73. Clarke PGH. Developmental cell death: Morphological diversity and multiple mechanisms. *Anat Embryol* 1990;181:195–213.

74. Pulsinelli WA, Brierley JB, Plum F. Temporal profile of neuronal damage in a model of transient forebrain ischemia. *Ann Neurol* 1982;11:491–498.

75. Cohen GM, Sun X-M, Snowden RT, Dinsdale D, Skilleter DN. Key morphological features of apoptosis may occur in the absence of internucleosomal DNA fragmentation. *Biochem J* 1992;286:331–334.

76. Charriaut-Marlangue C, Margaill I, Represa A, Popovici T, Plotkine M, Ben-Ari Y. Apoptosis and necrosis after reversible focal ischemia: An in situ DNA fragmentation analysis. *J Cereb Blood Flow Metab* 1996;16:186–194.

77. Tominaga T, Kure S, Narisawa K, Yoshimoto T. Endonuclease activation following focal ischemic injury in the rat brain. *Brain Res* 1993;608:21–26.

78. Li Y, Sharov VG, Jiang N, Zaloga C, Sabbah HN, Chopp M. Ultrastructural and light microscopic evidence of apoptosis after middle cerebral artery occlusion in the rat. *Am J Pathol* 1995;146:1045–1051.

79. MacManus JP, Hill IE, Huang Z-G, Rasquinha I, Xue D, Buchan AM. DNA damage consistent with apoptosis in transient focal ischaemic neocortex. *NeuroReport* 1994;5:493–496.

80. van Lookeren Campagne M, Gill R. Ultrastructural morphological changes are not characteristic of apoptotic cell death following focal cerebral ischaemia in the rat. *Neurosci Lett* 1996;213:111–114.

81. Zhongting H, Kazunari Y, Hitoshi O, Haiping L, Mitsuhiro K. The in vivo time course for elimination of adrenalectomy-induced apoptotic profiles from the granule cell layer of the rat hippocampus. *J Neurosci* 1997;17:3981–3989.

82. Liu XZ, Xu XM, Hu R, Du C, Zhang SX, McDonald JW, Dong HX, Wu YJ, Fan GS, Jacquin MF, Hsu CY, Choi DW. Neuronal and glial apoptosis after traumatic spinal cord injury. *J Neurosci* 1997;17:5395–5406.

83. Goto K, Ishige A, Sekigushi K, Izuka S, Sugimoto A, Yuzurihara M, Aburada M, Hosoya E, Kogure K. Effects of cycloheximide on delayed neuronal death in rat hippocampus. *Brain Research* 1990;534:299–302.
84. Ames AI, Wright LW, Kowada M, Thurston JM, Majno G. Cerebral ischemia. II. The no-reflow phenomenon. *Am J Pathol* 1968;52:437–447.
85. Schmid-Schönbein GW. Capillary plugging by granulocytes and the no-reflow phenomenon in the microcirculation. *Proc Fed Amer Soc Exp Biol* 1987;46:2397–2401.
86. Harlan JM, Vedder NB, Winn RK, Rice CL. Mechanisms and consequences of leukocyte-endothelial interaction. *West J Med* 1991;155:365–369.
87. Hallenbeck JM, Dutka AJ, Tanishima T, Kochanek PM, Kumaroo KK, Thompson CB, Obrenovitch TP, Contreras TJ. Polymorphonuclear leukocyte accumulation in brain regions with low blood flow during the early postischemic period. *Stroke* 1986;17:246–253.
88. Menger MD, Lehr H-A, Messmer K. Role of oxygen radicals in the microcirculatory manifestations of postischemic injury. *Klin Wochenschr* 1991;69:1050–1055.
89. del Zoppo G, Schmid-Schönbein GW, Mori E, Copeland BR, Chang C-M. Polymorphonuclear leukocytes occlude capillaries following middle cerebral artery occlusion and reperfusion in baboons. *Stroke* 1991;22:1276–1283.
90. Zhang RL, Chopp M, Li Y, Zaloga C, Jiang N, Jones ML, Miyasaka M, Ward PA. Anti-ICAM-1 antibody reduces ischemic cell damage after transient middle cerebral artery occlusion in the rat. *Neurology* 1994;44:1747–1751.
91. Bowes MP, Zivin JA, Rothlein R. Monoclonal antibody to the ICAM-1 adhesion site reduces neurological damage in a rabbit cerebral embolism stroke model. *Exp Neurol* 1993;119:215–219.
92. Clark WM, Madden KP, Rothlein R, Zivin JA. Reduction of central nervous system ischemic injury by monoclonal antibody to intercellular adhesion molecule. *J Neurosurg* 1991;75:623–627.
93. Rod MR, Auer RN. Combination therapy with nimodipine and dizocilpine in a rat model of transient forebrain ischemia. *Stroke* 1992;23:725–732.
94. Uematsu D, Araki N, Greenberg JH, Sladky J, Reivich M. Combined therapy with MK-801 and nimodipine for protection of ischemic brain damage. *Neurology* 1991;41:88–94.
95. Zivin JA, Mazzarella V. Tissue plasminogen activator plus glutamate antagonist improves outcome after embolic stroke. *Arch Neurol* 1991;48:1235–1238.
96. Auer RN. Combination therapy with U74006F (tirilazad mesylate), MK-801, insulin and diazepam in transient forebrain ischaemia. *Neurol Res* 1995;17:132–136.
97. Bowes MP, Rothlein R, Fagan SC, Zivin JA. Monoclonal antibodies preventing leukocyte activation reduce experimental neurologic injury and enhance efficacy of thrombolytic therapy. *Neurology* 1995;45:815–819.
98. American Heart Association. Heart and stroke facts and figures. Dallas: American Heart Association, 1992:
99. Lyden PD, Rapp K, Babcock T, Rothrock J. Ultra-rapid identification, triage, and enrollment of stroke patients into clinical trials. *J Stroke Cerebrovasc Dis* 1994;4:106–113.
100. Lyden PD, Zivin JA. Hemorrhagic transformation after cerebral ischemia: Mechanisms and incidence. *Cerebrovasc Brain Met Rev* 1993;5:1–16.
101. Kaufman HH. Intracerebral hematomas. New York: Raven Press, 1992:1–240.
102. Kanno T, Sano H, Shinomiyo Y, Katada K, Nagata J, Hoshino M, Mitsuyama F. Role of surgery in hypertensive intracerebral hematoma. *J Neurosurg* 1985;61:1091–1099.
103. Broderick J, Brott T, Tomsick T, Tew J, Duldner J, Huster G. Management of intracerebral hemorrhage in a large metropolitan population. *Neurosurgery* 1994;34:882–887.
104. Lisk DR, Pasteur W, Rhoades H, Putnam RD, Grotta JC. Early presentation of hemispheric intracerebral hemorrhage: prediction of outcome and guidelines for treatment allocation. *Neurology* 1994;44:133–139.

105. Yang G-Y, Betz AL, Chenevert TL, Brunberg JA, Hoff JT. Experimental intracerebral hemorrhage: relationship between brain edema, blood flow, and blood-brain barrier permeability in rats. *J Neurosurg* 1994;81:93–102.

106. Brott TG, Haley EC, Jr, Levy DE, Barsan W, Broderick J, Sheppard GL, Spilker J, Kongable GL, Massey S, Reed R, Marler JR. Urgent therapy for stroke: Part 1. Pilot study of tissue plasminogen activator administered within 90 minutes. *Stroke* 1992;23:632–640.

107. Hommel M, Boissel JP, Cornu C, Boutitle F, Lees KR, Besson G, Leys D, Amarenco P, Bogaert M. Termination of streptokinase in severe acute ischaemic stroke. *Lancet* 1995;345:57.

108. NINDS rt-PA Stroke Study Group. Tissue plasminogen activator for acute ischemic stroke. *N Engl J Med* 1995;333:1581–1587.

II   SCIENTIFIC RATIONALE
AND CLINICAL TRIALS

4

Pre-Clinical Testing
of Thrombolytic Therapy for Stroke

Anne M. Guyot, MD
and Steven R. Levine, MD

CONTENTS

INTRODUCTION
EARLY EXPERIMENTAL STUDIES OF THROMBOLYSIS
    FOR STROKE USING PLASMIN, UROKINASE, OR STREPTOKINASE
PRECLINICAL TRIALS OF T-PA
T-PA ANALOGS
GLOBAL ISCHEMIA
SUMMARY AND CONCLUSIONS
REFERENCES

INTRODUCTION

Prior to definitive human trials, considerable effort was expended in the laboratory to study and perfect thrombolytic therapy. Here we wish to summarize the essential literature that provided the experimental impetus for proceeding to human trials. From this experience, two important lessons emerged. First, thorough exploration of drug risks and benefits should be performed in animal models prior to human trials. Second, animal models can predict human results accurately, but only if the correct models are chosen, and the results handled rigorously. For example, the experimental data clearly predicted the efficacy, and the side effects, of thrombolytic therapy. Furthermore, the excessive risk associated with streptokinase was predicted by the animal models. These data serve to illuminate an approach to studying putative stroke therapies in the future.

From: *Thrombolytic Therapy for Stroke*
Edited by: P. D. Lyden © Humana Press Inc., Totowa, NJ

EARLY EXPERIMENTAL STUDIES OF THROMBOLYSIS FOR STROKE USING PLASMIN, UROKINASE, OR STREPTOKINASE

Table 1 *(5,11–18)* shows the experimental and basic studies of thrombolytics for ischemic stroke. Meyer et al. *(3)* created pumice emboli with subsequent platelet and thrombi adherence to the regions of damaged endothelium in cats and monkeys. Intravenous or intra-arterial injection of either bovine or human plasmin resulted in lysis of the thrombi in every experiment. Intra-arterial infusion caused more rapid clot dissolution and the streptokinase-activated human plasmin was believed to be minimally more effective than the bovine-fibrinolysin. Clot lysis began 4 to 18 min after intra-arterial infusion and 8 to 30 min after dosing. Hemorrhagic infarction did not appear to be increased by fibrinolytic therapy. However, 2 to 4 h postfibrinolysis infusion the thrombus usually started to reform and propagate. This did not occur if heparin was given $\frac{1}{2}$ to 1 h before fibrinolytics. Distal emboli resulting from the parent clot dissolution was documented in five experiments. These smaller emboli were then also dissolved.

Del Zoppo et al. *(5)* demonstrated that after 3 h of reversible eccentric balloon (inflatable silastic placed transorbitally) compression of the baboon middle cerebral artery (MCA) proximal to take off the lenticulostriate arteries ($n = 5$), intracarotid urokinase (12×106 IU over 1 h begun 30 min after balloon deflation), improved neurological function and reduced infarct size without evidence of macroscopic intracranial hemorrhage (ICH) compared with untreated animals ($n = 6$).

DeLey et al. *(19)* showed that very early treatment with intracarotid streptokinase (500,000 IU) in conjunction with flunarizine prevented the lowering of the cerebral metabolic rate of oxygen as determined by positron emission tomography (PET) scanning in a dog MCA occlusion (autologous blot clot) model.

PRECLINICAL TRIALS OF t-PA

Table 2 shows the experimental and basic studies of thrombolytics for ischemic stroke. There has been intense interest in establishing the efficacy of thrombolytics, especially tissue plasminogen activator (t-PA) for experimental cerebral ischemia, primarily using the autologous clot cerebral embolism model in rabbits *(20–22)*.

If t-PA is administered immediately after experimental embolic occlusion, significant reduction in neurological damage occurs *(20)*. t-PA may reduce neurological damage in rabbit embolic stroke models as late as 45 min after the cerebral embolic occlusion *(7)*. t-PA-related ICH hemorrhage did not occur when therapy was started 4 h after the onset of vascular occlusion. However, there was no benefit when treatment was delayed for 1 h *(7)*. In both a small- and a large-clot rabbit embolic stroke model, there was no evidence that t-PA changed the histological appearance of lesions compared with untreated controls. Zivin et al.

Table 1
Experimental and Basic Studies of Thrombolytics for Ischemic Stroke

Author	Year	Urokinase/Streptokinase/ Plasmin Animal Model	Main results (Compared with Controls when Applicable)
Whisnant (11)	1960	Clot in Internal Carotid Artery	No increased risk of hemorrhagic infarction compared with controls
Centero (12)	1985	Rabbit autologous clot	Variable and no statistical differences with controls, no gross ICH
Del Zoppo (5)	1986	Baboon MCA balloon	Improved neurologic function, reduced infarct size, no macroscopic ICH
Hirschberg (13–15)	1987	Dog MCA occlusion	Thrombolysis, no ICH 5 petechial hemorrhages
Slivka (16)	1987	Rabbit CCA/MCA occlusion	Two gross ICH; petechial hemorrhage same as controls
Deley (17)	1988	Dog MCA clot	Thrombolysis without improved tissue perfusion or infarct reduction if treatment 30 min after 3-h-old clot injected. If treatment within 5 min of insult: normalization of cerebral blood flow and salvaged tissue
Clark (18)	1989	Rabbit autologous clot	>50% hemorrhage

Abbreviations: ICH, intracranial hemorrhage; MCA, Middle Cerebral Artery; CCA, Common Carotid Artery.

Table 2
Experimental and Basic Studies of Thrombolytics for Ischemic Stroke: t-PA

Author	Year	Animal model	Treatment onset	Main results (Compared with Controls when Applicable)
Zivin (20)	1985	Rabbit autologous clot	<2 min up to 45 min, 1 h	Neurologic improvement, no large ICH, no protection
Del Zoppo (22)	1986	Baboon reversible MCA occlusion	3 h	Improved neurological function
Penar (23)	1987	Rat autologous clot	—	No effect on vessel patency, no ICH, less "low flow" regions, untreated groups, no change in fibrinogen
Kissel (24)	1987	Rabbit autologous clot	—	Improved cerebral blood flow at 90 min but not at 30 minutes
Watson (25)	1987	Rat with laser-induced thrombosis	—	Segmental recanalization, decreased lesion volume in 6/9, no ICH
Papadopolous (26)	1987	Rat with human clot	2 h	Increased CBF, within 30 min, improved EEG, thrombolysis achieved, no ICH
Slivka (16)	1987	Rabbit CCA/MCA occlusion	24 h	3/4 ICH
Chehrazi (27)	1988	Rabbit autologous clot	30 min, 2 h, 4 h	Reduced infarct size in 20 min treatment onset group, no ICH
Philips (28,29)	1988	Rabbit autologous clot	15 min	Rapid reperfusion, no macroscopic ICH, no difference in infarct extent
Clark (18)	1989	Rabbit autologous clot	≤60 min, 6 h	14% hemorrhage (37% in controls) 30 hemorrhage (21 in controls)
Lyden (9)	1989	Rabbit embolism	10 min	100% lysis at 5 mg/kg, no increased ICH
Bednar (30)	1990	Rabbit embolism	<60 min	Restored CBF, reduced final infarct size
Benes (10)	1990	Rabbit embolism	30 min	Reduced infarct incidence, no ICH
Terashi (6)	1990	Hypertensive rats given	t-PA preischemia	Higher brain ATP and lower lactate in t-PA than vehicle treated rats, no hemorrhagic lesions, no arterial platelet in t-PA treated rats

Abbreviations: ICH, intracranial hemorrhage; MCA, Middle Cerebral Artery; CBF, cerebral blood flow; EEG, electroencephalogram; CCA, Common Carotid Artery; ATP, adenosine triphosphate.

(20) documented for the first time that t-PA could, in fact, substantially improve neurological function after embolization with artificially made clots.

Using awake baboons, Del Zoppo et al. *(33)* studied t-PA-induced hemorrhage transformation of ischemic brain within 3.5 h after MCA occlusion and 30 min of reperfusion. Three doses of t-PA (0.3 mg/kg, $n = 6$; 1.5 mg/kg, $n = 6$) were infused over 1 h and compared with normal saline infusion ($n = 12$). Peripheral (nonintracranial) hemorrhages were related to t-PA dose, significant for the two highest doses. Peak plasma recombinant tissue plasminogen activator (rt-PA) levels were directly related to dose. No significant differences in the incidences or volumes of infarction-related hemorrhages occurred in any group compared with saline-treated animals that were sacrificed at 14 d. Their data suggest that t-PA alone does not increase the risk (incidence or volume) of hemorrhagic infarction if administered within 3.5 h after MCA occlusion and reperfusion in baboons. Their data also suggest that t-PA does not substantially decrease the infarct volume at any of the doses administered early after symptom onset.

t-PA administered later *(16)* rather than earlier *(7)*, albeit in different models, was more often associated with ICH. Lyden et al. *(9)* found no difference in the frequency of ischemic brain hemorrhage transformation if t-PA was administered 10 min, 8 h, or 24 h after injection of autologous emboli.

Vaugh et al. *(34)* demonstrated that t-PA combined with iv aspirin synergistically and markedly prolonged the template bleeding time with a significant bleeding tendency. Administering reactivated t-PAI-1 can rapidly reverse this bleeding time prolongation.

Del Zoppo et al. *(5)* infused rt-PA (0.3 mg/kg or 1.5 mg/kg) in baboons following 3 h of reversible acute MCA occlusion. Five of six animals at each dose (10 of 12 total) had petechial hemorrhagic infarction at 14 d compared with 7 of 12 control animals and infarct size did not differ between treated and untreated animals.

Slivka and Pulsinella *(16)* investigated the hemorrhagic potential of both t-PA (200,000 U; 10% bolus remainder over 4 h) and streptokinase (10,000 U/kg bolus or 32,000 U/kg bolus, remainder over 4 h) initiated 24 h after experimental stroke in rabbits using a tandem common carotid and ipsilateral MCA occlusions with 2 h of halothane. In addition, six rabbits were administered streptokinase (10,000 U/kg bolus) 1 h after occlusion. Microscopic hemorrhage was frequently present in infarct tissue irrespective of treatment. Gross hemorrhagic infarction did not occur in rabbits either untreated or administered streptokinase 1 h after occlusion but did occur in the other groups of treated animals. Two of 12 animals administered streptokinase 24 h after injection had gross hemorrhages within the infarct. Only the t-PA treated rabbits showed a significantly greater incidence of gross hemorrhage than controls. Their data suggest that the use of thrombolytic agents may increase the risk of microscopic hemorrhage unless the agents are administered early enough after onset of the insult.

In pioneering work that set the stage for well-conducted clinical trials, Zivin et al. *(7)* found that rt-PA-induced ICH did not occur more commonly than controls when therapy was started within 4 h after the onset of vascular occlusion in rabbit emboli model of ischemic stroke. rt-PA was administered at 1.0 mg/kg at 15, 30, or 60 min after small-clot embolization (24-h aged clot) and at 2 mg/kg at 45 and 60 min after small-clot embolization. rt-PA was also administered 30 min or 4 h after large-clot (1 mm^3) embolization. Evaluations were performed "blinded" to the treatment group. The effective dose of clots required to produce a clinically apparent neurological disorder in 50% of a group of animals was significantly greater in the rt-PA-treated rabbits when t-PA was administered at 15, 30, or 45 min but not at 60 min postembolization in either the 1 mg/kg or 2 mg/kg dose. In controls, grossly apparent ICH was present in 3 of 10 (30%) animals.

When t-PA was administered 30 min after embolization, 8 of 14 rabbits had gross hemorrhage. When t-PA was delayed 4 h, 2 of 10 animals had such hemorrhages (p = NS). In the small-clot model, ICH was uncommon, visible only microscopically, and only found in association with relatively large infarcts. The presence of microscopically visible intravascular clots was a function of the time between clot injection and animal death. In the large-clot model, the microscopy of the lesions in control- and t-PA-treated rabbits was indistinguishable, and no difference was noted in neurological functions *(8,9)*.

Lyden et al. *(9)* demonstrated in the rabbit emboli stroke model that ICH rates in the t-PA – (3 mg/kg or 5 mg/kg) or saline-treated group did not differ. t-PA was infused 10 min, 8 h, and 24 h after emboli were instilled. Lyden et al. *(8)* also evaluated saline, t-PA, or streptokinase infusion in a similar rabbit embolic stroke model at various times of infusion to assess the rate of thrombolysis and cerebral hemorrhage 24 h later. Only streptokinase was associated with a significant increase in the rate of cerebral hemorrhage compared with the saline controls. In animals administered 3 mg/kg, 5 mg/kg, or 10 mg/kg of t-PA, there was no clear dose response for hemorrhage, but there was for thrombolysis. However, only in rabbits who achieved thrombolysis was t-PA associated with twice (24%) the hemorrhage rate as saline controls (12%), whereas the hemorrhage were nearly identical in animals without thrombolysis.

Benes et al. *(10)* found that treatment with either t-PA or urokinase significantly reduced the number of emboli present in a rabbit stroke model but only t-PA significantly reduced the incidence of infarction. No animal suffered an ICH.

In summary, the studies by Phillips et al. *(28,29)* Zivin et al. *(7,20)* Kissel et al. *(24)* Del Zoppo et al. *(22)* and Papadopolous et al. *(26)* taken together suggest that t-PA reliably opens cerebral arteries occluded with either autologous or nonautologous embolic clots. Further, there is preliminary experimental data to suggest that t-PA is more effective in inducing thrombolysis within precerebral vessels than systemic vessels *(35)*.

t-PA ANALOGS

Analogs to rt-PA are available through recombinant DNA technologies and offer the possibility of an active portion of molecule that may have better fibrin specificity and penetration and a longer in vivo half-life than rt-PA *(2)*.

Phillips et al. *(172,173)* investigated the effects of a t-PA analog, Fb-Fb-CF, in a rabbit embolic model. This analog consisted of the catalytic fragment of t-PA and a dimer of the B fragment of staphylococcal protein A (Fb-Fb-CF) and has a longer serum half-life (90 min) than rt-PA (3 min). When Fb-Fb-CF was given as a bolus ($n = 10$) 15 min after embolization, cerebral reperfusion, documented angiographically, occurred in 48 ± 21 min (range 30–90 min) while controls (saline treated, $n = 8$) did not reperfuse by 180 min ($p < 0.01$). Furthermore, reperfusion was demonstrated at 66 ± 32 min posttreatment (range 30–90 min, $n = 11$) when the treatment was delayed 90 min after embolization (control = 100 ± 25 min; $n = 12$); two spontaneous lyses occurred in controls ($p < 0.01$). One small macroscopic hemorrhage within an infarct was observed in the Fb-Fb-CF 15-min treated group (none in controls). In the 90-min group, microscopic hemorrhage was observed in four t-PA-analog and three saline-treated animals. Plasma fibrinogen levels decreased 16% immediately after and 19% by 180 min following Fb-Fb-CF treatment ($n = 7$). No macroscopic or microscopic ICH was observed in noninfarcted brain regions although intraventricular hemorrhages occurred on one Fb-Fb-CF and two control animals only in the 90-min group.

An rt-PA analog (0.8 mg/kg, 1 mg = 500,000 IU) was given in a rabbit autologous clot cerebral embolization model *(28)*, either 15 min or 90 min after embolization, in conjunction with serial angiography *(38)*. Reperfusion was documented in both the 15- and 90-min groups treated with rt-PA analogs (different than controls) without a difference in median time to reperfusion in the two groups. In the 15-min group, 0 of 8 controls reperfused and in the 90-min group, 2 of 12 controls spontaneously reperfused. One small hemorrhage into a zone of infarction was observed in the 15-min rt-PA analog-treated group (0 in controls) and four hemorrhages into infarcts were observed in the 90-min group (three in controls), such that the risk of hemorrhage was essentially the same for rt-PA analog-treated rabbits and saline-treated rabbits.

Using the model developed by Lyden and Zivin, further studies of mutant t-PA, known as TNK-t-PA are now underway. As of this writing, data have only appeared in abstract form. TNK, a genetically modified form of wild-type t-PA with a longer biological half-life and greater fibrin specificity, could have greater safety and/or efficacy. Hemorrhage was detected in 26% (6/23) of the control group, 80% (16/20) of the wild-type t-PA group, 57% (12/21) in the 0.6 mg/kg TNK group, and 73% (8/11) in the 1.5 mg/kg TNK group ($p < 0.01$, chi square). TNK shows comparable rates of recanalization, and may cause fewer hemorrhages, compared to wild-type t-PA in a model of embolic stroke.

GLOBAL ISCHEMIA

Moritomo et al. *(39)* studied heparin (100 U/kg) plus urokinase (3000 U/kg IV) given 15 min of complete *global* ischemia for 6 h in dogs. The studied group experienced up to 70% improvement in postischemic hypoperfusion CBF with significantly improved neurological outcome, suggesting that these two drugs together might improve impaired microcirculation.

SUMMARY AND CONCLUSIONS

Data from experimental cerebral ischemia studies have pointed to the need to treat acute clinical stroke within a few hours or less to effectively reduce stroke morbidity and mortality *(40–42)*. Specifically, with reversible MCA occlusion models of focal cerebral ischemia (dogs and cats), the animals uniformly survive without neurologic deficit if the occlusion is for less than 2 to 3 h *(43)*. Similarly in primates, MCA occlusion for 3 h or less will lead to clinical improvement and a decrease in infarct size, with complete recovery generally associated with less than 2 h of MCA occlusion *(44–46)*. Therefore, it appears unlikely that ischemic brain can be salvaged if vascular occlusion persists longer than 4 to 6 h (similar to the pathophysiology of myocardial ischemia). If t-PA is administered immediately after experimental embolic occlusion, significant reduction in neurologic damage occurs *(20)*. Microscopic transformation was increased in treated experimental animals, whereas macroscopic transformation ICH occurred more frequently in subjects given the higher doses of t-PA and in subjects who underwent delayed treatment *(16)*.

REFERENCES

1. Brott T. Thrombolytic therapy for stroke. *Cerebrovascular Brain Metab Rev* 1991;3:91–113.
2. Fears R. Biochemical pharmacology and therapeutic aspects of thrombolytic agents. *Pharmacol Rev* 1990;42:202–222.
3. Meyer JS, Gilroy J, Barnhart ME, et al. Therapeutic thrombolysis in cerebral thromboembolism. In: *Cerebral Vascular Diseases*, Siekert W, Whisnant JP, eds. Grune & Stratton: Philadelphia. 1963; pp. 160–175.
4. Sussman BJ, Fitch TSP. Thrombolysis with fibrinolysin in cerebral arterial occlusion. *JAMA* 1958;167:1705–1709.
5. Del Zoppo GJ, Copeland BR, Waltz TA, et al. The beneficial effect of intracarotid urokinase on acute stroke in a baboon model. *Stroke* 1986;17:638–643.
6. Terashi A, Kobayashi Y, Katayama Y, et al. Clinical effects and basic studies of thrombolytic therapy on cerebral thrombosis. *Semin Thromb Hemost* 1990;16:236–241.
7. Zivin JA, Lyden PD, DeGirolami U, et al. Tissue plasminogen activator. Reduction of neurologic damage after experimental embolic stroke. *Arch Neurol* 1988;45:387–391.
8. Lyden PD, Madden KP, Clark WM, et al. Incidence of cerebral hemorrhage after antifibrinolytic treatment for embolic stroke. *Stroke* 1990;21:1589–1593.
9. Lyden PD, Zivin JA, Clark WA, et al. Tissue plasminogen activator-mediated thrombolysis of cerebral emboli and its effect on hemorrhagic infarction in rabbits. *Neurology* 1989;39:703–708.

10. Benes V, Zabranski JM, Boston M, et al. Effect of intraarterial antifibrinolytic agents on autologous arterial emboli in the cerebral circulation of rabbits. *Stroke* 1990;21:1594–1599.

11. Whisnant JP, Millikan CH, Seikert RG. *Cerebral infarction and fibrinolytic agents.* Roberts HR, Gevatz JD, eds. Proceedings of the Conference on Thrombolytic Agents, Chicago. 1970; pp. 235–245.

12. Centeno RS, Hackney PB, Rothsock Jr. Streptokinase clot lysis in acute occlusions of the cranial circulation: Study in rabbits. *Am J Neuroradiol* 1985;6:589–594.

13. Hirschberg M, Hofferberth B. Rapid fibrinolysis at different time intervals in a canine model of acute stroke. *Stroke* 1987;18:292, (abstr).

14. Hirschberg M, Hofferberth B. Thrombolytic therapy with urokinase and prourokinase in a canine model of acute stroke. *Neurology* 1987;37:133, (abstr).

15. Hirschberg M, Korves M, Koc I, et al. Thrombolysis of cerebral thromboembolism by urokinase in an animal model. *Schweiz Med Wochenschr* 1987;117:1811–1813.

16. Slivka A, Pulsinelli W. Hemorrhagic complications of thrombolytic therapy in experimental stroke. *Stroke* 1987;18:1148–1156.

17. DeLey G, Weyne J, Demeester G, et al. Experimental thromboembolic stroke by positron emission tomography: Immediate versus delayed reperfusion by fibrinolysis. *J Cereb Blood Flow Metab* 1988;8:539–545.

18. Clark WM, Madden KP, Zivin ZA, et al. Intracerebral Hemorrhage: tPA versus streptokinase thrombolytic therapy. *Neurology* 1989;39:183, (abstr).

19. DeLey G, Weyne I, Demeester G, et al. Streptokinase treatment versus calcium overload blockade in experimental thromboembolic stroke. *Stroke* 1989;20:357–361.

20. Zivin JA, Fisher M, DeGirolami U, et al. Tissue plasminogen activator reduces neurological damage after cerebral embolism. *Science* 1985;230:1289–1292.

21. Zivin JA. Thrombolytic therapy for stroke. In: *Current Neurosurgical Practice,* Weinstein PR, Faden AL, eds. Protection of the brain from ischemia. Williams & Wilkins: Baltimore. 1990; pp. 231–236.

22. Del Zoppo GJ, Copeland BR, Hacke W, et al. Intracerebral hemorrhage following rt-PA infusion in a primate stroke model. *Stroke* 1988;19:134, (abstr).

23. Penar PL, Greer CA. The effect of intravenous tissue-type plasminogen activator in a rat model of embolic cerebral ischemia. *Yale J Biol Med* 1987;60:233–243.

24. Kissel P, Chchrazi B, Seibert JA, et al. Digital angiographic quantification of blood flow dynamics in embolic stroke treated with tissue-type plasminogen activator. *J Neurosurg* 1987;67:399–405.

25. Watson BD, Prado R, Dietrich W, et al. Mitigation of evolving cortical infarction in rats by recombinant tissue plasminogen activator following photochemically induced thrombosis. Raichle ME, Powers WJ eds. Cerebrovascular Diseases. New York: Raven 1987;317–330.

26. Papadopulous SM, Chandler WF, Salamat MS, et al. Recombinant human tissue-type plasminogen activator therapy in acute thromboembolic stroke. *J Neurosurg* 1987;67:394–398.

27. Chechraza BB, Seibert JA, Kissel P. Evaluation of recombinant tissue plasminogen activator in embolic stroke. *Neurosurgery* 1989;24:355–360.

28. Phillips DA, Fisher M, Smith TW, et al. The safety and angiographic efficacy of tissue plasminogen activator in a cerebral embolization model. *Ann Neurol* 1988;23:391–394.

29. Phillips DA, Davis MA, Fisher M. Selective embolization and clot dissolution with tPA in the internal carotid artery circulation of the rabbit. *Am J Neuradiol* 1988;9:899–902.

30. Bednar MM, McAuliffe M, Raymond S, et al. Tissue plasminogen activator reduces brain injury in a rabbit model of thromboembolic stroke. *Stroke* 1990;21:1705–1709.

31. Sloan MA. Thrombolytic therapy in experimental focal ischemia. Sawaya R, ed. Fibrinolysis and the Central Nervous System. Philadelphia:Hanley and Belfus. 1990;177–188.

32. Jang IK, Gold HK, Ziskind AA, et al. Differential sensitivity of erythrocyte-rich and platelet-rich arterial thrombi to lysis with recombinant tissue-type plasminogen activator: *Circulation* 1989;79:920–928.

33. Del Zoppo GJ, Copeland BR, Andercheck K, et al. Hemorrhagic transformation following tissue plasminogen activator in experimental cerebral infarction. *Stroke* 1990;21:596–601.

34. Vaughn DF, DeClerck PJ, De Mol, et al. Recombinant plasminogen activator inhibitor-1 reverses the bleeding tendency associated with the combined administration of tissue-type plasminogen activator and aspirin in rabbits. *J Clin Invest* 1989;84:586–591.

35. Chehrazi BB, Seibert JA, Hein L, et al. Differential effect of tPA induced thrombolysis in the CNS and the systemic arteries. *Stroke* 1989;20:153, (abstr).

36. Phillips DA, Fisher M, Smith TW, et al. The effects of a new tissue plasminogen activator analogue Fb-Fb-CF, on cerebral reperfusion in a rabbit embolic stroke model. *Ann Neurol* 1989;25:281–285.

37. Phillips DA, Fisher M, Davis MA, et al. Delayed treatment with a tPA analogue and streptokinase in a rabbit embolic stroke model. *Stroke* 1990;21:602–605.

38. Fisher M, Phillips DA, Smith TW, et al. Early and delayed thrombolytic therapy in rabbit cerebral embolization model using a tPA analogue. In: *Cerebrovascular Disease*, Ginsberg MD, Dietrich WD, eds. Raven: New York. 1989; pp. 29–32.

39. Morimoto N, Hashimoto H, Kosaka F. Effect of heparin-urokinase on brain damage induced by cerebral ischemia in dogs. *Stroke* 1989;20:154, (abstr).

40. Barsan WG, Brott TG, Olinger CP, et al. Identification and entry of the patient with acute cerebral infarction. *Ann Emerg Med* 1988;17:1192–1195.

41. Alexander, LF, Yamamoto Y. Ayoubi S. et al. Efficacy of tissue plasminogen activator in the lysis of thrombosis of the cerebral venous sinus. *Neurosurgery* 1990;26:559–564.

42. Segal R, Dejouny M, Nelson D, et al. Local urokinase treatment for spontaneous intracerebral hematoma. *Clin Res* 1982;30:412A, (abstr).

43. Weinstein PR, Anderson GG, Telles DA. Neurological deficit and cerebral infarction after temporary middle cerebral artery occlusion in unanesthesized cats. *Stroke* 1986;17:318–324.

44. Boisvert DP, Gelb AW, Tang C, et al. Brain tolerance to middle cerebral artery occlusion during hypotension in primates. *Surg Neurol* 1989;31:6–13.

45. Collins RC, Dobkin BH, Choi DW. Selective vulnerability of the brain: New insights into the pathophysiology of stroke. *Ann Intern Med* 1989;110:992–1000.

46. Crowell RM, Olsson Y, Klatzo I et al. Temporary occlusion of the middle cerebral artery in the monkey: Clinical and pathological observations. *Stroke* 1970;1:439–448.

5

Combination
of Thrombolytic Therapy
with Neuroprotectants

James C. Grotta, MD

CONTENTS

INTRODUCTION
RATIONALE FOR COMBINATION THROMBOLYSIS
    AND NEUROPROTECTION
LABORATORY STUDIES OF COMBINED NEUROPROTECTION
    AND THROMBOLYSIS
CLINICAL STUDIES OF COMBINED NEUROPROTECTION
    AND THROMBOLYSIS
CONCLUSION
REFERENCES

INTRODUCTION

Thrombolysis is the first scientifically established treatment for acute ischemic stroke, but we now need to build on that success. One possible way this might be accomplished is by combining thrombolysis with neuroprotection (see Chapter 3). Such "combination therapy" might reduce complications of thrombolysis, especially hemorrhage, by protecting damaged endothelium or reducing the volume of tissue necrosis. It might also prevent secondary injury associated with reperfusion. Finally, it might augment the benefit of thrombolysis by extending the time window before irreversible damage occurs. This chapter will explore the rationale behind combination therapy and describe laboratory and clinical results to date.

From: *Thrombolytic Therapy for Stroke*
Edited by: P. D. Lyden © Humana Press Inc., Totowa, NJ

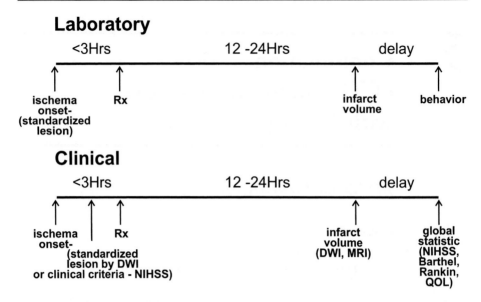

Fig. 1. Idealized clinical trial algorithm based on typical laboratory paradigm for testing neuroprotective drugs.

RATIONALE FOR COMBINATION THROMBOLYSIS AND NEUROPROTECTION

Failure of Neuroprotective Drugs Alone in Clinical Trials

Despite their consistent positive effect when used in animal models of focal ischemia, when used alone in clinical trials, neuroprotective drugs have so far been ineffective. There are many explanations for these failures, the most obvious being excessive delay to starting therapy, poor selection of patients, inadequate doses, insufficient statistical power, and unfortunate selection of end points. As depicted in Fig. 1 (top), in laboratory studies of neuroprotective drugs in animal stroke models, we produce a standardized amount of injury. We start therapy within 3 h, usually within an hour or so. We use large doses since our models may be insensitive to side effects that may limit dosing in elderly fragile stroke patients. We measure infarct volume, and then we employ a battery of behavioral outcomes. Our clinical trials should follow the same paradigm (Fig. 1, bottom), but so far have failed to do so. Let us examine these differences between the laboratory and clinical trials more closely.

The most important lesson of our attempts to model stroke in the lab and then investigate experimental therapies is the brief time window we have for effective neuronal salvage by either reperfusion or neuroprotection. The only conclusive positive clinical study of reperfusion (the National Institute of Neurological

Disorders and Stroke [NINDS] recombinant tissue plasminogen activator [rt-PA] trial) was exactly predicted by animal models; reperfusion must occur and therefore the patient must be treated within 3 h. All studies with longer time windows have failed. With regards to neuroprotection, calcium influx into neurons, as detected by its binding to calmodulin, correlates very well with ultimate cell death and functional outcome, and has been the target of many of our neuroprotective therapies. In all of our models, calcium binding to calmodulin becomes maximal within 2 h, so that the time window at least for the early events related to calcium after ischemia is very short *(1)*. All of the various drugs we have tested in the laboratory need to be started early in order to produce neuroprotection. In the case of lubeluzole, when started 15 or 30 min after occlusion, or even up to an hour, we found some benefit. Beyond that there was no effect. With *N*-tert-butyl-alpha-phenylnitrone (PBN), a very effective spintrap agent, we can get some effect up to 2 h, and some combinations of neuroprotective drugs can be effective when started out to 2 h after stroke onset. There are over 100 studies in the literature that show the efficacy of the glutamate antagonist MK801. A random sampling of these could find none in which MK801 could be given beyond 2 h and still reduce damage. Yet in no clinical trial of neuroprotection yet carried out has the drug been started within 4 h except in a handful of patients. Most trials have recruited patients 4–24 h after stroke onset.

In addition to starting our therapies earlier, we need to focus our clinical trials on those populations of patients that we think are going to respond to therapy, and then we can expand our indications beyond that point. That was the successful strategy employed by the NINDS rt-PA investigators by demonstrating efficacy in the best candidates, i.e., those treated within 3 h. In addition to those arriving in time to receive treatment early, other good candidates for neuroprotection, as in the lab, are those with a standardized amount of brain injury. Standardizing the infarct might be done through imaging, but right now, the easiest way to standardize our patient population is through putting limits on the National Institutes of Health (NIH) stroke scale that we use to allow patients into the trial, excluding those with mild strokes who are likely to recover spontaneously, and those with devastatingly severe strokes who are not likely to improve. Depending on the mechanism of action of the drug (i.e., antagonists of receptors not present in white matter), we might also try to exclude subcortical strokes.

The choice of end points is also critical. Whether infarct volume will be a surrogate measure of outcome remains to be seen. However, now that we have effective therapy, it's interesting to look back and compare the responses of rt-PA in animals compared to humans. There are some striking similarities. Work from Zhang and colleagues *(2)* found that in a rat model, rt-PA is associated with a 56% improvement in the neurological score. In the NINDS trial in stroke patients, the drug was associated with a 62% improvement in functional outcome. In the laboratory studies, rt-PA reduced infarct volume by about 33% and

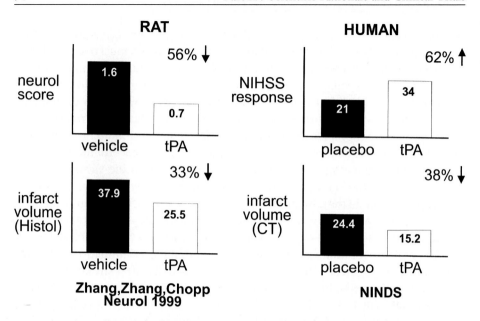

Fig. 2. Comparison of the clinical effect of tPA on the neurological score and on infarct volume, in experimental studies in rat (Zhang et al. *[2]*) vs clinical trials in human stroke patients.

in the NINDS clinical trial, rt-PA reduced infarct volume by about 38% (Fig. 2). It's going to be very important, as we develop positive therapies, to look back at what our experience was in the laboratory and see what parts of the laboratory experience were most useful in deciding whether these drugs work or not. The rt-PA data suggest that our laboratory models are accurate not only in predicting the time window for effective treatment, but also for predicting the relative magnitude of effect. Furthermore, it appears that our behavioral and functional outcomes are at least as good and probably even more sensitive at detecting response to therapy than just simply measuring infarct volume.

In the laboratory, we use a battery of functional outcomes. The only trial to employ this approach was also the only positive trial, i.e., the NINDS rt-PA study. In that trial we used the global statistic, which combines a number of different outcome measures. The global statistic is not that difficult to understand *(3)*. Consider a portrait artist; each angle gives a different perspective of the subject. One wouldn't consider completing a portrait by painting from only one angle. Similarly, a global test that combines several different measures, each one evaluating a different but related response to therapy, is likely to give a more complete (and perhaps more sensitive) representation of the results.

Even if we take into consideration all these features of our clinical trials, and do post-hoc analyses of the neuroprotective trials carried out to date, it is clear that when used alone, neuroprotective drugs produce at best only a "weak signal." In many of the trials with 6 h time windows (the shortest time windows yet studied with reasonably large numbers of patients), most notably the trials of aptiganel, clomethiazole, and lubeluzole, there was at best only a suggestion of benefit at the highest dose levels when imbalances in stroke severity were corrected by limiting analysis to those patients with more standardized insults. Attempting to make any extrapolations about efficacy from the Phase II data in relatively small numbers of patients has proved consistently misleading when the Phase III data were examined. These observations indicate that the effect of any one of these drugs alone is likely to be small, requiring a large sample size to detect a small difference between groups, and that this difference might be easily overwhelmed by small flaws in the study design or imbalances in the type of patients randomized.

An analogy would be a weak radio signal. Imagine yourself on a remote country road late at night trying to pull in a distant radio station. The music fades in and out. How might the reception be made clearer? One way of course is to drive closer to the signal. In a clinical trial, the analogy would be by moving the treatment closer to the time of onset, i.e., shortening the time window. Only as you move closer to the signal and the music gets clearer do you realize that what you had thought was reasonably good reception was really filled with interference. The other way to make the music clearer is to make the signal stronger; in that way the music may be clear at a greater distance. The clinical trial analogy would be by making the treatment more powerful. One way to do this is to combine treatments together, in this case to combine neuroprotective drugs together or with thrombolysis.

In order to justify combination therapy, the two treatments must have advantages over either one alone. There are at least three reasons why adding reperfusion might increase the effect of neuroprotection over what is achieved by neuroprotection alone. First, by increasing blood flow to threatened penumbral regions, reperfusion therapies might increase the delivery of concomitantly administered neuroprotective drugs to these target regions. Second, the fate of penumbral tissue is proportional to the depth and duration of blood flow reduction. By limiting the depth of hypoperfusion early after the onset of ischemic injury, reperfusion therapies might reduce cellular necrosis and maintain a larger amount of ischemic brain tissue in a penumbral or salvageable state, which might be ameliorated by concomitant neuroprotective drugs. Finally, since reperfusion and neuroprotection are complementary in their mechanisms of action, adding reperfusion might produce a therapeutic effect that could not be achieved even with maximal doses of neuroprotectives.

Reperfusion Injury

Just as concomitant thrombolysis might uncover the therapeutic efficacy of neuroprotective drugs, adding neuroprotective drugs to thrombolytics might reduce side effects and secondary injury associated with reperfusion.

Although their overall effect is positive, drugs that produce reperfusion, especially thrombolytics, have well-known adverse effects. These include bleeding into ischemic regions or aggravation of infarct-related cerebral edema, both likely the result of increased hydrostatic pressure applied to a damaged blood-brain barrier (Fig. 3). These devastating side effects of thrombolysis might be prevented or reduced by drugs that protect the integrity of the vascular endothelium. Such drugs might include free radical scavengers or anti-adhesion molecules, which prevent leukocyte-mediated injury.

A less well-understood adverse consequence of reperfusion is cytotoxicity associated with reperfusion of moderately injured brain tissue. There are several explanations for this so-called "reperfusion injury." First, it has been shown that reperfusion is associated with a secondary wave of glutamate and other neurotransmitter release and consequent movement of calcium intracellularly resulting in excitotoxicity *(4)*. Second, restoration of blood flow may be sufficient to allow synthesis of damaging proteins and other cytokines. Third, reperfusion may supply oxygen to ischemic regions which provides a substrate for peroxidation of lipids and free radical formation *(5)*.

We have been able to demonstrate reperfusion injury in a rat model of moderate ischemia produced by tandem occlusion of the ipsilateral common carotid and middle cerebral arteries (MCA) (Fig. 4) *(6)*. The figure shows that opening the MCA up and allowing reperfusion following 2–5 h of MCA occlusion is associated with substantial infarction when measured after 24 h, whereas leaving the MCA permanently occluded was associated with very little damage even if histological evaluation was deferred up to a week to allow for the appearance of delayed cell death. This reperfusion injury could be ameliorated by lubeluzole, but even more strikingly by the spin-trap agent PBN and the protein synthesis inhibitor cyclohexamide. These results suggest that reperfusion injury may have an inflammatory basis and suggest that combining reperfusion with appropriate neuroprotective agents, which achieve therapeutic levels by the time the artery recanalizes, might improve the outcome beyond what can be achieved by thrombolysis alone.

LABORATORY STUDIES OF COMBINED NEUROPROTECTION AND THROMBOLYSIS

One of the first studies of combination neuroprotection with reperfusion showed that calcium entry into neurons continued and actually increased upon reopening the MCA after 60 min of occlusion. The noncompetitive glutamate

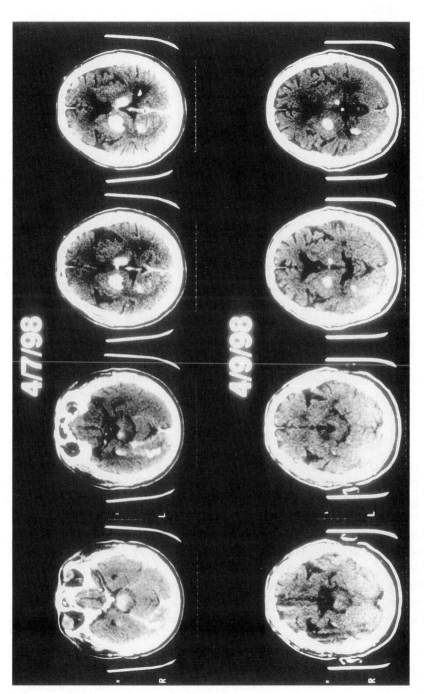

Fig. 3. CT scan in patient immediately after (top) and 2 d after (bottom) intra-arterial thrombolysis of a basilar artery thrombosis. Note the enhancement from the arteriographic contrast in the pons, thalami, and right occipital lobe in the post-treatment scan. On follow up study 2 d later, hemorrhagic transformation is seen in the latter two areas possibly representing reperfusion injury in regions of ischemia and initially disrupted blood-brain barrier.

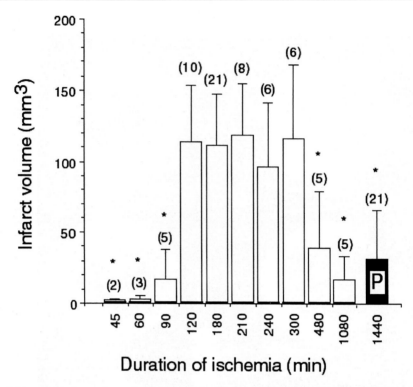

Fig. 4. Duration of transient middle cerebral artery occlusion (TMCAo) vs infarct volume 24 h later. TMCAo of 120–300 min followed by reperfusion produces more damage than longer or permanent MCAO. P, permanent. *See* ref. *6.*

antagonist MK 801, which blocks the NMDA-associated ion channel, partially but incompletely reduced calcium influx, and the combination of MK 801 and the voltage gated ion channel blocker nimodipine completely normalized the intracellular calcium signal (Fig. 5) *(7).*

We have studied the combination of reperfusion and neuroprotection as well. In our model, reperfusion is augmented after temporary MCA occlusion by administering diaspirin crosslinked hemoglobin (DCLHb). DCLHb is an ideal hemodiluting agent. It is a stable dimer of human hemoglobin that does not dissociate and has an oxygen affinity similar to blood, but does not increase whole blood viscosity as does a comparable volume of red blood cells. It can be given as an intravenous infusion.

In our model, blood is exchanged for DCLHb to achieve a hematocrit reduction to about 30%. Treating animals with DCLHb beginning 15 min after various durations of MCA occlusion followed by reperfusion doubled the time the MCA could be occluded without resulting in ischemic damage (Fig. 6) *(8).* Adding

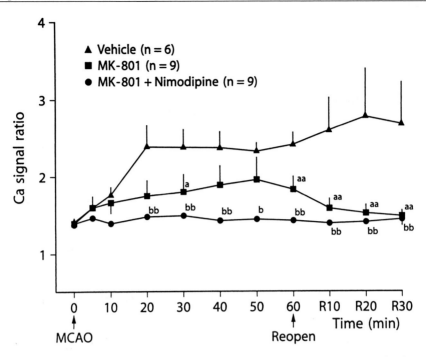

Fig. 5. Intracellular calcium at various intervals after transient middle cerebral artery occlusion. The increase in calcium is partially prevented by MK-801 and completely prevented by the combination of MK-801 and nimodipine (*see* ref. *7*).

lubeluzole, which limits the production of nitric oxide (NO) following glutamate release, decreased the volume of infarct eventually produced, regardless of the duration of ischemia.

This experiment demonstrates the effect of adding complementary therapies. DCLHb, which increased perfusion and oxygenation after an infarct, increased the therapeutic window by maintaining injured tissue in a reversible "penumbral" state for a longer period of time. Lubeluzole blocked some of the key intracellular perturbations leading to irreversible injury in this penumbral region, thus reducing the ultimate volume of infarcted tissue.

Other studies have more directly examined the role of combining neuroprotection with thrombolysis. Such studies are limited by the paucity of autologous clot animal models in which to test thrombolytic drugs. One of the first such studies was carried out by Zivin and colleagues *(9,10)* in the rabbit embolism model. The rabbit model involves a simple cutdown in the neck, occlusion of the external carotid artery, and implanting a cannula in the common carotid artery to inject particles. After the surgery is complete, the animal is awake and unanesthetized, so many aspects of physiology that might influence neuroprotection,

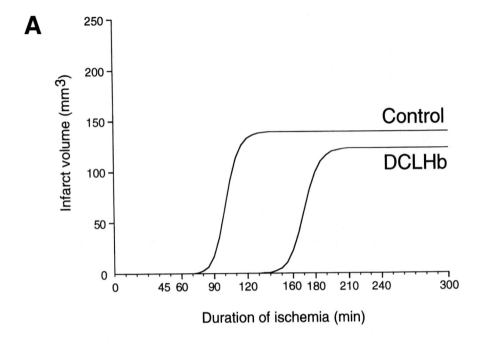

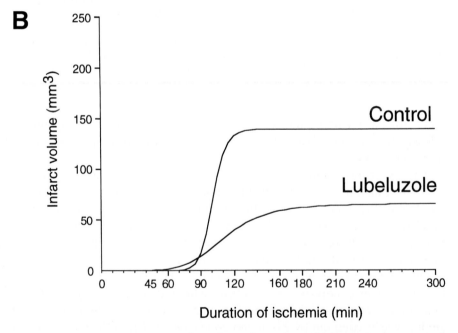

Fig. 6. Infarct volume after variable durations of transient middle cerebral artery occlusion (TMCAo) in rats treated with diaspirin cross-linked hemoglobin (DCCHb), lubeluzole, or the combination compared to controls. DCCHb prolongs the time animals can tolerate TMACo before infarction occurs (**A**), while lubeluzole reduces the size of the infarct (**B**).

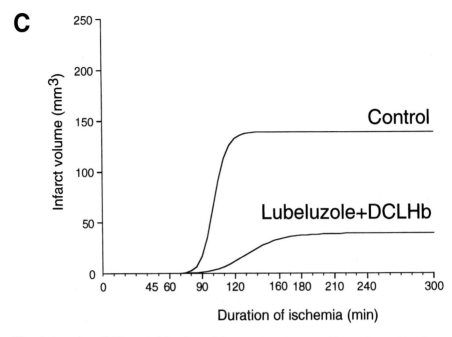

Fig. 6. *(continued)* The combination of the two treatments achieves both objectives **(C)**.

such as a blood pressure, body temperature, and blood gases, are under normal physiologic regulation.

To study ischemic stroke, blood is taken from a donor animal, allowed to form clots, and injected into the carotid circulation. This produces clots in end vessels in the brain. Tracer amounts of radioactive microspheres are injected with the clots and are used to measure the specific activity of the brain and to determine how many clots lodge in the brain. The result is small infarcts in random locations throughout the brain.

Data are analyzed by plotting the weight of microspheres, which is a measure of the amount of clot in the brain, vs percentage of animals displaying neurologic deficits (Fig. 7). There are two parameters of interest in this curve. One is the position parameter, which is the mean weight of clots the animal can tolerate. The other is the slope parameter, which is an estimate of the population variance. If the curve shifts to the right, it implies that the animals can tolerate more clots. A change in the slope of the curve means that something else has happened. Shifts in the slope typically occur when two effects are taking place at the same time. For example, a drug might provide neuroprotection but simultaneously alters blood pressure. One problem with this model is that there is a ceiling effect. Animals given high doses of clots often die before they can be treated.

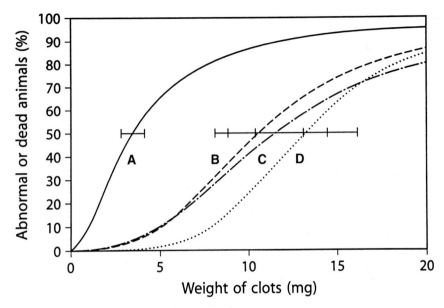

Fig. 7. Paradigm for testing the effect of drugs in the microembolism model. Increasing amounts of emboli are injected until all animals die. TPA started 15, 45, and 30 min after clot injection (**B, C,** and **D**) all increase the amount of clot tolerated compared to controls (**A**).

Figure 7 illustrates the effect of rt-PA alone in this model *(9)*. Curve A is the control and shows that the untreated animals tolerated about 3 mg of clots. Curves B, C, and D are the results of treating with rt-PA at 15, 45, and 30 min after clots were injected. They show that the treated animals tolerated about three times more clots than the control animals. However, if treatment was delayed for 1 h, the curve was not significantly different from the control curve. This was the first demonstration in a clinically applicable model that rt-PA reduced neurologic damage.

This model was used in a study of rt-PA and MK-801, which is a glutamate antagonist *(10)*. MK-801 was given at 1 mg/kg 5 min after embolization. rt-PA was given at 1 mg/kg at various later times. MK-801 alone had no significant effect. rt-PA alone at 60 min after embolization nearly doubled the amount of clots the animal could tolerate (Table 1). Giving both drugs at 60 min was more effective than rt-PA alone, even though MK-801 was ineffective alone. Delaying rt-PA treatment to 90 min did not produce a therapeutic effect.

This model was also used to study combination therapy with an anti-ICAM monoclonal antibody plus rt-PA *(11)*. Whereas the rt-PA/MK-801 study was designed to increase the amount of clot the animal could tolerate, the rt-PA/anti-

Table 1
Effect of t-PA and MK-801 on Neurologic Function (from *10*)

Drug	Dose (mg/kg)	t-PA treatment (min)	$ES_{50} \pm SE$ (mg)[a]	n
Saline			5.34 ± 0.99	25
MK-801	1		2.46 ± 4.04	17
t-PA	1	60	$9.09 \pm 1.23*$	11
MK-801 + t-PA	1 + 1	60	$12.32 \pm 0.95**$	12
MK-801 + t-PA	1 + 1	90	8.44 ± 1.88	12

[a]ES_{50} is the amount of microspheres resulting in death of 50% of animals.
*Significantly different from control.
**Significantly different from t-PA alone.

Table 2
Interaction of Anti-ICAM and t-PA (from *11*)

Group	Dose (mg/kg)	Time (min)	n	$ES_{50} \pm SE$ (mg)[a]
Control			24	2.61 ± 0.18
Anti-ICAM	2	15	17	3.03 ± 0.37
t-PA	3	120	27	3.90 ± 0.87
Anti-ICAM + t-PA	2 + 3	15+ 120	19	$4.61 \pm 0.68*$

[a]ES_{50} is the amount of microspheres resulting in death of 50% of animals.
*Significantly different from control.

ICAM study attempted to increase the window of time until start of treatment. Data showed that the combination could extend the time window to 2 h, whereas neither drug alone was effective when treatment was initiated at 2 h. This is evidence for a positive interaction of the combination (Table 2).

More recently, Zhang and colleagues *(2)* have developed an autologous clot occlusion of the MCA in rats. Treatment with rt-PA alone improved neurologic deficits and reduced mean infarct volume compared to controls when the drug was started within 2 h of arterial occlusion, but had no benefit when treatment was delayed out to 4 h. The anti-CD18 antibody, which presumably prevents white blood cell adhesion to ischemic endothelium and consequent inflammatory damage to surrounding brain regions, had no effect when administered alone at either time point. However, when both rt-PA and the anti-CD18 antibody were given together, there was substantial reduction of neurologic deficit even when combined treatment was delayed out to 4 h *(2)*. Thus, the synergism of this particular combination was especially notable in extending the time window of effective therapy.

CLINICAL STUDIES OF COMBINED NEUROPROTECTION AND THROMBOLYSIS

To date, only two studies designed to evaluate the effect of combining thrombolysis and neuroprotection have been carried out, and one was terminated prematurely. In patients given intravenous rt-PA within 3 h of stroke onset according to the NINDS protocol, lubeluzole had to be started within 1 h of starting rt-PA, i.e., before the rt-PA infusion was completed. The lubeluzole was administered as a bolus followed by continuous infusion so that therapeutic blood levels would be achieved by the time reperfusion from the rt-PA was likely to occur. The study was designed to evaluate the safety of the combination, particularly to ensure that the incidence of hemorrhage was not increased (and perhaps decreased), and was a companion to a larger evaluation of lubeluzole given as monotherapy out to 8 h following stroke onset. When the larger 8-h study was completed and found to be negative, the combination trial was terminated after 80–90 patients had been enrolled. Although the number treated was too small to draw definite conclusions, there was no evidence of benefit. However, the study demonstrated that such a trial design is feasible *(12)*.

Further trials are needed to confirm this. This approach has been taken with recent studies of clomethiazole. Whereas a large study of monotherapy compared to placebo was conducted, a smaller study was designed to test the combination of rt-PA given within 3 h, and clomethiazole given within 8 h *(13)*. The study included 97 patients given clomethiazole and 93 patients given placebo; all patients received t-PA first according to NINDS protocol. Overall, there was no benefit seen. In the patients with the worst strokes however, there was a possible beneficial effect. These results suggest that clomethiazole may augment the beneficial effect of t-PA in patient with large strokes.

Other neuroprotective trials are now being carried out that allow treatment with rt-PA if clinically indicated, so that some patients in these studies will receive combination therapy. However, since only a minority of stroke patients arrive in time to receive treatment within 3 h, these studies are not likely to have sufficient numbers of patients to evaluate the effect of combination treatment vs monotherapy. This can only be done if such studies are formally stratified, thereby forcing substantial numbers of patients into the combined treatment group.

CONCLUSION

Although still unproven as a means to improve on results obtained with thrombolytic therapy alone, combination therapy of thrombolysis with neuroprotective drugs has a sound theoretical and experimental basis. Although one possible benefit of such an approach may be to extend the therapeutic time window, any such combination should be started as early as possible after the onset of stroke symptoms, and it is likely that the neuroprotective agent will be most effective if it is administered before or along with lytic therapy.

REFERENCES

1. DeGraba T, Ostrow P, Grotta J. Threshold of calcium disturbances after focal cerebral ischemia in rats—implications of the window of therapeutic opportunity. *Stroke* 1993;24:1212–1217.
2. Zhang RL, Zhang ZG, Chopp M. Increased therapeutic efficacy with rt-PA and anti-CD18 antibody treatment of stroke in the rat. *Neurology* 1999;52:273–279.
3. Tilley B, Marler J, Geller N, Lu M, Legler J, Brott T, Lyden P, Grotta J, for the NINDS rt-PA Stroke Trial Study Group. Use of a global test for multiple outcomes in stroke trials with application to the National Institute of Neurological Disorders and Stroke t-PA Trial. *Stroke* 1996;27:2136–2142.
4. Matsumoto K, Lo EH, Pierce AR, Halpern EF, Newcomb R. Secondary elevation of extracellular neurotransmitter amino acids in the reperfusion phase following focal cerebral ischemia. *J Cereb Blood Flow Metab* 1996;16:114–124.
5. Traystman RJ, Kirsch JR, Koehler RC. Oxygen radical mechanism of brain injury following ischemia and reperfusion. *J Appl Physiol* 1991;71:1185–1195.
6. Aronowski J, Strong R, Grotta J. Reperfusion injury: demonstration of brain damage produced by reperfusion after transient focal ischemia in rats. *J Cereb Blood Flow Metab* 1997;17:1048–1056.
7. Uematsu D, Greenberg JH, Reivich M, Karp A. In vivo measurement of cytosolic free calcium during cerebral ischemia and reperfusion. *Ann Neurol* 1988;24:420–428.
8. Aronowski J, Strong R, Grotta JC. Combined neuroprotection and reperfusion therapy for stroke: the effect of lubeluzole and diaspirin crosslinked hemoglobin in experimental focal ischemia. *Stroke* 1996;27:1571–1576.
9. Zivin JA, deGirolami U, Kochhar A, et al. A model for quantitative evaluation of embolic stroke therapy. *Brain Res* 1987;435:305–309.
10. Zivin JA, Mazzarella V. Tissue plasminogen activator plus glutamate antagonist improves outcome after embolic stroke. *Arch Neurol* 1991;48:1235–1238.
11. Bowes MP, Rothlein R, Fagan SC, et al. Monoclonal antibodies preventing leukocyte activation reduce experimental neurologic injury and enhance efficacy of thrombolytic therapy. *Neurology* 1995;45:815–819.
12. Grotta JC. Combination therapy stroke trial: rt-PA +/- lubeluzole. *Stroke* 2000;31:278.
13. Lyden PD, Ashwood T, et al. The Clomethiazole Acute Stroke Study in Ischemic, Hemorrhage, and t-PA Treated Stroke: Design of a Phase III Trial in the United States and Canada. *The Journal of Stroke and Cerebrovascular Diseases* 1998; 7: No.6:435–441.

6

Early Studies
of Thrombolytic Therapy for Stroke

Anne M. Guyot, MD, Luchi Quinones, MD,
and Steven R. Levine, MD

CONTENTS

INTRODUCTION
INITIAL STUDIES OF THROMBOLYTIC
    FOR "ACUTE" ISCHEMIC CEREBROVASCULAR DISEASE
EARLY POST-CT STUDIES
BRAIN HEMORRHAGIC COMPLICATIONS
THROMBOLYTIC THERAPY
    FOR CEREBRAL VENOUS/SINUS THROMBOSIS
THROMBOLYTIC AGENTS IN THE TREATMENT
    OF HEMORRHAGIC CEREBROVASCULAR DISEASES:
    EARLIER STUDIES
SUMMARY AND CONCLUSIONS
REFERENCES

INTRODUCTION

The demonstration that t-PA is clinically effective for acute ischemic stroke treated within three hours of symptom onset was based upon many important studies over the past two decades that then lead to groundbreaking preliminary clinical trials *(1–3)*. This chapter will highlight and discuss this historical aspect of investigations and their results so as to place the current state-of-the-art in perspective. Thrombolytic therapy is an inherently attractive treatment for ischemic stroke based on the known pathologic and angiographic substrates of ischemic cerebrovascular disease. The majority of acute ischemic strokes are the direct consequences of atherothrombosis or thromboembolism of a cerebral or

From: *Thrombolytic Therapy for Stroke*
Edited by: P. D. Lyden © Humana Press Inc., Totowa, NJ

precerebral artery (*see* Chapter 2) *(4–6)*. The critical event is usually the formation of an acute thrombus *(6)*. The basis for thrombolytic treatment is to achieve arterial recanalization with a relatively safe agent soon enough to improve patient outcome.

There is currently one proven therapy (that is, FDA-approved) for the treatment of acute human ischemic stroke. Therefore, there is a great need for potentially safer thrombolytic agents that offer the greatest potential in a risk-benefit analysis. Stroke is a serious health care problem worldwide and is the third leading cause of death in the United States, following myocardial infarction (MI) and cancer. Only recently have physicians attempted to intervene in acute ischemic stroke with the sense of critical urgency that experimental ischemic models have suggested it is necessary for the beneficial outcome *(7–13)*.

Timing of use of thrombolytics is key because a therapeutic window, measured in hours, is available for reperfusion-enhancing agents to maximize both efficacy and safety in the treatment of acute ischemic stroke *(9–13)*. This has already been demonstrated for the treatment of MI with thrombolytic agents. Furthermore, data from acute coronary artery thrombolysis studies suggest that recanalization occurs independent of the location of the thrombotic occlusion *(14,15)*.

Because the preponderance of all strokes are caused by the acute thromboembolic occlusion of the cerebral artery, the majority of acute stroke victims may benefit from rapid implementation of thrombolytic therapy. Correlation of the occlusive cerebral arterial lesion with clinical deficit has been noted in nearly 61 of 81 (75%) patients documented to have cerebral hemisphere infarctions studied within 6 h of symptom onset with cerebral angiography *(6)*. Furthermore, the outcome of patients with angiographically proven middle cerebral artery (MCA) occlusions is poor when managed conservatively *(16)*, as 30% die within 3 mo and an additional 38% survive with severe neurological deficits. Clearly, aggressive strategies for the treatment of human stroke are necessary as there is a severe lack of tolerance of the brain to focal ischemia *(9–11)*. Harvey and Rasmussen *(17)* found that the maximum time of proximal (1 cm from origin) MCA occlusion in the monkey that still allowed a reduction in infarct size on reperfusion was 50 min. Temporary occlusion for greater than 1 h resulted in the same infarct size as permanent MCA occlusion.

As knowledge of the intrinsic fibrinolytic system has increased *(18–23)*, use of newly developed fibrinolytic agents in the therapy of acute MI has continued *(22,24)*. Given that the model of myocardial ischemia—an occluded artery resulting in infarcted tissue—is similar, knowledge concerning fibrinolytic therapy at the proper dose and time for myocardial ischemia should have application when lysing clot in the cerebral circulation.

Although thrombolytic or fibrinolytic therapy was attempted in cerebrovascular disease approx three decades ago during the pre-computed tomography

Table 1
Limitations of Pre-CT Era Stroke Thrombolysis Trials

Lack of adequate control groups
No direct imaging of pathologic process (ICH not definitively excluded)
Prolonged time of symptom onset to treatment
A small number of angiographic studies (to assess recanalization)
Few objective patient inclusion/exclusion criteria
Limited publication of demographic information, concurrent pathology, medication
Significant variability from patient to patient in:
    Nature and dose of thrombolytic agent
    Ancillary therapy
    Time frame for inclusion in the study

(CT) era, less than beneficial outcome was observed *(25–36)*. The pre-CT clinical studies of intravenous (iv) thrombolytic therapy for stroke *(25,28,29,31,35,36)* were limited because they did not investigate truly acute ischemic stroke, assess recanalization, or assess clinical outcome independent of intracranial hemorrhage (ICH) *(37)*. A detailed review of these studies is presented as they are instructive via their limitations and results. The more recent studies are then presented, including the recent preliminary data on t-PA *(2)* for ischemic stroke that has led to today's "gold standard": the placebo-controlled, randomized clinical trial. Hemorrhagic complications are discussed as the results of thrombolytic therapy for cerebrovascular diseases other than ischemic stroke: cerebral venous thrombosis, intracerebral and intraventricular hematoma, and subarachnoid hemorrhage. The relevant experimental studies of thrombolytic therapy are also detailed.

INITIAL STUDIES OF THROMBOLYTIC
FOR "ACUTE" ISCHEMIC CEREBROVASCULAR DISEASE

Clinical Studies: Pre-CT

During the initial use of thrombolytic therapy for ischemic stroke *(31–34)* cerebrospinal fluid (CSF) analysis was used in most studies to exclude cerebral hemorrhage; however, ICH could not be definitely excluded on the basis of CSF analysis alone. In general, results of these trials were highly variable and frequently reported unacceptable rates of hemorrhage and death. Limitations of these pre-CT studies are summarized in Table 1. Summarizing all these trials, only 33 of 265 patients studied underwent pre- and posttreatment cerebral angiography. The size of the clot was unchanged in 13 patients *(25,36,38,40)*, although only a small fraction of arteries totally recanalized *(27,36)*. Only two of the eight early trials used a placebo group that would help distinguish between spontaneous and therapeutic thrombolysis *(27,36)*.

The first attempt to treat ischemic stroke using a thrombolysis was reported in 1958 by Sussman and Fitch *(39)*. They treated three patients with plasmin Fibrinolysin; one patient had moderate clinical improvement with recanalization of the MCA. The other two patients did not improve clinically despite one case of large cerebral vessel recanalization. Sussman and Fitch *(39)* may have been the first to observe that those patients presenting early after the onset of stroke symptoms were the most likely to benefit from thrombolytic therapy. Clifton *(34)* reported a 45-yr-old woman with a hemiplegia of 3 d duration from a post-operative carotid artery thrombosis. The clot was lysed after 15 min of plasmin therapy, but she died 48 h later (on Dicumarol and heparin) owing to a tracheal obstruction from a hematoma. Clifton also mentions that two cases of cerebral thrombosis were treated with plasmin (inadequate doses) without success. In 1958, Clifton was given credit *(41)* for being the first to use purified activated plasminogen with favorable results in thrombotic cerebral circulatory disorders. Two years later, Herndon et al. *(42)* treated 13 patients within 3 d of presumed ischemic stroke onset (clear CSF) with bovine thrombolysin and anticoagulants. Eight (62%) patients improved. None of the four patients who had cerebral angiography performed were found to have complete occlusions. Five patients died; however, there was no evidence for hemorrhagic infarction or ICH found at postmortem examinations.

Herndon et al. *(43)* then reported 27 cases given fibrinolytic therapy for cerebral artery occlusion (CSF with >3000 red blood cells as a contraindication); diagnosis was confirmed by autopsy in 6 cases and by arteriography in 16 (Table 2). In addition, one case of retinal vein thrombosis and one case of bilateral cavernous sinus thrombosis were treated with fibrinolytic agents. Two of three patients treated "early" (within 6 h) died (at 31 h and 3 d), both of whom had basilar artery thrombosis, whereas the third patient improved.

Ten patients with cerebrovascular thrombotic events treated with fibrinolytic agents (Table 2) were reported by Clark and Clifton *(31)*. Of the three patients treated by intra-arterial instillation of fibrinolysin directly into the occluded carotid artery, all showed complete recanalization of the vessel with normal blood flow. One of these showed good clinical response (out of coma and motion of the paralyzed extremities) but the other two died of local hematoma or a rebleeding aneurysm. Lysis of the carotid thrombus in the aneurysm patient occurred with the administration of 200,000 U of fibrinolysin with return of function in the paralyzed extremity and definite clearing of coma. Systemic instillation of the fibrinolytic agent was performed in seven cases; two (29%) completely recovered, three improved, and two were unchanged.

Meyer et al. *(28)* used intra-arterial human thrombolysin, iv bovine thrombolysin, and anticoagulants in 14 patients. Four of seven patients with internal carotid artery (ICA)-MCA distribution infarcts improved, 2 were unchanged, and 1 died. Of the 5 patients with vertebrobasilar disease, 2 improved (one then died of medical

Table 2
Thrombolytic Therapy for Presumed Ischemic Cerebrovascular Disease Pre-CT: Major Series of Patients

Author	Reference number	n	Thrombolytic agent	Ancillary	Outcome
Herndon*	(43)	27	Fibrinolysin over 3 d iv	Heparin, Dicoumarol	15% involved, 33% died, 4 systemic hemorrhages
	(25)	50	Bovine fibrinolysin or human plasmin		31% died, 16% progressed/unchanged, 52% improved
Clark & Clifton†	(31)	10	Fibrinolysin up to 4 d		2 rapid complete recovery, 3 rapid improvement, 2 died
Meyer‡	(36)	40 (randomized to thrombolytic or placebo	Thrombolysin (iv plasmin) over 3 d	Anticoagulants	45% improved in each group, 35% died in each group
Meyer‡	(27)	73 (randomized to thrombolytic or placebo, both administered heparin stroke-in-progression	SK iv	Heparin	43% SK treated improved, 35% SK treated died
Fletcher§	(35)	31	Urokinase iv	Hyperbaric Oxygen	"No improvement," 4 with clinical ICH
Larcan	(47)	36	Urokinase		52% died

Abbreviations: IV, intravenous; SK, streptokinase; ICH, intracranial hemorrhage.
*Duration symptoms: 2 h to 1 mo (3 treated ≤ 6 h).
†Only 1/10 treated ≤ 6 h, duration of symptoms = 3 h – 1 mo.
‡All treated ≤ 72 h after symptom onset.
§All treated ≤ 36 h after stroke onset (range 8–34 h).
75% death rate in similar patients treated symptomatically or only with hyperbaric oxygen.

complications), and 2 were unchanged. Eleven of 14 patients underwent cerebral angiography; 3 showed clot dissolution, and 1 had presumed clot dissolution.

A pilot study was then reported by Meyer et al. *(36)* who randomized 40 patients with occlusion of the carotid or MCA tree in a placebo-controlled trial using iv plasmin (thrombolysin) (Table 2). Thirty-four (85%) had angiography before treatment and eight (20%) had repeat arteriograms before hospital discharge. The plasmin dose was 200,000 U administered over 4 h daily for 3 d. All cases were also treated with subcutaneous heparin that was then followed with oral warfarin therapy. At 10 d there was no difference in outcome between placebo- and plasmin-treated groups when the subgroup with proven occlusive disease of the large vessels was analyzed. Of those 8 patients with repeat angiography, 6 had no change, and 2 had partial recanalization (one in each treatment group). One patient who was administered plasmin and died 48 h after beginning treatment from a large hemorrhagic infarction had been given a loading dose of warfarin (30 mg) for 2 d in error.

Meyer et al. *(27,29)* reported 73 patients with progressive stroke treated within 72 h of onset of symptoms with heparin ($n = 36$) or heparin plus streptokinase ($n = 37$) (6 h infusions, individually dosed after a dose-prediction test) in a randomized protocol (Table 2). Patients had to have a clear CSF and systolic BP less than 180 mm Hg before inclusion. Improvement or deterioration was assessed "quantitatively" (no further details) at baseline and 10 d later. Arteriography was obtained on admission (demonstrating an occluded vessel in 35) and repeated at 10 d if an occluded vessel was found initially. Twenty-one (58%) of 36 heparin-treated patients and (43%) of 37 streptokinase- and heparin-treated patients improved, whereas four (11%) and 13 (35%) of the two groups, respectively, died. Statistical analysis was not performed. Clot lysis was demonstrated by repeat angiography or at autopsy in 10 patients (three heparin treated, seven treated with heparin plus streptokinase). Autopsies on 13 of 17 who died (three controls, 10 in the streptokinase group) showed three cerebral hemorrhages (all streptokinase treated), one hemorrhagic infarction (streptokinase treated), and nine "anemic" infarctions (all three controls and six streptokinase treated).

Fletcher et al. *(35)* reported results of a pilot study of iv urokinase in cerebral infarction involving 31 patients treated either with a single- or double-infusion period, each of 10 to 12 h (Table 2). Patients enrolled in the study had more severe neurological deficits than the average stroke patient observed at their institution. Angiography was performed before urokinase treatment in seven patients. One had no vascular lesion noted, and in two others the examination was unsatisfactory. Four patients had stenotic disease or occlusion of the MCA. One patient died from complication of a neck hematoma following traumatic carotid angiography. The investigators stated "it was our clinical impression that no instance of unequivocal clinical improvement, attributable to treatment, was observed." The investigators concluded that the number of patients treated with urokinase was so small that neither assessment of overall treatment efficacy nor response comparisons among urokinase dosages could be made. Anecdotal pre-CT reports of thrombolytics for cerebrovascular disease continued *(44–46)* as did a larger series with urokinase *(47)*.

Fletcher et al. *(48)* also showed that plasma plasminogen was higher in patients with cerebral infarction than controls. However, endogenous fibrinolysis develops slowly following stroke *(49)* and is associated with increased relative activity of thrombin.

In summary, arterial recanalization was shown in 31% to 100% of the patients in whom pre- and posttreatment angiography was performed. However, because of a discouraging number of ICH, enthusiasm for these agents dissipated *(50)*.

EARLY POST-CT STUDIES

Advances in clinical and neuroimaging assessment of ischemic cerebrovascular disease combined with the expanding knowledge of the pathophysiology of human brain infarction *(13)* led to a resurgence of enthusiasm for newer potentially safer thrombolytic agents and techniques in human ischemic stroke (Table 3) *(51)*.

Early reestablishment of cerebral blood flow (CBF) has been demonstrated experimentally *(52)* to limit the extent of brain infarction. Previous studies likely initiated treatment too late, i.e., longer than 6 to 8 h after the onset of symptoms and as long as beyond 2–3 d after the onset of symptoms. Beginning with the early 1980s, case reports again appeared that reported clinical improvement from ischemic stroke following cerebral arterial recanalization with intra-arterial thrombolytic agents *(53–64)*.

Streptokinase/Urokinase

Larger early series post-head CT. Otomo et al. *(65)* studied 359 stroke patients using urokinase (60,000 IU/d) for 7 d or placebo in a double-blind protocol. Improvement in two of three clinical outcome scales was noted in the urokinase-treated group. Fujishima et al. *(66)* reported on 143 patients with cerebral infarction treated with either urokinase (2.83×10^5 U V I over 6 h [$n = 81$] or a combination of urokinase-dextran sulfate (DS), 2.84×10^5 U plus 300 mg DS over 1 d [$n = 62$]) in a multicenter cooperative study (Table 3). Only 89% of the cases had head CT performed for stroke diagnosis and 30% had spinal taps. The clinical assessment was based on a qualitative scale of deficit severity—severe, moderate, mild, or normal. Therapeutic usefulness, as assessed by overall clinical improvement rate and safety rating, was obtained in 74% of urokinase-treated patients and 84% of the urokinase-dextran-treated patients.

From 1983 to May 1986, Hacke et al. *(67)* reported their experience with 43 prospectively studied patients given either local intra-arterial urokinase or streptokinase for angiographically documented vertebrobasilar artery territory throm-

Table 3

Thrombolytic Stroke Trials Incorporating Neuroimaging: Post-CT Series

Author	Year	n	Thrombolytic agent	Ancillary Therapy	Outcome
Matsou (68)	1979	33	Low-dose UK	–	No improvement
Hossman (69)	1983	15	Ancrod	LMW dextran, mannitol	Improvement in neurologic deficit, no ICH, 60% 1-yr survival (47% in control group)
Fijishima (66)	1988	143	IV UK for 1 to 7 d	62 also received DS	Moderate to marked improvement in 31% UK treated, in 61% UK + DS treated hemorrhagic events in 3.2% of UK + DS treated mortality 1.6%/2.5%
del Zoppo (63)	1988	20	IA, UK, or SK up to 4 h	Heparin, hydroxyethyl starch in some patients	75% complete recanalization, 20% hemorrhagic transformation
Hacke (67)	1988	43	IA, UK, or SK up to 48 h	Heparin, hydroxyethyl starch	44% recanalized, 46% persistent occlusion, 9.3% hemorrhagic transformation
Mori (70)	1988	22	IA, UK	Variable: hypervolemic or isovolemic hemodilution, 10% IV glycerol, aspirin, heparin, or combination	45% immediate recanalization, 18% hemorrhagic infarction
Terashi (71)	1990	364	t-PA	–	No difference between groups
Haley (72)	1990	21	IV t-PA	–	9% fatal ICH, 15% improves during the infusion
Pollak (73)	1990	20	Ancrod	–	Greater stroke scale improvement compared with controls
Brott (2)	1990	74	IV t-PA	–	50% 2-h improvement, 4% symptomatic ICH
rt-PA acute stroke study group	1991	104	IV t-PA	–	31% partial recanalization, 4% complete recanalization, 22% hemorrhagic infarction, 9.6% ICH

Abbreviations: UK, urokinase; LMW, low molecular weight; ICH, intracranial hemorrhage; IV, intravenous; DS, dextran sulfate; IA, intra-arterial; SK, streptokinase.

bosis (Table 3). Recanalization of the cerebral artery following thrombolytic treatment correlated significantly with clinical outcome. All infusions were via a superselective catheter located as close as possible to the occlusive lesion. Heparin, 300 U/h, was routinely administered simultaneously with the thrombolytic agents and then administered at 1000 U/h iv with hydroxylethyl starch. All patients without recanalization died, whereas 14 (74%) of 19 who recanalized survived (p = 0.000007), 10 with a "favorable" outcome. Patients (with two exceptions) were not administered thrombolysis if the initial head CT showed hypodense areas in the brain stem or cerebellum. Twenty-nine (67%) of the 43 patients were treated within 24 h after symptom onset, but only 6 of 8 patients with acute symptoms were treated within 6 h. Twenty-five patients had a progressive initial clinical course, and roughly half had recanalization of the vessel after therapy. However, 7 of 8 patients with acute clinical onset did not recanalize. When patients were awake or somnolent, 15 cases recanalized and 13 did not; in contrast, of patients who were stuporous or comatose, 4 cases recanalized and 11 did not. Six of 9 more rostral occlusions recanalized, as did 5 of 11 more caudal occlusions. Only 5 of 15 mid-basilar occlusions recanalized. No significant difference emerged in the distribution of occlusive lesions that did or did not recanalize. Four of the 43 cases developed hemorrhagic transformation: 1 was detected on routine CT, 4 d after treatment, and 3 were noted after clinical deterioration. Three of the ICH were located in the pons with variable extension into cerebellar structures. Two of the four died from ICH. Fibrinogen, aPTT, and fibrin split product measurement in the patients with hemorrhagic events were not different from the patients without ICH. Three of the four patients received urokinase in extended infusion (8.6 to 16.2×10^5 U total over 11 to 24 h). All received iv heparin. Two of four with hemorrhagic infarction did not show recanalization. This has also been documented in infarcts not treated with thrombolytic agents *(74)*. One patient with a massive ICH was treated over 72 h after symptom onset and recanalized. The investigators concluded in this very promising study (albeit neither randomized, angiographically blinded, nor adequately controlled), that technically successful thrombolysis of vertebrobasilar artery occlusions is associated with beneficial clinical outcome. Their expanded experience with 66 patients was also reported *(75)*. Harenberg et al. *(76)* also reported a similar experience with urokinase for basilar artery occlusion.

Data on local intra-arterial urokinase or streptokinase for acute carotid territory stroke was reported by Del Zoppo et al. *(63)* from a prospective, angiographically based, two-center open-pilot study (Table 3). Twenty patients age 28 to 80 yr (average 54 yr) were studied. Seventy-five percent (15 of 20) with acute stable symptoms (mean treatment onset interval 7.6 h) demonstrated complete recanalization (unblinded evaluation) with 10 of 15 exhibiting clinical improvement by the time of hospital discharge. Hemorrhagic transformation within the infarct was not accompanied by clinical worsening. Enrollment symptoms were unilateral motor deficits with or without aphasia occurring within 6 to 8 h before treatment initiation. Complete occlusion of a major brain-supplying artery in the carotid artery distribution appropriate to the acute symptoms demonstrated by angiography was required before treatment initiation. Cerebral arterial disease locations included ICA siphon ($n = 2$), intracranial carotid bifurcation ($n = 3$), ipsilateral ICA + MCA embolus ($n = 3$), MCA ($n = 5$) and/or MCA branch ($n = 6$), and PCA ($n = 1$). All but two cases demonstrated at least partial recanalization. The longest time from symptom onset to treatment time with complete recanalization was 10 h. All 4 with hemorrhagic transformation had complete recanalization and were treated 6–10 h post symptom onset (all were also treated with heparin and hydroxyethyl starch). Three of these four patients showed clinical improvement. Deterioration or death occurred in 3 other patients, all with proximal MCA occlusion, 2 with mass effect. Nine of 10 patients demonstrating clinical improvement received the intra-arterial treatment within 4 to 8 h after symptom onset. All three patients who suffered strokes as complications of interventional angiographic procedures were treated within 1 h of symptom onset, had complete recanalization, and did *not* show clinical improvement. All four hemorrhagic transformations occurred in the deep gray matter of the affected hemisphere. These data are often cited to support a claim that patients should not receive thrombolytic therapy beyond 6 h following stroke onset. However, 3 of the 4 hemorrhage patients treated late actually improved.

Mori et al. *(70)* reported 22 patients who received intracarotid urokinase for evolving cerebral infarction due to angiographically documented thromboembolic occlusion of the MCA or its major branches (Table 3). The recanalized group more commonly had noncardiac (intra-arterial) source of embolism (possibly smaller clot) than the nonrecanalized group. Five of 6 with "excellent" outcome were in the recanalized group, and the volume of CT infarction (mL) was significantly less in the recanalized group (35.5 ± 55.4) compared with the nonrecanalized group (172.8 ± 122.6) ($p < 0.01$). The volume of CT infarction also correlated with the initial neurological state ($r = 0.76$, $p < 0.001$) and outcome ($r = 0.95$, $p < 0.001$). Prognosis was also correlated with restoration of blood flow ($r = 0.60$, $p = 0.003$). There was no correlation between initial neurological state and recanalization. Neither interval from onset to infusion nor dose of urokinase correlated with prognosis.

Mori et al. *(70)* reported on large volume clots that were less likely to be lysed. When thrombi are large enough to be visualized on CT *(77)*, there was generally a lack of major clinical improvement and these patients often developed a large volume infarct on follow-up CT scan, suggesting that recanalization did not occur with treatment (iv t-PA).

t-PA Preliminary Trials

Terashi et al. *(71)* treated 364 stroke patients with either t-PA ($n = 171$) or urokinase in a double-blinded protocol. Of the total number of patients, 36%

started treatment within 24 h and 70% within 48 h. There were no statistically significant differences between the two groups at the 7-d clinical evaluation. "Adverse effects" were noted in approx 10% of each group, and the incidence of hemorrhagic infarction was less than 5% in each group.

In an open-labeled safety/efficacy multicenter trial of rt-PA in acute stroke *(3)*, patients were treated after CT and angiography (required to demonstrate a cerebral artery occlusion consistent with the focal neurological deficit) within 8 h of symptom onset with a single preassigned dose of iv t-PA. Preliminary data following completion of this dose-escalation trial was reported for 104 of 139 (75%) patients undergoing angiography who received 1 of 8 t-PA dose rates. Ninety-four patients were included. Partial (29/94 or 31%) and/or complete (4/94 or 4%) recanalization was noted at all dose rates, most consistently in patients who had distal cerebral arterial branch occlusion. There was a 22% rate of hemorrhagic infarction. Intracerebral hemorrhage occurred in 9.6%, with deterioration in 60% of these. Hemorrhagic infarction and ICH were significantly ($2p = 0.006$) associated with treatment beginning after 6 h but were not associated with t-PA dose, recanalization, presence of CT abnormality, hypertension, or aspirin use. A dose rate for t-PA providing consistent recanalization was not achieved.

A second dose-escalation safety study of t-PA was completed, with early treatment emphasized *(2)*. Initiation of iv t-PA was required within 90 min of symptom onset. Pretreatment angiography was not required, and patients were not excluded on the basis of ischemic stroke subtype (e.g., small vessel obstruction). Seventy-four patients were treated with 1 of 7 t-PA doses. Symptomatic ICH occurred in three patients (4%) and was associated with higher doses of t-PA. One patient died, and another patient required neurosurgical evacuation, (that patient's ICH occurred in the cerebellum even though his acute infarction involved the right cerebral hemisphere). All three patients became symptomatic within 3 h following cessation of t-PA in the absence of anticoagulation therapy. A second cohort of 21 patients was treated under the same protocol but at 90 to 180 min from symptom onset *(72)*. Two patients sustained ICH (9%), both fatal. For all patients, clinical improvement during the t-PA infusion occurred in 20 treated within 90 min (27%) and in 3 treated at 90 to 180 min (15%). Improvement was not related to t-PA dose, severity of the original neurological deficit, nor location or presumed mechanism of infarction. As control patients were not included in these safety studies, conclusions regarding efficacy could not be drawn. Very early treatment was shown to be feasible, and the clinical outcomes were not inconsistent with an advantage for urgent therapy.

Mori et al. *(72)* reported the results of a randomized double-blind, placebo-controlled trial of t-PA in acute carotid stroke using angiographically confirmed occlusion of the internal carotid artery of the MCA within 6 h of symptom onset. t-PA was administered (20 or 30 MIU dosing) iv over 1 h. Angiography was performed pre- and posttreatment. Recanalization occurred in 3 of 12 (25%)

placebo, 4 of 9 (44%) 20 MIU t-PA, and 5 of 19 (50%) 30 MIU t-PA-treated patients (placebo vs drug, $p = 0.1$). Patients receiving t-PA showed better improvement in the neurological scale than the placebo group. Hemorrhagic transformation (generally mild) occurred in 5 placebo-treated patients and 5 of 12 placebo, 6 of 9 twenty MIU t-PA, and 4 of 10 thirty MIU t-PA-treated groups.

Small Series and Case Reports

Malinouski and Nikota *(41)* reviewed data from Russia on fibrinolytic therapy for cerebral thromboembolism, including a young woman, age 27, with cerebral emboli following surgery for mitral stenosis and intra-atrial thrombosis. Streptokinase was given 2.5 h postoperatively. Six hours later she showed signs of improvement but then deteriorated and died 4 wk later. Cerebral arteries were patent at autopsy.

Zeumer et al. *(53)* reported a 27-yr-old woman who received streptokinase followed by heparin via a catheter in the vertebral artery after sustaining an acute rostral basilar artery occlusion. There was rapid and "impressive" improvement in the clinical, electrophysiological, and radiographic findings.

Henze et al. *(78)* described a 64-yr-old woman who became suddenly comatose and was admitted to the hospital 50 min later. One hundred thirty minutes after symptom onset angiography showed a rostral basilar artery occlusion. Immediately after informed consent, 15 mg t-PA was administered as bolus followed by 50 mg t-PA infusion over 30 min via intravertebral artery catheter, and then 35 mg t-PA over the following 1 h (total dose 1.5 mg/kg). Angiography 1.5 and 20 h after the start of thrombolytic therapy showed recanalization of the entire basilar artery. No hemorrhage was observed on CT. The patient was left with mild neurological deficits.

Jafar et al. *(79)* treated an MCA embolus with iv t-PA that occurred during catheterization to treat a cerebral arteriovenous malformation that had bled 3 wk earlier. The patient's aphasia and hemiplegia predominantly resolved, then recurred, was treated again with iv t-PA and iv heparin, and the patient returned neurologically to normal; repeat angiography showed flow through the previously occluded MCA.

These preliminary data (summarized in Tables 3 and 4) *(2,3,53,58,63,65,73, 78–91)* suggest that some patients may make clinical neurological improvements following thrombolytic therapy for ischemic stroke with only a small incidence of ICH as a complication. When streptokinase was administered intra-arterially to acute stroke patients within 6 h of stroke symptom onset, 90% had angiographically proven effective recanalization and 60% had clinical improvement *(56)*. Other small series of truly acute patients have had clinical improvement after treatment with fibrinolytic agents (urokinase, streptokinase) *(54,85)*. Therefore, placebo-controlled, randomized studies (*see* Chapter 7) are critical to determine the benefit of thrombolytics in acute clinical ischemic stroke.

Table 4
Small Series and Case Reports Post-CT

Author	Year	n	Thrombolytic agent	Ancillary therapy	Outcome
Kaufman (46)	1977	1	IV thrombolysin	Decadron, mannitol, stellate ganglion block	Improved
Abe (81)	1979	6	UK	–	Two improved
Zeumer (53)	1982	1	IA SK	Heparin	Rapid improvement
Nenci (85)	1983	4	IU, SK, or UK	IV prednisolone	Variable: improvement or death, no bleeding
Henze (78)	1987	1	IA t-PA	–	Clinical improvement and recanalization
Zeumer (58)	1989	7	IA UK	Heparin in some	2/7 died, 1 locked-in, 4 with excellent "outcome" ICH in at least 1
Jungreis (86)	1989	1	IA UK	–	Clot lysis with subsequent reocclusion, no bleeding
Morgan (87)	1990	1	IA UK	Heparin	Recanalization and gradual recovery
Jafar (79)	1991	1	IV t-PA	Heparin	Resolved aphasia and hemiplegia, rapid MCA embolus lysis (occurred twice)
Herderschee (88)	1991	2	IV t-PA	–	1 died, 1 remarkable and sudden improvement with recanalized basilar artery

Abbreviations: IV-intravenous; UK- urokinase; IA-intra-arterial; SK- streptokinase; ICH- hemorrhage; MCA-middle cerebral artery.

Newer techniques, such as a *trans*-thrombus bolus of fibrinolytic agent to accelerate thrombolysis *(92)*, may eventually aid in the clinical treatment of cerebrovascular occlusions, although the risk of distal embolization may be greater.

BRAIN HEMORRHAGIC COMPLICATIONS

Clinical Studies

Table 5 summarizes the reports of cerebral hemorrhagic complications of thrombolytic therapy *(62,98–119)*. Tables 6–12 summarize strokes complicating therapy in the MI trials. The risk of ICH during or subsequent to iv streptokinase or urokinase in patients unselected for cerebral disease (e.g., acute MI) has been approx 1% *(62,100,120,121)*.

Thrombolytics for MI

Strokes (combined ischemic and hemorrhagic) complicating MI have, in general, become less common in the thrombolytic era compared with the prethrombolytic era *(121)*. Initial rates for ICH in MI patients treated with streptokinase and rt-PA were estimated at 2.2 per 1000 and 1 per 200, respectively *(121)*.

As a rule, ICH-complicating thrombolytic therapy for MI occurs within 24 h of treatment and at times during treatment. When ICH occurs, it is generally not in the deep cerebral gray matter characteristic of hypertensive ICH, but rather it is in the lobar/subcortical white matter in up to 70% of the cases *(122)*, and it may be multiple in up to one-third of the patients. Approximately one-fourth to one-half of patients with ICH complicating thrombolytic therapy for MI will die from their stroke *(121)*.

The International Study Group *(123)* found more strokes in t-PA-treated MI patients (1.3%) than in streptokinase-treated MI patients (1%), combining over 20,000 patients from Gruppo Italiano Per Lo Studies Della Stepto Chinasi Nell' Infarctomiocardico (GISSI)-2 and elsewhere.

Coller *(23)* reviewed the clinical studies using antiplatelet agents with thrombolytic therapy. In the second International Study of Infarct Survival (ISIS-2) trial, the absolute total number of strokes was reduced approx 50% and 25% in the aspirin plus streptokinase group compared with the placebo group and streptokinase only group, respectively. The total number of hemorrhagic strokes in the streptokinase groups was higher 1 d after treatment compared with the placebo group; however, it was lower after 1 d resulting in a lower total number of strokes overall. The combination of antiplatelet and thrombolytic agents appears to reduce the overall risk of stroke despite an increase in hemorrhagic strokes presumably by limiting the extent of myocardial wall damage (potential subsequent cardioembolic stroke source) and inhibiting the thrombotic process.

The Anglo-Scandinavian study of early thrombolysis (ASSET) *(111)* reported that 1.1% of the patients receiving rt-PA in the MI group had strokes, of whom 11 of the 28 stroke patients died, for a total risk of death from stroke of 0.4%. In the placebo group there were 25 strokes and 6 deaths, giving a stroke incidence of 1% and a risk of death from stroke of 0.2%. However, the strokes in the rt-PA group occurred during the first 24 h of therapy. Fatal hemorrhagic strokes primarily occurred during infusion of the rt-PA. However, postinfusion strokes were more commonly embolic, with 8 of 11 occurring in this period. This compared with two fatal hemorrhagic strokes occurring in the postinfusion period on placebo, and 15 of 17 embolic strokes occurring in the postinfusion period.

Fennerty et al. *(124)* rigorously reviewed reports of hemorrhagic complications of thrombolytic therapy for the treatment of MI and venous thromboembolism. The event was classified as a cerebral hemorrhage if a patient developed a cerebrovascular event during therapy, and an associated CT was not described. They found no cerebral hemorrhages reported in the GISSI trial *(125)*. However, there were 9 central nervous system (CNS) hemorrhages (0.1%) of 8377 patients treated with streptokinase vs one patient who developed a CNS hemorrhage in the placebo group. None of the cerebral hemorrhages were fatal.

In the trial reported by Topel et al. *(126)*, there was no obvious relationship to the risk of hemorrhage and the dose of fibrinolytic therapy. However, there was apparently a relationship to the degree of systemic fibrinogenolysis. The authors found in their review that in the noninvasive streptokinase trials, there was a graded major hemorrhage rate of 0.8% and a 0.1% rate of cerebral hemorrhage and a 0.02% rate of fatal hemorrhage in over 15,000 patients who received streptokinase. In the streptokinase invasive studies, there were no CNS or fatal hemorrhages in over 400 patients. In the t-PA trials for MI, the incidence of major hemorrhage was approx 12%; in invasive studies involving over 1900 patients, the rate of major hemorrhage was 12.7%, the rate of cerebral hemorrhage 0.6%, and fatal hemorrhage 0.1%. These rates were similar to those observed in the invasive studies with streptokinase. The authors believed, although this opinion is based on only two randomized studies comparing streptokinase and t-PA, that there is no evidence to support the conclusion that current rt-PA dose regimens were associated with less hemorrhagic side effects than streptokinase.

Intravenous and intracoronary routes of streptokinase administration appeared to have similar hemorrhagic complications. Confounding the risk of CNS hemorrhage from thrombolytic agents is the concomitant or subsequent use of anticoagulant (heparin or warfarin) therapy. As many as 1.7% of MI patients administered thrombolytic therapy with heparin may develop ICH *(100,127)*, although the partial thromboplastin times (PTTs) are frequently prolonged from the heparin *(103)*.

Price *(107)* reviewed the data on the frequency of stroke in six recent placebo-controlled trials of thrombolytic therapy (3 streptokinase, 3 rt-PA) for acute MI

Table 5
Clinical Studies: Cerebral Hemorrhagic Complications of Thrombolytic Therapy

Author	Year	n	Indication	Agent	Cerebral hemorrhagic event(s) outcome
Hass (98)	1966	1	MCA occlusion	IV UK	Fatal hemorrhage infarction
Hannaway (99)	1976	4	Ischemic stroke	IV UK	4 ICH, 3 fatal
Aldrich (100)	1985	2	Digital, arterial occlusion, MI	IV SK	ICH
Aldrich	1985	1996	Retrospective review of SK therapy		0.7% ICH
AIMS (101)	1986	624	MI	APSAC	2 hemorrhagic strokes
Sato (117)	1986	9	Acute cerebral embolism	IV, UK	56% CT hemorrhagic infarction
BMJ (37)	1986	3768			1.7% ICH
FDA	1986		—	80–100 mg, t-PA	0.4% ICH
del Zoppo (62)	1986	1099	DVT Peripheral, arterial thrombosis	SK or UK	0.27% ICH
				SK or UK	1% ICH
Braunwald (105)	1987		Acute MI	150 mg IV t-PA	1.5%–2.0% ICH
TIMI15 (105)	1987		Acute MI	150 mg IV t-PA	1.6% ICH
				150 mg IV t-PA	0.6% ICH
TAMI (108)	1987	386	MI		0.05% ICH, 0.025% fatal ICH
ISIS-2 (106)	1988	8377	Acute MI	IV SK	0.1% ICH (0.01% ICH in controls)
Carlson (109)	1988	450	MIMI	t-PA	0.44% ICH with heparin
ASSET (111)	1988		MI	IV t-PA	1.1% stroke, 0.4% fatal stroke
ECSG (112)	1998		Acute MI	IV t-PA	1.4% ICH (all administered aspirin and heparin)
Carlson (109) review	1988	5258 (AIMS+ISIS+GISSI)	MI	t-PA	0.68% ICH
		2975	MI	t-PA	88 strokes of unknown type
					9 ICH (with heparin) 11 strokes of unknown type

Hirshberg (118)	1989	122	Occluded peripheral arteries or grafts	IA SK or UK	3 ICH, 2 fatal
Price (107)	1990	14,957	MI	SK	15 ICH
Kase (102,103)	1990	6	MI	t-PA	ICH, 67% fatal patients without CT scans
GISSI-II (110)	1990	>20,000	MI		
Ramsey (114)	1990	1	MI	IV SK	ICH + SHD with cerebral amyloid angiopathy
Eleff (119)	1990	1	Superior Vena Cava Syndrome	IV SK	Epidural hematoma 7 h after IV SK stopped and IV heparin started
		1	Peripheral vascular occlusive disease	IA UK (with heparin)	ICH + SAH, fatal
Proner (115)	1990	1	MI	t-PA, heparin	ICH from AVM
ISIS-3 (116)	1991	46,092	MI	SK, t-PA	0.6% ICH
Pendleburg (113)	1991	1	MI	IV t-PA (with heparin)	ICH with cerebral amyloid angiopathy

Note: Many of the ICH associated with thrombolytic agents have been complicated by concomitant heparin use with prolonged PTTs, aspirin use, or hyofibrinogenemia (120).

Abbreviations: MCA, middle cerebral artery; IV, intravenous; UK, urokinase; ICH, intracranial hemorrhage; SK, streptokinase; MI myocardial infarction; CT, computed tomography; DVT, deep venous thrombosis; IA, intra-arterial; SDH, subdural hematoma; SAH, subarachnoid hemorrhage; AVM, arteriovenous malformation.

Table 6
Stroke in ISIS–2 Study

		D 0–1 Treatment					
ISIS-2	n	Hemorrhagic stroke	Other stroke	After D 1	Total strokes	Fatal strokes	Baseline stroke
Placebo	4300	0	9	36	45	18	15
Aspirin	4295	0	4	18	28	8	8
SK	4300	4	11	21	36	12	8
Aspirin and SK	4292	6	6	13	25	12	8

Table 7
Stroke in Streptokinase for MI Studies

	n	All strokes	Hemorrhagic	Nonhemorrhagic	Unknown type
ISIS-2					
SK	8595	61	7	–	54
Placebo	8595	67	0	–	67
AIMS					
SK	502	2	–	–	2
Placebo	502	5	–	–	5
GISSI					
SK	5860	59	8	9	42
Placebo	5860	40	0	7	33

Table 8
TIMI-II Associated ICH

TIMI-11	n	ICH
rt-PA (150 mg) and heparin	980	12 (1.3%)
rt-PA (100 mg) and heparin	3016	11 (0.4%) (p < 0.01)

(heparin use variable). In the three streptokinase trials (AIMS, ISIS, GISSI), 14,957 patients in the thrombolytic group suffered 112 strokes (0.75%), of which 15 were ICH, 9 were ischemic, and 88 were unknown type. In the placebo arms of these trials, 112 (0.75%) of 14,949 suffered strokes, none documented as ICH, 7 ischemic, and 105 unknown type. In the three rt-PA trials (ASSET, TAMI, Australia) (heparin administered), 36 (1.21%) of 2975 patients administered rt-PA had strokes, 9 ICH, 16 ischemic, and 11 of unknown type. In the placebo arms of these three trials, 30 (1.05%) of 2868 patients had stroke, 4 ICH, 19 ischemic, and 7 unknown type. Conclusions are difficult in these six studies

Table 9
Stroke in rt-PA for MI Studies

	n	All strokes	Hemorrhagic	Nonhemorrhagic
TIMI I, II, III rt-PA				
With or without UK	708	13 (1.8%)	4	9

Table 10
Strokes in GISSI–2 Study

	n	All strokes	Hemorrhagic	Nonhemorrhagic
GISSI-2				
t-PA	6182	70 (1.1%)	19 (0.3%)	28 (0.4%)
SK	6199	54 (0.87%)	15 (0.25%)	24 (0.4%)

Table 11
Strokes in ASSET Study

Asset	n	All Strokes	Hemorrhagic	Nonhemorrhagic	Unknown Type
t-PA	1518	28	7	11	10
Placebo	2495	25	2	17	6
TAMI					
t-PA	386	6	2	4	0
Placebo	302	4	2	2	0
Australia t-PA		2	–	1	1
Placebo	71	1	–	–	1

Table 12
Strokes in ISIS-3 Study

Isis-3	All studies	Hemorrhagic	Nonhemorrhagic
Eminase	1.5%	0.6%	0.9%
SK	1.1%	0.3%	0.8%
t-PA	1.5%	0.7%	0.8%

concerning risk of stroke subtype, although more patients administered strep-tokinase appeared to develop ICH, despite the total number of strokes not differing between thrombolytic-treated patients and placebo-treated patients. Only one fatal systemic hemorrhage was reported in these trials (128). The most common time of ICH was within the first 6 h after treatment. Data from the GISSI trial *(125,129)* suggest that streptokinase-treated patients develop more ischemic strokes during the first 2 d, and then the rate decreases with time. The GISSI-II study, involving more that 20,000 patients with MI had only a 0.3% rate of ICH *(122,127)*. Heparin use did not increase the risk of stroke. Many of the patients did not have CT scans however. In the TIMI-II trial (all patients treated with rt-PA, heparin [with bolus], and aspirin), age correlated with increased risk of ICH. Of the ICH patients who were administered the 150-mg rt-PA dose, 67% had no recovery, 25% had major residual, and 8% had minor residual compared with 36%, 9%, and 38%, respectively, in the 100-mg rt-PA treated group.

Ischemic Complications of Thrombolytic Therapy

O'Connor et al. *(140)* found ischemic stroke complicating thrombolytic therapy for MI in the TAMI I, II, and III trials to be related to the presence of a large anterior wall MI (greatest chance of intraventricular clot infarction), and mortality associated with ischemic stroke was 11%.

Transient ischemic attack of cardioembolic source has been reported at the end of a 3-h infusion of streptokinase (1,500,000 IU) for thrombosis on an artificial (Bjork-Shiley) mitral valve *(141)*. Successful thrombolysis of thrombi adherent to artificial heart valves has been reported *(142,143)* and may be a reasonable treatment in this group of patients at very high risk of stroke, but may also potentially lead to separation of the clot from the valve and subsequent embolic stroke or systemic emboli.

Cranston et al. *(144)* reported a 42-yr-old man with an acute anterior wall MI who was administered rt-PA by a heparin drip. He had a large hypokinetic area involving the entire superior and anterior wall and apex and a dyskinetic area at the apex and distal inferior wall. On d 2 he underwent successful percutaneous transluminal coronary angioplasty (PTCA), heparin was stopped, and aspirin was started. On d 8 he developed a new anterolateral wall MI and within 2 h was administered rt-PA. Three hours after onset of rt-PA, he developed a large right cerebral infarct possibly because of partial lysis of the left ventricular thrombus by rt-PA with subsequent embolization. Others have observed similar phenomena *(145)*.

Aldrich et al. *(100)* reported a patient who developed an occluded right carotid to brachial artery umbilical vein bypass graft (for right subclavian stenosis) 10 d after surgery. Streptokinase (250,000 U) and heparin 10,000 U iv (then 1000 U/h) were administered and 5 h later, she developed an MCA infarct, presumably from graft clot lysis and distal embolization.

Fatal ischemic cerebral edema may follow reperfusion after treatment with rt-PA. Koudstaal et al. *(146)* reported two patients with presumed MCA occlusions treated within 4 h of stroke onset with t-PA. These were the first 2 of 10 patients to be studied in a pilot study of thrombolysis with t-PA and acute stroke in the Netherlands. After a baseline CT, both patients received 100 mg of t-PA (10-mg bolus followed by a 50-mg infusion over the first hour and 40 mg over the second hour). The first patient manifested a sudden onset of paralysis of the left arm and leg and an inability to speak and initially demonstrated remarkable improvement. A few hours after infusion the patient again became mute and vomited twice. Repeat CT showed a massive infarction with edema in the anterior cerebral and MCA territories. The patient had pronounced systemic fibrinolysis and α_2-antiplasmin consumption. The patient deteriorated and died between 2 and 3 d after the onset of stroke. Presumably this patient developed cerebral arterial reocclusion to explain the improvement and subsequent decline with thrombosis into the internal carotid artery system based on CT findings. The second patient developed a global aphasia, forced deviation of his head and eyes to the left with a right hemianopia, and paralysis at the right arm and face. Baseline CT was normal and following t-PA the patient failed to improve. Repeat CT showed multiple infarctions and the patient died 1 wk after the onset of symptoms. Unfortunately, neither angiographic nor pathological confirmation was provided. Despite the concern introduced by this report, no other reports of reperfusion cerebral edema have appeared.

THROMBOLYTIC THERAPY
FOR CEREBRAL VENOUS/SINUS THROMBOSIS

A slowly growing number of reports have anecdotally suggested thrombolytic agents are of benefit for cerebral venous occlusive disease (148–150). These studies are summarized in Table 13 (151–178). Clearly time to treatment is critical as diagnosis is less straightforward than for arterial stroke and venous stroke is much less common. Meyer briefly mentioned that a group of patients with venous thrombosis in both his and the Washington University's group treated with streptokinase did extremely well (30).

In patients with central venous thrombosis (CVT) treated with thrombolytic agents, a review of the literature reveals a total of 119 cases, ranging from case reports to a series of 49 patients by Tsai. Ages of the patients range from 6 d to 71-yr-of-age. Urokinase was used in 98 patients, in doses ranging from 20,000 units to a total of 13.79 million units. Nine cases were treated with alteplase, 2 with rt-PA, 3 with thrombectomy followed by rt-PA, and 6 treated with thrombectomy alone. All were treated with heparin following the initial intervention. Onset of symptoms to treatment ranged from 1 d to 10 d, with one case having symptoms for years preceding treatment. Most reported good outcomes following clot lysis. There were no double-blind placebo-controlled studies reported.

Table 13
Thrombolytic Therapy for Cerebral Venous/Sinus Thrombosis

Author	Year	n	Type Of Cerebral Venous/Sinus Thrombosis	Treatment	Major Results/Outcome
Clinical Herndon (151,152)	1960	1	Bilateral cavernous sinus thrombosis	Thrombolysin	Improved
Bowell (153)	1970	8	Central retinal vein occlusion	Ancrod	Improved if treatment within 4 d of onset
Vines (154) and Fletcher	1971 1977	5	Cerebral venous occlusive	UK	Successful
Harvey (155)	1974	1	Bilateral septic cavernous sinus thrombosis	IV SK	Residual thrombus
Kohner (156)	1976	20	Central retinal vein occlusion within 7 d of symptoms	IV SK, anticoagulants	Improved visual acuity compared with randomized controls, early vitreous hemorrhage in 3 SK treated patients, not improved
Gettelfinger (157)	1977	1	Cerebral venous occlusive disease	–	Not improved
Rousseaux (158)	1978	1	Cerebral venous occlusive disease	–	Not improved
DiRocco (159)	1981	5	Aseptic cerebral dural sinus, cavernous, transverse sinus thrombosis	IV UK (with heparin)	Patency in 4, minor bleeding in 3
Zeumer (56)	1985	4	Cerebral venous thrombosis	Intra-carotid fibrinolytics	All recanalized
Bogdahn (160) (review)	1988	194	Cerebral venous thrombosis	Not specified	Full neurological recovery in 77%

Scott (161)	1988	1	Cerebral venous thrombosis	IV–UK	Reperfusion, hemorrhagic infarct, improved clinically
Higashida (162)	1989	1	Left transverse sinus thrombosis	IV UK	Full neurological improvement with normal growth development at 3 yr; Patency of the sinuses on repeat venogram
Persson (163)	1990	1	Superior sagittal sinus, bilateral transverse sinus, galeric venous system	Surgical thrombectomy, IV SK	Significant improvement with partial recanalization
Alexander (164)	1990	8	Rabbit-induced cerebral dural venous thromboses	IV t-PA	7/8 total lysis; 1/8 partial lysis
Barnwell (165)	1991	3	Dural sinus thrombosis Experimental	IV SK	2/3 improved with recanalization
Manthous (166)	1992	1	Superior sagittal sinus thrombosis	IV UK	Improved with no neurologic residua; Repeat cerebral angiogram revealed partial sagittal sinus recanalization and improved cortical vein filling
Smith (167)	1994	7	Dural sinus thrombosis	Local urokinase infusion	Improved neurological condition
Khoo (168)	1995	1	Superior sagittal, both transverse sinuses, and straight sinus thromboses	IV UK	Recovered with no neurological sequela; Rapid dissolution of thrombus in the sagittal and straight sinuses
Horowitz (169)	1995	12	Superior sagittal sinus, transverse sinus, straight sinus, internal cerebral veins, and vein of Galen thromboses	Direct UK infusion to sinuses and veins	8 fully recovered; 3 recovered with some sequela; and 1 died from pulmonary emboli; 11 patients had partial to complete patency of the sinuses and 1 patient had no change from pretreatment
Smith (170)	1997	1	Straight sinus, left transverse and sigmoid sinuses	Direct SSS infusion of UK	Complete neurological recovery; patent veins and sinuses

(continued)

Table 13 (*continued*)

Author	Year	n	Type Of Cerebral Venous/Sinus Thrombosis	Treatment	Major Results/Outcome
		1	Thrombosis of the superior sagittal sinus, straight sinus, right sigmoid, and transverse sinuses; internal cerebral veins, the vein of Galen	Direct infusion of UK to the sinuses	Full neurological recovery; patent straight sinus while posterior transverse, sigmoid, and posterior
Rael (171)	1996	1	Superior sagittal sinus and transverse sinuses thrombosis	Direct injection to the sinuses of rt-PA	Improved with no focal neurological deficit; Follow-up MR venogram showed flow signal throughout the superior sagittal sinus
Renowden (172)	1997	1	Superior sagittal and right transverse sinuses	IV alteplase	Improved neurological Status and complete recovery of visual acuity; Almost complete recanalization of the sinuses
Sun (173)	1997	9	Superior sagittal, straight, and transverse sinuses	Local injection of t-PA	Improvement of symptoms and improved recanalization in all cases
Niwa (174)	1997	1	Superior sagittal sinus	Direct sinus infusion of UK	Improved without any neurological deficits
Bagley (175)	1997	1	Superior sagittal, straight, and transverse sinuses	Direct sinus infusion of UK	Complete resolution of headache and partial improvement of visual acuity; MR venography showed dural sinus patency
Gertszten (176)	1997	1	Straight and right transverse sinuses	Direct sinus infusion of UK	Gradual neurological improvement; Continued patency of sinuses and veins
Kuether (177)	1998	1	Superior sagittal, right transverse, and right sigmoid sinuses	Direct sinus infusion of UK	Rapid improvement of the neurological status and normal patency of the sinuses
D'Alise (178)	1998	1	Superior sagittal and transverse sinus thrombosis	Direct sinus infusion of UK	Full neurological recovery; MRI showed patency of the sinuses

Abbreviations: UK, urokinase; IV, intravenous; SK, streptokinase.

THROMBOLYTIC AGENTS IN THE TREATMENT OF HEMORRHAGIC CEREBROVASCULAR DISEASES: EARLIER STUDIES

Intracerebral Hemorrhage

In 1982, Segal et al. *(165)* reported local urokinase treatment for experimental spontaneous ICH in adult macaques. Autologous clots (6 cm^3) were injected into the right internal capsule. Two animals received 5000 U urokinase in 0.1 μL of saline injected into the ICH 3 h after placement. The animals regained partial motor function whereas all three control animals remained hemiplegic. The CT in the urokinase-treated group had normal density at the ICH site at 3 and 7 d. Narayan and Narayan *(180,181)* were able to demonstrate ICH clot dissolution with urokinase in a rabbit model. Kaufman et al. *(182)* injected t-PA in rat brains without subsequent hemorrhage or inflammation.

In 51 humans with ICH, Matsumoto and Hondo *(183)* used urokinase without apparent clinical benefit and without complications attributed to the drug, although two patients rebled. Mohadjer et al. *(184)* used urokinase under CT guidance for fibrinolytic removal of cerebellar ICH in 14 patients. One patient died in the direct postoperative period, whereas the others had good to very good quality of life 6 mo post-ICH. Thrombolysis of brain parenchymal clot appears to be promising, relatively safe, less invasive approach to the management of ICH. Further clinical studies are clearly indicated.

Subarachnoid Hemorrhage

Several investigators have used fibrinolytic therapy to dissolve subarachnoid clot with the idea of reducing the secondary vasospastic complications *(185–192)*. The cerebral spinal fluid's natural fibrinolytic activity is insufficient to adequately lyse the subarachnoid fibrin thrombus *(188,189)*. Early reports *(190)* of cisterna magna injections of streptokinase and streptodornase were able to lyse clots in a cat subarachnoid hemorrhage (SAH) model, but also produced brain and meningeal inflammation.

Several studies have suggested benefit, albeit without rigorous methodology, of urokinase given intrathecally or intracisternally for SAH clot dissolution *(191,192)*. Alksne et al. *(193,194)* demonstrated that plasmin administered within the CSF in experimental pig SAH reduced histological evidence of vasospasm.

Seifert *(195)* demonstrated the efficacy of two boluses of intracisternal t-PA (25 μg) to completely prevent angiographic and pathological evidence of vasospasm 48 h and 6 h after two injections of blood in the two hemorrhage model of cerebral vasospasm in dogs.

Findlay et al. *(196)* found that t-PA administered intracisternally 2 h after SAH in primates could uniformly lyse clot and almost totally eliminated vasospasm at 1 wk. Side effects were minimal.

Shiobara *(192)* and Kodama *(197)* were probably the first to use intrathecal fibrinolytic therapy for human SAH. When urokinase and ascorbic acid were continuously infused in the basal cisterns of patients with severe SAH who underwent early aneurysm clipping, there appeared to be reduced cerebral vasospasm-related ischemic stroke.

Saito et al. *(198)* found that cisternal irrigation up to 15 d with 24,000 U urokinase (and 40 mg of gentamycin) in patients with SAH ($n = 25$) was associated with postoperative vasospasm in 6 (24%), restricted only, however, to the peripheral branches of the cerebral vessels (M2 or M3 or A2 portions of the middle and anterior cerebral arteries, respectively). Clinical studies with thrombolytic therapy for SAH have been underway for the past decade *(199)*, and this form of therapy appears promising. Seifert and Stolke *(200)* mention disappearance of intracisternal blood at 12 h and at 24 h following 10 mg of t-PA injected into the cerebral basal cisterns.

Intraventricular Hemorrhage

Pang et al. *(201–203)* used intraventricular urokinase in a dog model of experimental intraventricular hemorrhage (IVH). Dogs treated with urokinase had faster clot lysis and more clinical improvement compared with control dogs. No treatment hemorrhages occurred. Todo et al. *(199)* treated 6 patients with large bilateral IVH with urokinase instilled directly into the cerebral ventricles started 1 to 7 d after symptoms. Five of the six patients showed very good or excellent clinical outcome and the size of the clot was reduced. The time to clear the third and fourth ventricles of blood ranged from 2 to 10 d (mean 4.2 d). Two developed delayed obstructive hydrocephalus. Rebleeding did not occur. Five controls were selected retrospectively. Direct ventricular infusion of t-PA to treat IVH has also been anecdotally reported *(191)*. The patient suffered IVH secondary to ruptured aneurysm and the IVH persisted causing increased intracranial pressure after evaluation of the frontal ICH. The intraventricular hematoma was partially lysed with 8 mg of t-PA injected on d 1 and 2 postoperatively. The patient improved, although was not fully independent. The time to clear the third and fourth ventricles of blood ranged from 2 to 10 d (mean 4.2 d). Two developed delayed obstructive hydrocephalus. Rebleeding did not occur. Five controls were selected retrospectively. Direct ventricular infusion of t-PA to treat IVH has also been anecdotally reported *(191)*. The patient suffered IVH secondary to ruptured aneurysm and the IVH persisted causing increased intracranial pressure after evaluation of the frontal ICH. The intraventricular hematoma was partially lysed with 8 mg of t-PA injected on d 1 and 2 postoperatively. The patient improved, although was not fully independent. A pilot clinical study of thrombolysis of IVH is now underway.

Table 14
Factors Thought to be Related
to Successful Outcome After Thrombolytic Therapy

- Time from arterial obstruction to treatment
- Severity of the ischemia
- Volume of ischemic region
- Type of thrombolytic agent used
- Dose of thrombolytic agent used
- Adjunctive therapy used as anticoagulants, aspirin

SUMMARY AND CONCLUSIONS

The knowledge obtained from these earlier studies set the stage for the larger, more recent randomized clinical trials reported in this book. They also led to the awareness for the clearly mandated rapid, aggressive team approach needed to truly treat acute ischemic stroke successfully *(206)*. Furthermore, at least one-third of ischemic stroke patients reperfuse spontaneously (and obviously too late) within 48 h of stroke onset *(210)*. Several factors believed to be related to successful outcome after thrombolytic therapy are summarized in Table 14.

Zivin *(211)* succinctly reviewed thrombolysis for stroke, both experimental and clinical, and summarized some of the difficulties of the early clinical stroke trials with thrombolytic agents and speculated about future prospects *(212)*. Although hemorrhagic complications of t-PA in-clinical and experimental stroke have been consistently reported and remain a major concern of thrombolytic therapy *(107,109,121,213–215)*. Zivin foresaw t-PA proving valuable in the treatment of some forms of thromboembolic stroke.

REFERENCES

1. Brott T. Thrombolytic therapy for stroke. *Cerebrovascular Brain Metab Rev* 1991;3:91–113.
2. Brott TG, Haley EC, Levy D, et al. Safety and Potential Efficacy of Tissue Plasminogen Activator (tPA) for stroke. *Stroke* 1990;21:181 (abstr).
3. The rt-PA/Acute Stroke Study Group. An open safety/efficacy trial of rt-PA in acute thromboembolic stroke: Final report. *Stroke* 1991;22:153.
4. Solis O, Robertson GR, Taveras JM, et al. Cerebral angiography in acute cerebral infarction. *Rev Interam Radial* 1977;2:19–25.
5. Hacke W, Del Zoppo GJ, Harker LA. Thrombosis and cerebrovascular disease. In: *Recent Advances in Diagnosis and Management of Stroke*, Poeck K, Ringelstein EB, Tacke W, eds. Springer-Verlag: New York. 1987; pp. 59–64.
6. Fieschi C, Argentino C, Lenzi GL, et al. Clinical and instrumental evaluation of patients with ischemic stroke within the first six hours. *J Neurol Sci* 1989;91:311–321.
7. Barsan WG, Brott TG, Olinger CP, et al. Identification and entry of the patient with acute cerebral infarction. *Ann Emerg Med* 1988;17:1192–1195.

8. Barsan WG, Brott TG, Olinger CP, et al. Early treatment for acute ischemic stroke. *Ann Intern Med* 1989;11:449–451.

9. Boisvert DP, Gelb AW, Tang C, et al. Brain tolerance to middle cerebral artery occlusion during hypotension in primates. *Surg Neurol* 1989;31:6–13.

10. Collins RC, Dobkin BH, Choi, DW. Selective vulnerability of the brain: New insights into the pathophysiology of stroke. *Ann Intern Med* 1989;110:992–1000.

11. Crowell RM, Olson Y, Klatzo I, et al. Temporary occlusion of the middle cerebral artery in the monkey: Clinical and pathological observations. *Stroke* 1970;1:439–448.

12. Shiraishi K, Sharp FR, Simon RP. Sequential metabolic changes in rat brain following middle cerebral artery occlusion: A 2-deoxyglucose study. *J. Cereb Blood Flow Metab* 1989;9:765–773.

12a. Astrup J, Siesjo B, Symon L. Thresholds in cerebral ischemia: The ischemic penumbra. *Stroke* 1981;12:723–725.

13. Welch KMA, Levine SR, Ewing JR. Viewing stroke pathophysiology: Analysis of contemporary methods. *Stroke* 1986;17:1071–1076.

14. Kambara H, Kawai C. Thrombolytic therapy in Japan: Urokinase infusion for acute myocardial infarction. In: *Tissue Plasminogen Activator in Thrombolytic Therapy*, Sobel BE, Collen D, Grossbard EB, eds. Dekker: New York. 1987; pp. 223–235.

15. TIMI Study Group. Special Report. The thrombolysis in myocardial infarction (TIMI) trial. *N Engl J Med* 1985;312:932–936.

16. Saito I, Segawa H, Shiokawa Y, et al. Middle cerebral artery occlusion: Correlation of computed tomography and angiography and clinical outcome. *Stroke* 1987;18:863–868.

17. Harvey JE, Ramussen T. Occlusion of the middle cerebral artery. An experimental study. *Arch Neurol Psychiatr* 1951;66:20–29.

18. Sloan MA. Thrombolysis and stroke: Past and future. *Arch Neurol* 1987;44:748–768.

19. Loscalzo J, Braunwald E. Tissue plasminogen activator. *N Engl J Med* 1988;319:925–931.

20. Verstraete M, Colled D. Thrombolytic therapy in the eighties. *Blood* 1986;67:1529–1541.

21. Verstaete M. Biochemical and clinical aspects of thrombolysis. *Semin Hematol* 1978;15:35–54.

22. Marder VJ, Sherry S. Thrombolytic therapy: Current status. *N Engl J Med* 1988;318:12–20,1585–1595.

23. Coller BS. Platelets and thrombolytic therapy. *N Engl J Med* 1990;322:33–42.

24. Fears R. Biochemical pharmacology and therapeutic aspects of thrombolytic agents. *Pharmacol Rev* 1990;42:202–222.

25. Herndon RM, Nelson JN, Johnson JF, et al. Thrombolytic treatment in cerebrovascular thrombosis. In: *Anticoagulants and Fibrinolysis*, MacMillan RL, Mustard JF, eds. Lea & Febiger: Philadelphia. 1961; pp. 154–164.

26. Meyer JS. Controlled clinical trials of cerebral thrombolysis: A voice from the past. In: *Cerebrovascular Disease*, Raichle ME, Powers WJ, eds. Raven: New York. 1987; pp. 343–349.

27. Meyer JS, Gilroy J. Barnhart ME, et al. Anticoagulants plus streptokinase therapy in progressive stroke. *JAMA* 1963;189:373.

28. Meyer JS, Gilroy J, Barnhart ME, et al. Therapeutic thrombolysis in cerebral thromboembolism. Randomized evaluation of intravenous streptokinase. In: *Cerebral Vascular Diseases*, Millikan CH, Siekert W, Whisnant JP, eds. Grune & Stratton: Philadelphia. 1963; pp. 160–175.

29. Meyer JS, Herndon RM, Gotoh F, et al. Therapeutic thrombolysis. In: *Cerebral Vascular Diseases*. Fourth Princeton Conference. Millikan CHG, Siekert RG, Whisnant JP, eds. Grune & Stratton: Philadelphia. 1965; pp. 200–213.

30. Meyer JS. Controlled clinical trials of cerebral thrombolysis: A voice from the past. In: *Cerebrovascular Diseases*, Raichle ME, Powers WJ, eds. Raven: New York. 1987; pp. 343–347.

31. Clarke RL, Clifton EE. The treatment of cerebrovascular thrombosis and embolism with fibrinolytic agents. *Am J Cardiol* 1960;30:546–551.
32. Clifton EE. Early experience with fibrinolysin. *Angiology* 1959;10:244–252.
33. Clifton EE. The use of plasmin in humans. *Ann NY Acad Sci* 1957;68:209–229.
34. Clifton EE. The use of plasmin in the treatment of intravascular thrombosis. *J Am Geriatr Soc* 1958;6:118–127.
35. Fletcher AP, Alkajaersig N, Lewis M, et al. A pilot study of urokinase therapy in cerebral infarction: *Stroke* 1976;7:135–142.
36. Meyer JS, Gilroy J, Barnhart MI, et al. Therapeutic thrombolysis in cerebral thromboembolism. Double-blind evaluation of intravenous plasmin therapy in carotid and middle cerebral arterial occlusion. *Neurology* 1963;13:927–937.
37. NIH Consensus Conference: Thrombolytic therapy in treatment. *Br Med J* 1980;280: 1585–1587.
38. Brooks J, Davis D, Devivo G. Blood syndromes: Its control with urokinase therapy. *J Clin Med* 1970;76:879,880.
39. Sussman BJ, Fitch TSP. Thrombolysis with fibrinolysin in cerebral arterial occlusion. *JAMA* 1958;167:1705–1709.
40. Sussman BJ, Fitch TSP. Thrombolysis with fibrinolysin in cerebral arterial occlusion: The role of angiography. Angiology 1959;10:268–282.
41. Malinovsky I, Nikola IN. Embolism of the cerebral arteries. In: *Anticoagulant and Thrombolytic therapy in Surgery*, Malinovski I, Nikola IN, eds. Mosby: St Louis. 1979; pp. 239–250.
42. Herndon RM, Meyer JS, Johnson JF. Treatment of cerebrovascular thrombosis with fibrinolysin. *Am J Cardiol* 1960;30:540–555.
43. Herndon RM, Meyer JS, Johnson JF. Fibrinolysin therapy in thrombotic diseases of the nervous system. *J Mich St Med Soc* 1960;59:1684–1692.
44. Amias AG. Streptokinase, cerebral vascular disease and triplets. *Br Med J* 1977;11: 1414,1415.
45. Atkin N, Nitzberg S, Dorsey J. Lysis of intracerebral thromboembolism with fibrinolysin: Report of a case. *Angiology* 1964;15:436–439.
46. Kaufman HH, Lind TA, Clark DS. Non penetrating trauma to the carotid artery with secondary thrombosis and embolism: Treatment by thrombolysin. *Acta Neurochir (Wien)* 1977;37:219–244.
47. Larcan A, Laprevote-Heully MC, Lambert H, et al. Indications des thrombolytiques au cours des accidents vasculaires cerebraux thrombosants traites par aillers par O.H.B. (2ATA). *Therapie* 1977;32:259–270.
48. Fletcher AP, Alkjaersig N, Devies A, et al. Blood coagulation and plasma fibrinolytic enzyme system pathophysiology in stroke. *Stroke* 1976;7:337–348.
49. Feinberg WM, Bruck DC, Ring ME, et al. Hemostatic markers in acute stroke. *Stroke* 1989;20:592–597.
50. Marder VJ. Fibrinolytic agents: Are they feasible for stroke therapy. In: *Cerebrovascular Disease*, Plum F, Pulsimeli W, eds. Raven: New York. 1985; pp. 241–247.
51. Theron J, Courteoux P, Casasco A, et al. Local intraarterial fibrinolysis in the carotid territory. *Am J Neuroradiol* 1989;10:753–765.
52. Hossman K-A, Zimmerman V. Resuscitation of the monkey brain after incomplete ischemia. I. Physiological and morphological observations. *Brain Res* 1974;81:59–74.
53. Zeumer H, Hacke W, Kolman HL, et al. Lokale Fibrinolysetherapie bei Basilaris-thrombose. *Dtsch Med Wochenschr* 1982;97:728–731.
54. Zeumer H, Hacke W, Ringelstein EB. Local intraarterial thrombolysis in vertebrobasilar thromboembolic disease. *Am J Neuroradiol* 1983;4:401–404.

55. Zeumer H, Hundgen R, Ferbert A, et al. Local intraarterial fibrinolytic therapy in inaccessible internal carotid occlusion. *Neuroradiology* 1984;26:315– 317.

56. Zeumer H. Survey of progress: Vascular recanalizing techniques in interventional neuroradiology. *J Neurol* 1985;231:287–294.

57. Zeumer H, Hacke W, Ringelsrein EF. Local intraarterial thrombolysis in vertebrobasilar thromboembolic disease. *Am J Neuroradiol* 1983;4:401–404.

58. Zeumer H, Freitag HJ, Grzyska V, et al. Interventional neuroradiology: Local intraarterial fibrinolysis in acute vertebrobasilar occlusion: Technical developments and recent results. *Neuroradiology* 1989;31:336–340.

59. del Zoppo GJ. t-PA and scupa: New concepts in the treatment of acute stroke. In: *Recent Advances in Diagnosis and Management of Stroke*, Poeck K, Ringelstein EB, Tacke W, eds. Springer-Verlag: New York. 1987; pp. 115–127.

60. del Zoppo GJ, Copeland BR, Waltz TA, et al. The beneficial effect of intracarotid urokinase on acute stroke in a baboon model. *Stroke* 1986;17:638–643.

61. del Zoppo GJ. Thrombolytic therapy in cerebrovascular disease stroke. *Stroke* 1988;19: 1174–1179.

62. del Zoppo GJ, Zeumer H, Harker LA. Thrombolytic therapy in stroke: Possibilities and hazards. *Stroke* 1986;17:595–607.

63. del Zoppo GJ, Ferbert A, Otis S, et al. Local intra-arterial fibrinolytic therapy in acute carotid territory stroke. A Pilot Study. *Stroke* 1988;19:307–313.

64. Hacke W, Berg-Dammer E, Zeumer H. Evoked potential monitoring during acute occlusion of the basilar artery and selective local thrombolytic therapy. *Arch Psychiatr Nervenkr* 1982;2322:541–548.

65. Otomo E, Tohgi H, Hirai T, et al. Clinical efficacy of AK-124 (tissue plasminogen activator) in the treatment of cerebral thrombosis-dose finding study by means of multicenter double-blind comparison. *JPN Pharmacol Ther* 1988;16:2207–2233.

66. Fujishima M, Omae T, Tanaka K, et al. Controlled trial of combined urokinase and dextran sulfate therapy in patients with acute cerebral infarction. *Angiology* 1986;37:487–498.

67. Hacke W, Zeumer H, Ferbert A, et al. Intra-arterial thrombolytic therapy improves outcome in patients with acute vertebrobasilar occlusive disease. *Stroke* 1988;21:1216–1222.

68. Matsuo O, Kosugi T, Mihara, et al. Retrospective study on the efficacy of using urokinase therapy. *Acta Haematol Jap* 1979;42:684–688.

69. Hossman V, Heiss W-D, Bewermeyer H, et al. Controlled trial of Ancrod in ischemic stroke. *Arch Neurol* 1983;40:803.

70. Mori E, Tabuchi M, Tyoshida T, et al. Intracarotid urokinase with thromboembolic occlusion of the middle cerebral artery. *Stroke* 1988;19:802–812.

71. Terashi A, Kobayashi Y, Katayama Y, et al. Clinical effects and basic studies of thrombolytic therapy on cerebral thrombosis. *Semin Thromb Hemost* 1990;16:236–241.

72. Haley EC Jr, Levy D, Sheppard G, et al. A dose escalation safety study of intravenous tissue plasminogen activator in patients treated from 90 to 180 minutes from onset of acute ischemic stroke. *Ann Neurol* 1990;28:225 (abstr).

72a. Mori E, Yoneda Y, Ohksawa S, et al. Double-blind, placebo controlled trial of recombinant tissue plasminogen activator (rt-PA) in acute carotid stroke. *Neurology* 1991;41:347 (suppl 1).

73. Pollak VE, Glas-Greenwalt P, Olinger CP, et al. Ancrod causes rapid thrombolysis in patients with acute strokes. *Am J Med Sci* 1990;299:319–325.

74. Ogata J, Yutaui L, Imakita M, et al. Hemorrhagic infarct of the brain without a re-opening of the occluded arteries in cardioembolic stroke. *Stroke* 1989;20:876–883.

75. Bruckmann H, Ferbert A, del Zoppo GJ, et al. Acute vertebral basilar thrombosis: Angiologic-clinical comparison and therapeutic implications. *Acta Radiol* 1987;369:38–42.

76. Harenberg J, Zimmermann R, Heuck CC, et al. Fibrinolysis of basilar artery thrombosis. Serono symposium, No 31. Tilsner V, Lenau H, eds. Fibrinolysis and Urokinase. San Diego: Academic. 1980; 391–404.

77. Tomsick T, Brott T, Barsan W, et al. Thrombus localization with emergency cerebral computed tomography. *Stroke* 1990;21:180 (abstr).

78. Henze T, Boerr A, Tebbe U, et al. Lysis of basilar artery occlusion with tissue plasminogen activator. *Lancet* 1987;2:1391 (letter)

79. Jafar JJ, Tan WS, Crowell RM. Tissue plasminogen activator thrombolysis of a middle cerebral artery embolus in a patient with an arteriovenous malformation. *J Neurosurg* 1991;74:808–812.

80. Otomo E, Araki G, Itoh E, et al. Clinical efficacy of urokinase in the treatment of cerebral thrombosis: Multicenter double-blind study in comparison with placebo. *Clin Eval* 1985;13:711–751.

81. Abe T, Kazama M. Thrombolytic therapy of cerebrovascular occlusive disease. In: *Prophylactic Approach to Hypertensive Disease*, Yamori Y, Lovenberg W, Freis E, eds. Raven: New York. 1979; pp. 441–447.

82. Abe T, Kazawa M, Naito I. Clinical evaluation for efficacy of tissue culture urokinase (TCUK) on cerebral thrombosis by means of multicenter double-blind study. *Blood Vessels* 1981;12:321–341.

83. Abe T, Kazawa M, Naito I. Clinical features of urokinase (60,01) 0 units/day) on cerebral infarction: Comparative study by means of multicenter double-blind test. *Blood Vessels* 1981;18:342–358.

84. Adachi K, Sahashi K, Fujii K, et al. A significance of urokinase treatment in acute cerebral infarction: Assessment from neurological signs and CT findings. *J Aichi Med Univ Assoc* 1980;8:305.

85. Nenci GG, Gresek P, Taramelli M, et al. Thrombolytic therapy for thromboembolism of vertebrobasilar artery. *Angiology* 1984;34:561–571.

86. Jungreis CA, Wechsler LR, Horton JA. Intracranial thrombolysis via a catheter embedded in the clot. *Stroke* 1989;20:1578–1580.

87. Morgan JK, Sadasivan B, Ausman JI, et al. Thrombolytic therapy and posterior circulation extracranial-intracranial bypass for acute basilar artery thrombosis. Case report. *Surg Neurol* 1990;33:43–47.

88. Herderschee D, Limburg M, Hijdra A, et al. Recombinant tissue plasminogen activator in two patients with basilar artery occlusion. J *Neurol Neurosurg Psychiatry* 1991;54:71–73.

89. Buteux G, Jubault V, Suisse A. Local recombinant tissue plasminogen activator to clear cerebral artery thrombosis development soon after surgery. *Lancet* 1988;2:1143,1144.

90. Bruckman HJ, Ringelstein EB, Buchner H, et al. Vascular recanalizing techniques in the hindbrain. *Circ Neurosurg Rev* 1987;10:197–199.

91. Courtheoux P, Theron J, Derloh JM, et al. In situ fibrinolysis in supra-aortic main vessels. *J Neuroradiol* 1986;13:111–124.

92. Sullivan KL, Gardiner GA, Shapiro MJ, et al. Transthrombus bolus of fibrinolytic agents. *Radiology* 1989;173:805–808.

93. Feldmann E, Sousa JM, Brass LM, et al. Factors delaying evaluation of acute stroke. *Neurology* 1990;40:145 (abstr).

94. Broderick J, Brott T, Barsan W, et al. Blood pressure during the 1st hours of acute focal cerebral ischemia. *Neurology* 1990;40:145 (abstr).

95. Dalal PM, Shah PM, Sheth SL, et al. Cerebral embolism: Angiographic observation on spontaneous lot lysis. *Lancet* 1965;1:61–64.

96. Irino T, Taneda M, Minami T. Angiographic manifestations in post-recanalized cerebral infarction. *Neurology* 1977;27:471–475.

97. Lodder J, Krijne-Kubat B, Vanderlugt PJM. Timing of autopsy. Confirmed hemorrhagic infarction with reference to cardioembolic stroke. *Stroke* 1988;19:1482–1484.

98. Hass WK, Clauss RM, Goldberg AF. Special problems associated with surgical and thrombolytic treatment of strokes. *Arch Surg* 1986;92:27–31.

99. Hanaway J, Torack R, Fletcher AP, et al. Intracranial bleeding associated with urokinase therapy for acute ischemic hemispheral stroke. *Stroke* 1976;7:143–146.

100. Aldrich MS, Sherman SA, Greenberg HS. Cerebrovascular complications of streptokinase infusion. *JAMA* 1985;253:1777–1779.

101. AIMS Trial Study Group: Effect of intravenous APSAC on mortality after acute myocardial infarction. Preliminary report of a placebo-controlled clinical trial. *Lancet* 1988;2:545–549.

102. Kase CS, Pessin MS, Zivin JA, et al. and the tPA Acute Stroke Study Group. Intracranial hemorrhage following thrombolysis with tissue plasminogen activator. *Neurology* 1990;40:191 (abstr).

103. Kase CS, O'Neal AM, Fisher M, et al. Intracranial hemorrhage after use of tissue plasminogen activator for coronary thrombolysis. *Ann Intern Med* 1990;12:17–21.

104. Bruckmann H, Ferbert A. Putaminal hemorrhage after recanalization of an embolic MCA occlusion treated with tissue plasminogen activator. *Neuroradiology* 1989;31:95–97.

105. Braunwald E, Knatterud GL, Passamani E, et al. Update for the thrombolysis in myocardial infarction trial. *J Am Coll Cardiol* 1987;10:1970 (abstr).

106. ISIS-2 Collaborative Group: Randomized trial of intravenous streptokinase, oral aspirin, both or neither among 17, 187 cases of suspected acute myocardial infarction. *Lancet* 1988;2:349–360.

107. Price TR. Stroke in patients treated with thrombolytic therapy for acute myocardial infarction. The thrombosis in myocardial infarction clinical trial and a review of placebo-controlled trials. *Stroke* 1990; 21:111-8–111-9 (suppl 3).

108. Califf RM, Topol EJ, George BS, et al. Thrombolysis and Angioplasty in Myocardial Infarction Study Group: Hemorrhage complications associated with the use of intravenous tissue plasminogen activator in treatment of acute myocardial infarction. *Am J Med* 1988;85:353–359.

109. Carlson SE, Aldrich MS, Greenberg HS, et al. Intracerebral hemorrhage complicating intravenous tissue plasminogen activator treatment. *Arch Neurol* 1988;45:1070–1073.

110. GISSI-2: A factorial randomized trial of alteplase versus streptokinase and heparin versus no heparin among 12,490 patients with acute myocardial infarction. *Lancet* 1990;336:65–71.

111. The Anglo-Scandinavian study of early thrombolysis (ASSET). *Lancet* 1988;2:525–530.

112. Wilcox RG, yonder Lippe G, Olsson CG, et al. Trial of tissue plasminogen activator for mortality reduction in acute myocardial infarction. *Lancet* 1988;2:525–530.

113. Pendlebury WW, Iole ED, Tracy RP, et al. Intracerebral hemorrhage related to cerebral amyloid angiopathy and tPA treatment. *Ann Neurol* 1991; 29:210–213.

114. Ramsey DA, Penswick JL, Robertson DM. Fatal streptokinase-induced intracerebral hemorrhage in cerebral amyloid angiopathy. *Can J Neurol Sci* 1990;17:336–341.

115. Proner J, Rosenblum BR, Rothman A. Ruptured arteriovenous malformation complicating thrombolytic therapy with tissue plasminogen activator. *Arch Neurol* 1990;47:105,106.

116. Altman LK. Study of three drugs favors cheapest. New York Times, March 4, 1991, A14.

117. Sato Y, Mizoguchi K, Sato Y, et al. Anticoagulant and thrombolytic therapy for cerebral embolism of cardiac origin. *Kurume Med J* 1986;33:89–95.

118. Hirshberg A, Schneiderman J, Garnick A. Errors and pitfalls in intraarterial thrombolytic therapy. *J Vasc Surg* 1989;10:612–616.

119. Eleff SM, Borel C, Bell WR, et al. Acute management of intracranial hemorrhage in patients receiving thrombolytic therapy: Case reports. *Neurosurgery* 1990;26:867–869.

120. Sloan MA, Brott TG, Del Zoppo GJ. Thrombolysis and stroke. In: *Thrombolysis in Cardiovascular Disease*, Morris RM, Kubler W, Swan WJ, et al., eds. Dekker: New York. 1989; pp. 361–380.

121. Sloan MA, Plotnick GD. Stroke complicating thrombolytic therapy of acute myocardial infarction. *J Am Coll Cardiol* 1990;16:541–544.

122. Sloan MA, Price TR, Randall AM, et al. and the TIMI Investigators. Intracerebral hemorrhage after rt-PA and heparin for acute myocardial infarction: The TIMI II pilot and randomized trial combined experience. *Stroke* 1990;21:182 (abstr).

123. The International Study Group. In hospital mortality and clinical course of 20,891 patients with suspected acute myocardial infarction randomized between alteplase and streptokinase with or without heparin. *Lancet* 1990;336:7175.

124. Fennerty AG, Levine MN, Hirsh J. Hemorrhagic complications of thrombolytic therapy in the treatment of myocardial infarction and venous thromboembolism. *Chest* 1989;95(2): 88S–97S (suppl).

125. Gruppo Italiano Per Lo Studies Della Strepto Chinasi Nell' Infarto Miocardico (GISSI): Long term effects of intravenous thrombolysis in acute myocardial infarction: Final report of the GISSI study. *Lancet* 1987;2;871–874.

126. Topel EJ, Califf RM, George BS, et al. A randomized trial of immediate versus delayed elective angioplasty after intravenous tissue plasminogen activator in acute myocardial infarction. *N Engl J Med* 1987; 317:581–588.

127. Gore J, Sloan M, Price T, et al. Intracranial hemorrhage after rt-PA and heparin for acute myocardial infarction (The TIMI II pilot and randomized combined experience. *J Am Coll Cardiol* 1990;15:15A (abstr).

128. Safety of tissue plasminogen activator (moderator M.L. Dyken). *Stroke* 1990;21:IV;10-III-11 (suppl 4).

129. Maggioni AP, Farina ML, Franzoni MG for the GISSI Group. Stroke in the GISSI trial. *Circulation* 1989;80:11,350 (suppl 2) (abstr).

130. Dodson RF, Tagashira Y, Kawamura Y, et al. Morphological responses of cerebral tissues to temporary ischemia. *Can J Neurol Sci* 1975;2:173–177.

131. Petito CK. Early and late mechanisms of increased vascular permeability following experimental cerebral infarction. *J Neuropathol Exp Neurol* 1979;38:222–234.

132. Sane DC, Stump DC, Topol EJ, et al. Thrombolysis and Angioplasty in Myocardial Infarction Study Group: racial differences in response to thrombolytic therapy with recombinant tissue-type plasminogen activator. Increased fibrinogenolysis in blacks. *Circulation* 1991; 83:170–175.

133. Althouse R, Maynard C, Olsufka M, et al. Risk factor for hemorrhagic and ischemic stroke in myocardial infarct patients treated with tissue plasminogen activator. *J Am Coll Cardiol* 1989;13:153A (abstr).

134. Brott T. Thrombolysis and stroke in clinical practice: Past, present, and future, In: *Fibrinolysis and the Central Nervous System*, Sawaya R, ed. Hanley and Belfus: Philadelphia. 1990; pp. 179–197.

135. Sane DC, Califf RM, Topol EJ. Bleeding during thrombolytic therapy for acute myocardial infarction: Mechanisms and management. *Ann Intern Med* 1989;111:1010–1022.

136. Zivin JA, Lyden PD, DeGirolami U, et al. Tissue plasminogen activator. Reduction of neurologic damage after experimental embolic stroke. *Arch Neurol* 1988;45:387–391.

137. Lyden PD, Madden KP, Clark WM, et al. Incidence of cerebral hemorrhage after antifibrinolytic treatment for embolic stroke. *Stroke* 1990;21:1589–1593.

138. Lyden PD, Zivin JA, Clark WA, et al. Tissue plasminogen activator-mediated thrombolysis of cerebral emboli and its effect on hemorrhagic infarction in rabbits. *Neurology* 1989;39:703–708.

139. Benes V, Zabranski JM, Boston M, et al. Effect of intraarterial antifibrinolytic agents on autologous arterial emboli in the cerebral circulation of rabbits. *Stroke* 1990;2:1594–1599.

140. O'Connor CM, Califf RM, Massey EW, et al. Stroke and acute myocardial infarction in the thrombolytic era: Clinical correlates and long-term prognosis. *J Am Coll Cardiol* 1990;16:533–540.

141. Ortono F, Fortcuberta J, Pons-L Laurado G, et al. Successful treatment of prosthetic heart-valve thrombosis with high short-term doses of streptokinase. *Lancet* 1988;2:626 (letter to editor).

142. Cambier P, Mombaerts P, Degeast H, et al. Treatment of prosthetic tricuspid valve thrombosis with recombinant tissue-type plasminogen activator. *Eur Heart J* 1987;8:906–909.

143. Witchitz S, Veyrat C, Moisson P, et al. Fibrinolytic treatment of thrombus on prosthetic heart valves. *Br Heart J* 1980;44:545–554.

144. Cranston, RE, Wolfson MA, Buschbaum HW, et al. Plasminogen activator and cerebral infarction. *Am Intern Med* 1988;108:766 (letter).

145. Stafford PJ, Strachan CL, Vincent R, et al. Multiple microemboli after disintegration of clot during thrombolysis for acute myocardial infarction. *Br Med J* 1989;299:1310–1312.

146. Koudstaal PJ, Stibbe J, Vermeulen M. Fatal ischemic brain edema after early thrombolysis with tissue plasminogen activator in acute stroke. *Br Med J* 1988;297:1571–1574.

147. Cercek B, Lew AS, Hod H, et al. Enhancement of thrombolysis with tissue-type plasminogen activator by pretreatment with heparin. *Circulation* 1986;74:583–587.

148. Kwaan HC, Dobbie JG, Fetherhour LL. The use of anticoagulants and thrombolytic agents in occlusive retinal vascular disease. In: *Thrombosis and Urokinase*, Paoletti R. Sherry S, eds. Academic: San Diego. 1977; pp. 191–198.

149. Kwaan H. Thromboembolic disorders of the eye. In: *Thrombolytic Therapy*, Comerata AJ, ed. Grune & Stratton: Philadelphia. 1988; pp. 153–163.

150. Gent A, et al. Central retinal vein thrombosis: Serial treatment with defibrination, aspirin and plasminotropic drugs. *Thromb Res* 1979;14:61–66.

151. Herndon RM, Meyer JS, Johnson JF. Fibrinolysin therapy in thrombotic diseases of the nervous system. *J Mich St Med Soc* 1960; 59:1684–1692.

152. Herndon RM, Meyer JS, Johnson J, et al. Treatment of cerebrovascular thrombosis with fibrinolysin. Preliminary Report. Am J *Cardiol* 1960;30:540–545.

153. Bowell RE, Marmion VJ, McCarthy CF. Treatment of central retinal vein thrombosis with ancrod. *Lancet* 1970;1:173,174.

154. Vines FS, Davis DO. Clinical radiological correlation in cerebral venous occlusive disease. *Radiology* 1971; 98:9–21.

155. Harvey JE. Streptokinase therapy and cavernous sinus thrombosis. *Br Med J* 1974;5:46 (letter).

156. Kohner EM, Pettit JE, Hamilton AM, et al. Streptokinase in central retinal vein occlusion: A controlled clinical trial. *Br Med J* 1976; 1:550–553.

157. Gettelfinger DM, Kokmen E. Superior sagittal sinus thrombosis. *Arch Neurol* 1977;34:2–6.

158. Rousseaux P, Bernard MH, Scherpereel B, et al. Thrombose des sinus veineux intra-craniens (apropos de 22 cas). *Neurochirurgie* 1978;24:197–203.

159. DiRocco C, Iannelli A, Leone G, et al. Heparin urokinase treatment in aseptic aural sinus thrombosis. *Arch Neurol* 1981; 38:431–435.

160. Bogdahn V, Mulfinger L, Ratzka M, et al. Diagnostic and therapeutic approach to cerebral venous thrombosis. *Neurology* 1988; 38:342 (abstr).

161. Scott JA, Pascuzzi RM, Hall PV. Treatment of aural sinus thrombosis with local urokinase infusion. *J Neurosurg* 1988; 68:284–287.

162. Higashida, RT, Helmer E, Halbach VV, et al. Direct thrombolytic therapy for superior sagittal sinus thrombosis. *American Journal of Neuroradiolog* 1989;10:S4–S6.

163. Persson L, Lilja A. Extensive aural sinus thrombosis treated by surgical removal and local streptokinase infusion. *Neurosurgery* 1990;26:117–121.

164. Alexander LF, Yamamoto Y, Ayoubi S, et al. Efficacy of tissue plasminogen activator in the lysis of thrombosis of the cerebral venous sinus. *Neurosurgery* 1990;26:559–564.

165. Barnwell SL, Higashida RT, Halbach VV, et al. Direct endovascular thrombolytic therapy for dural sinus thrombosis. *J Neurosurg* 1991;28:135–142.

166. Manthous CA, Chen H. Case Report: Treatment of superior sagittal sinus thrombosis with urokinase. *Connecticut Medicine* 1992;56(10):529–530.

167. Smith TP, Higashida RT, Barnwell SL, et al. Treatment of dural sinus thrombosis by urokinase infusion. *American Journal of Neuroradiology* 1994;15:801–807.

168. Khoo KBK, Long FL, Tuck RR, et al. Cerebral venous sinus thrombosis associated with the primary antiphospholipid syndrome. *The Medical Journal of Australia* 1995;162:30–32.

169. Horowitz M, Purdy P, Unwin H, et al. Treatment of dural sinus thrombosis using selective catheterization and urokinase. *Annals of Neurology* 1995;38(1):58–67.

170. Smith GA, Cornblath WT, Deveikis JP. Local thrombolytic therapy in deep cerebral venous thrombosis. *Neurology* 1997;48:1613–1619.

171. Rael JR, Orrison WW, Baldwin N, et al. Direct thrombolysis of superior sagittal sinus thrombosis with coexisting intracranial hemorrhage. *American Journal of Neuroradiology* 1997;18:1238–1242.

172. Renowden SA, Oxbury J, and Molyneux AJ. Case Report: Venous sinus thrombosis: The use of thrombolysis. *Clinical Radiology* 1997;52:396–399.

173. Sun YK, Jung HS. Direct endovascular thrombolytic therapy for Dural sinus thrombosis: Infusion of alteplase. *American Journal of Neuroradiology* 1997;18:639–645.

174. Niwa J, Ohyama H, Matumura S, et al. Treatment of acute superior sagittal sinus thrombosis by t-PA infusion via venography—direct thrombolytic therapy in the acute phase. *Surg Neurol* 1998;49:425–429.

175. Bagley LJ, Hurst R, Galetta S, et al. Use of a microsnare to aid direct thrombolytic therapy of dural sinus thrombosis. *American Journal of Roentgenology* 1998;170:784–786.

176. Gerszten PC, Welch W, Spearman M, et al. Isolated deep cerebral venous thrombosis treated by direct endovascular thrombolysis. *Surg Neurol* 1997;48:261–266.

177. Kuether TA, O'Neill O, Nesbit G, et al. Endovascular treatment of traumatic dural sinus thrombosis: Case Report. *Neurosurgery* 1998;42(5):1163–1167.

178. D'Alise MD, Fichtel F, Horowitz M. Sagittal sinus thrombosis following minor head injury treated with continuous urokinase infusion. *Surg Neurol* 1998;49:430–435.

179. Segal R, Dujouny M, Nelson D, et al. Local urokinase treatment for spontaneous intracerebral hematoma. *Clin Res* 1982;30:412A (abstr).

180. Narayan RK, Narayan TM, Katz DA, et al. Lysis of intracranial hematomas with urokinase in a rabbit model. *J Neurosurg* 1985; 62:580–586.

181. Narayan RK, Narayan RK. Thrombolytic therapy of intracerebral hematomas. In: *Fibrinolysis and the Central Nervous System*, Sawaya R, ed. Hanley and Belfus: Philadelphia. 1990; pp. 198–202.

182. Kaufman HH, Schochet S, Koss W, et al. Efficacy and safety of tissue plasminogen activator. *Neurosurgery* 1987;20:403–407.

183. Matsumoto K, Hondo H. CT-guided stereotoxic evacuation of hypertensive intracerebral hematomas. *J Neurosurg* 1984;61:440–448.

184. Mohadjer M, Eggert R, May J, et al. CT-guided stereotactic fibrinolysis of spontaneous and hypertensive cerebellar hemorrhage: Long-term results. *J Neurosurg* 1990;73:217–222.

185. Findlay JM, Weir BKA, Gordon P, et al. Safety and efficacy of intrathecal thrombolytic therapy in a primate model of cerebral vasospasm. *Neurosurgery* 1989; 24:491–498.

186. Findlay JM. Intrathecal thrombolytic therapy in the prevention of vasospasm following subarachnoid hemorrhage. In: *Fibrinolysis and the Central Nervous System*, Sawaya R, ed. Hanley and Belfus: Philadelphia. 1990; pp. 203–212.

187. Findley JM, Weir BKA, Kanamaru K, et al. Intrathecal fibrinolytic therapy after subarachnoid hemorrhage: Dosage study in a primate model and review of the literature. *Can J Neurol Sci* 1989;16:28–40.

188. Porter JM, Acinapura AJ, Kapp JP, et al. Fibrinolysis in the central nervous system. *Neurology* 1969;19:47–52.

189. Porter JM, Acinapura AJ, Kapp JP, et al. Fibrinolytic activity of the spinal fluid and meninges. *Surg Forum* 1966;17:425–427.
190. Peterson EW, Choo SH, Lewis AJ, et al. Lysis of blood and experimental treatment of subarachnoid hemorrhage. In: *Cerebral Arterial Spasm*, Wilkins RH, ed. Williams & Wilkins: Baltimore. 1980; pp. 625–627.
191. Yoshida Y, Ueki S, Takahashi A, et al. Intrathecal irrigation with urokinase in ruptured cerebral aneurysm cases. Basic studies and clinical applications. *Neurol Med Chir* (Tokyo) 1985;25:989–997.
192. Shiobara R, Kawase T, Toya S, et al. Scavenger surgery" for subarachnoid hemorrhage (II) continuous ventriculocisternal perfusion using artificial cerebrospinal fluid with urokinase. Timing of Aneurysm Surgery. Hawthorne: De Gruyter. 1985;365–372.
193. Alksne JF, Branson J, Biley M. Modification of experimental post-subarachnoid hemorrhage vasculopathy with intracisternal plasmin. *Neurosurgery* 1986;19:20–25.
194. Alksne JF, Brauston PJ, Bailey M. Modification of experimental post-subarachnoid hemorrhage vasculopathy with intracisternal plasmin. *Neurosurgery* 1986;19:20–25.
195. Seifert V, Eisert WG, Stolke D, et al. Efficacy of single intracisternal bolus injection of recombinant tissue plasminogen activator to prevent delayed cerebral vasospasm after experimental hemorrhage. *Neurosurgery* 1989;25:590–598.
196. Findlay JM, Weir BKA, Steinke D, et al. Effect of intrathecal thrombolytic therapy on subarachnoid clot and chronic vasospasm in a primate model of SAH. *J Neurosurg* 1988;69:723–735.
197. Kodama N, Sasaki T, Yamanobe K, et al. Prevention of vasospasm: Cisternal irrigation therapy with urokinase and ascorbic acid. In: *Cerebral vasospasm*, Wilkins RH, ed. Raven: New York. 1988; p. 415.
198. Saito I, Segawa H, Nagayama I, et al. Prevention of postoperative vasospasm by cisternal irrigation, in timing of Aneurysm Surgery. Hawthorne: de Gruyter. 1985;587–594.
199. Lamond R. Cisternal recombinant tPA administration in aneurysm subarachnoid hemorrhage. *J Neurosurg* 1990;72:336A (abstr).
200. Seifert V, Stolke D. Injection of tissue plasminogen activator to prevent delayed vasospasm. *Neurosurg* 1990;26:549–550.
201. Pang D, Sclabassi RJ, Horton JA. Lysis of intraventricular blood clot with urokinase in a canine intraventricular blood clot model. *Neurosurgery* 1986;19:540–546.
202. Pang D, Sclabassi RJ, Horton JA. Lysis of intraventricular blood clot with urokinase in a canine model: Part 2. In vivo safety study of intraventricular urokinase. *Neurosurgery* 1986;19:547–552.
203. Pang D, Sclabassi RJ, Horton JA. Lysis of intraventricular blood clot with urokinase in a canine model: Part 3. Effects of intraventricular urokinase on clot lysis and post hemorrhagic hydrocephalus. *Neurosurgery* 1986;19:553–572.
204. Todo T, Usui M, Takakura K. Treatment of severe intraventricular hemorrhage by intraventricular infusion of urokinase. *J Neurosurg* 1991;74:81–86.
205. Findlay JM, Weir BKA, Stollery DE. Lysis of intraventricular hematoma with tissue plasminogen activator. *J Neurosurg* 1991;74:803–807.
206. Hedges JR. Session 3: Thrombolytic therapy for acute stroke. *Ann Emerg Med* 1988;17: 1190–1191.
207. Brott T, Haley EC, Levy DE, et al. The investigational use of tPA for stroke: *Ann Emerg Med* 1988;17:1202–1205.
208. Gotoh F, Fukuuchi Y, Amano T, et al. Effect of tissue plasminogen activator on microcirculation and size of infarction following MCA occlusion in cat. *J Cereb Blood Flow Metabol* 1989;9:59 (abstr).
209. Weinstein PR, Anderson GG, Telles DA. Neurological deficit and cerebral infarction after temporary middle cerebral artery occlusion in unanesthesized cats. *Stroke* 1986;17:318–324.

210. Hakim AM, Pokrupa RP, Villanueva J. The effect of spontaneous reperfusion on metabolic function in early human cerebral infarcts. *Ann Neurol* 1987;21:279–289.

211. Zivin JA. Thrombolytic therapy for stroke. In: *Protection of the brain from ischemia. Current Neurosurgical Practice*, Weinstein ZPR, Faden AL, eds. Williams & Wilkins: Baltimore. 1990; pp. 231–236.

212. Zivin JA. A Perspective on the future of thrombolytic stroke therapy. In: *Cerebrovascular Diseases*, Ginsberg MD, Dietrich WD, eds. Raven: New York. 1989; pp. 33–37.

213. Del Zoppo GJ. Investigational use of tPA in acute stroke: *Ann Emerg Med* 1988;17: 1196–1201.

214. Poeck K. Intraarterial thrombolytic therapy in acute stroke. *Acta Neurol Belg* 1988; 88:35–45.

215. Berridge DC, Makin GS, Hopkinson BR. Local low dose intraarterial thrombolytic therapy: The risk of stroke or major hemorrhage. *Br J Surg* 1989;76:1230–1233.

7

Phase 2 Experience with Intravenous Thrombolytic Therapy for Acute Ischemic Stroke

E. Clarke Haley, Jr., MD

CONTENTS

INTRODUCTION
EARLY STUDIES
INTRAVENOUS ADMINISTRATION: OPEN-LABEL TRIALS
INTRAVENOUS ADMINISTRATION: CONTROLLED TRIALS
SUMMARY
REFERENCES

INTRODUCTION

Intravenous thrombolytic therapy for stroke was first used in the late 1950s (1), but convincing evidence of its efficacy was not established until 1995 (2). Whereas the fundamental therapeutic concept (i.e., restoration of cerebral blood flow to ischemic brain by recanalizing acutely occluded arteries) remained unchanged over that span, the field was benefited from stepwise advances in neuroimaging, pharmacology, logistics of critical care, and clinical trials design. These advances were pilot tested in the Phase 2 experience with thrombolytic drugs, and combined to make the successful pivotal efficacy trials possible.

This chapter will review the modern safety and preliminary activity studies conducted for intravenous thrombolytic therapy for ischemic stroke. Taken together, they provide insights into the mechanisms of action, dose selection, and potential hazards of thrombolytic drugs, and establish the necessary preliminary clinical experience for the conduct of the pivotal Phase 3 efficacy trials.

From: *Thrombolytic Therapy for Stroke*
Edited by: P. D. Lyden © Humana Press Inc., Totowa, NJ

EARLY STUDIES

The pioneering work of the early investigators in thrombolytic therapy for ischemic stroke has been extensively reviewed elsewhere *(3–5)* (*see* Chapter 4 to 6). Early investigators were handicapped by not having access to pretreatment CT scanning and were not as appreciative of the importance of very early treatment to maximize benefit and reduce risk. Most of the initial reports were discouraging with little evidence for benefit, and major concerns were raised that the therapy might, in fact, be harmful. By 1982, although thrombolytic therapy was being embraced for other indications, such as acute pulmonary embolism, it was strongly contraindicated for acute ischemic stroke *(6)*.

INTRAVENOUS ADMINISTRATION: OPEN-LABEL TRIALS

Prompted by encouraging reports using intra-arterial thrombolytic therapy appearing in the mid-1980s *(7–12)*, studies reporting initial experience with intravenous agents again began to appear in the early 1990s (Table 1). All chose to study rt-PA because of its relative clot specificity and its theoretical promise of greater safety. Moreover, what distinguished these studies from the earlier efforts with intravenous therapy was the emphasis on ultra-early intervention (at most, 8 h from onset), and the requirement of urgent head computerized tomography (CT) scanning to exclude hemorrhage prior to treatment.

del Zoppo and colleagues *(13)* employed an open-label, dose escalation design to test whether a dose-response relationship existed for two-chain form rt-PA (duteplase) on cerebral artery recanalization rates. Prospectively established safety guidelines focused on the incidence of neurologic deterioration in association with hemorrhagic change, either hemorrhagic infarction or parenchymal hematoma as determined by follow-up CT scanning. The study was not designed to test the effect on clinical outcome. Eligible subjects were required to undergo pretreatment CT scanning and selective catheter cerebral angiography and begin treatment within 8 h of the onset of stroke symptoms. Cerebral angiography was repeated immediately after the 60 min rt-PA infusion. In 23 mo at 16 centers, 104 patients began treatment with study drug, while 93 patients completed their infusions. Nine escalating doses ranging from 0.12 million International Units (MIU)/kg to 0.75 MIU/kg (approx 0.21 mg/kg to 1.28 mg/kg in alteplase equivalents) were examined in cohort sizes ranging from 4 to 15 patients each. Systemic heparin administration was forbidden for 24 h.

Overall, either partial or complete recanalization was observed in 34%, and no dose response for recanalization was seen in the doses studied. However, the trial was discontinued prematurely because of withdrawal of the study drug following a patent dispute. Distal intracranial occlusions were more frequently recanalized than proximal internal carotid artery occlusions. The cumulative incidence of hemorrhagic transformation (either hemorrhagic infarction or parenchymal

Table 1
Intravenous Open Label Studies

Study	Agent	# Patients	Treatment window	Design	Results
del Zoppo (1992)	rt-PA (duteplase)	93	0–8 h	Dose escalation Control angiography	34% recanalized, 10% worsening with hemorrhage. No dose response.
Yamaguchi (1991)	rt-PA (duteplase)	58	0–6 h	3 doses Control angiography	Recanalization better in higher doses. 21% CT hemorrhage.
Brott (1992)	rt-PA (alteplase)	74	0–90 min	Dose escalation No angiography	Dose-related risk of symptomatic hemorrhage. Safe with <0.95 mg/kg.
Haley (1992)	rt-PA (alteplase)	20	91–180 min	Dose escalation No angiography	10% symptomatic hemorrhage; 15% sustained neurological improvement.
Hennerici (1991)	rt-PA (alteplase)	18	0–24 h	Single 70 mg dose plus heparin; Control angiography	22% recanalization; 1 fatal hemorrhage, 9 additional deaths.
Von Kummer (1992)	rt-PA (alteplase)	32	0–6 h	Single 100 mg dose plus heparin; Control angiography	34% immediate recanalization; 9% symptomatic hemorrhage.
Overgaard (1993)	rt-PA (alteplase)	23	0–6 h	Single 100 mg dose; Baseline and follow-up SPECT	1 symptomatic hemorrhage; reperfusion on SPECT correlated with neurological improvement

hematoma) was 31%, of which about one-third (10%) had associated neurological worsening. Neither hemorrhagic transformation nor associated neurological worsening were related to dose or recanalization. Patients with hemorrhagic transformation were treated 0.8 h later than patients without hemorrhage.

Yamaguchi and associates *(14)* also used either 10, 20, or 30 megaunits (MU) of duteplase intravenously over 1 h to treat 58 patients with angiographically documented occlusions in the carotid territory within 6 h of the onset of symptoms. How the patients were assigned their dose of treatment was not specified in the report. Only 18% of patients receiving 10 MU achieved complete or partial recanalization, whereas 57% and 42% were partly or completely recanalized with 20 or 30 MU, respectively. Clinical improvement appeared to be associated with recanalization, particularly if treatment was begun less than 2 h after onset. Hemorrhagic transformation was observed on follow-up CT scans in 21% of patients, but the incidence of associated neurological deterioration was not reported.

In a US study sponsored by the National Institutes of Neurological Disorders and Stroke (NINDS), investigators at three centers examined the safety and clinical outcome from treatment with escalating doses of intravenous single-chain rt-PA (alteplase) in patients with very early stroke symptoms *(15)*. Eligible patients had pretreatment evaluation, including CT scanning, and treatment begun within 90 min of stroke onset. Because of the stringent time restrictions, pretreatment angiography was not a requirement. Again, systemic heparin was prohibited for 24 h.

During 32 mo, 74 patients were studied with 7 doses, ranging from 0.35 mg/kg to 1.08 mg/kg given over 60 to 90 min, with cohorts ranging from 1 to 22 patients. Hemorrhagic transformation (either hemorrhagic infarction or parenchymal hematoma) was observed in 7%, of which nearly one-half (3%) were associated with neurological worsening. Symptomatic hemorrhages occurred predominately in involved vascular territories, but also occurred in brain remote from the infarct. There was a statistically significant relationship between the incidence of symptomatic intracerebral hemorrhage and the total dose of rt-PA administered. No symptomatic hemorrhages were observed in patients receiving less than 0.95 mg/kg. No dose response with major neurological improvement, defined as a 4 or more point improvement in the National Institutes of Health (NIH) Stroke Scale, was observed at either 2 or 24 h. Nevertheless, the fact that 55% of patients treated with 0.85 mg/kg (with 10% of the total dose given as an initial bolus) had major neurological improvement within 24 h was viewed as an encouraging sign.

As confidence grew in the safety of intravenous alteplase administered to patients within 90 min of stroke onset, it was elected to study an additional 20 patients treated from 91 to 180 min from onset to explore the safety of expanding the potential therapeutic window *(16)*. Three doses ranging from 0.6 mg/kg to

Table 2
Pilot NINDS Dose Escalation Studies: Combined Results

Dose (mg/kg)	Patients (n)	OTT[+] (n,%)	24 h[++] (n,%)	Symptomatic bleeding (n,%)
0.35	6	3 (50%)	2 (33%)	0
0.60	19	4 (21%)	5 (26%)	0
0.85	10	4 (40%)	4 (40%)	0
0.85*	27	3 (11%)	13 (48%)	1 (4%)
0.95**	28	10 (36%)	12 (43%)	3 (11%)
0.95*	3	0 (0%)	1 (33%)	2 (67%)
1.05	1	0 (0%)	1 (100%)	0
TOTAL	94	24 (26%)	38 (40%)	6 (6%)

* - 10% of dose given as initial bolus.
** - 90-min infusion.
[+] - OTT = "on-the-table improvement;" Improvement by 2 or more points on the NIH Stroke Scale at 2 hours compared to baseline.
[++] - 24 h = Improvement by four or more points on the NIHSS at 24 h compared to baseline, or return to normal.

0.95 mg/kg were tested. These 20 patients were more severely neurologically impaired at baseline than the patients treated within 90 min, and the results of treatment were not as good. Overall, hemorrhagic transformation was observed in 30% of patients, of which one-third (10%) were associated with neurological worsening and death. While 25% had major neurological improvement within 2 h, only 15% were improved at 24 h. One symptomatic intracerebral hemorrhage occurred in six patients treated with 0.85 mg/kg, a dose which appeared safe in patients treated within 90 min. The investigators concluded that the results might still represent an improvement over the natural history of the disease, but concerns were raised about potential decreases in both safety and efficacy if treatment with thrombolytic therapy was delayed even beyond 90 min. Stratification by time from onset to treatment was recommended for future randomized, placebo-controlled trials of thrombolytic therapy.

Table 2 depicts the combined dose-escalation experience from the pilot NINDS studies. A dose-response relationship with symptomatic hemorrhage is suggested although the numbers are small. Assessing early clinical activity of therapy was problematic for the investigators from the beginning. Initial experience with the compound was associated with observations of dramatic neurological improvement within hours of beginning treatment. Although it could not be determined whether the clinical improvement was associated with recanalization, the investigators (and their NINDS-appointed oversight committee) surmised that such a clinical response might be the most proximate marker for clinical activity of the drug that was available. Hence, efforts to quantitate and standardize the dramatic neurological improvement ensued. Initially, the so-called on-the-table response was defined as an improvement in the NIH Stroke Scale score by 2 or more points within 2 h of beginning treatment. Additionally, investigators prospectively rated patients at 24 h with respect to whether or not the treating investigator subjectively thought there had been major neurological improvement. Further experience disclosed that some patients who did not improve during the first two hours did have major neurological improvement by 24 h. Hence, after the two pilot studies were completed, a shift in emphasis on quantitation of major neurological improvement moved from the 2-h posttreatment examination to the 24-h examination. A *post hoc* analysis revealed that at 24 h, patients who were prospectively designated by the treating investigator as having had major neurological improvement had a minimum of 4 or more points improvement on the NIH Stroke Scale compared to baseline or had returned to normal. The threshold of 2 or more points originally selected for the 2-h examination was not appreciable, clinically, as major neurological improvement at 24 h, particularly in patients with extensive baseline deficits (high initial NIH Stroke Scale scores), and was discarded for future NINDS studies. The 4 point improvement criterion was retained, however, as a measure of early activity of the drug in future Phase 2 trials. Later experience in placebo-controlled trials has exposed that the 4 point threshold, although clinically detectable, is too easily reached by placebo-treated patients, as well *(17)*.

Hennerici et al. reported the results of administering 70 mg alteplase intravenously over 90 min in 19 patients with ischemic stroke of less than 24-h duration *(18)*. Full dose intravenous heparin was also administered. One patient was excluded after entry because his symptoms were later determined to be of greater than 24-h duration. Of the other 18 patients, one sustained a fatal intracerebral hemorrhage, and early arterial recanalization was achieved in only 25%. Nine additional patients died of complications of their entry strokes. The onset times of many of the patients could not be determined with certainty, and the authors proposed that delayed treatment may have contributed to the poor outcomes. They also suggested that the dose of alteplase was too low.

Later, von Kummer and associates *(19)* reported on 32 patients with severe hemispheric deficits treated with a 100 mg of alteplase administered over 90 min, combined with a 5000 unit bolus of intravenous heparin followed by a continuous infusion at 1000–1500 units/h, aiming to double the activated partial thromboplastin time in each patient. All patients were treated within 6 h (mean ± S.D. = 3.8 ± 1.1 h) of stroke onset, and all had pretreatment CT scanning and cerebral angiography. Partial or complete recanalization of the infarct-related artery was documented angiographically in 34% immediately after the rt-PA infusion, and in an additional 19% within 12–24 h by predominantly transcranial Doppler assessment. Hemorrhagic transformation was observed in 38%, of which one-fourth (9%) was associated with neurological deterioration and death. At 4 wk, clinical outcome was classified as good (ambulatory, NIH Stroke Scale score <13) in 44% and poor or dead in the remainder. Good outcomes were correlated with recanalization within 24 h. Reocclusion was reported in one patient despite the heparin treatment. The authors acknowledged that their results did not show a clear benefit of concomitant heparin therapy, but suggested that it did not appear to be substantially more dangerous than rt-PA alone.

Overgaard and colleagues *(20)* also used a standard 100 mg dose of single-chain rt-PA in 23 patients treated within 6 h of stroke onset. Heparin was prohibited for the first 24 h. One patient died from an intracerebral hemorrhage, but that patient was also treated with heparin in violation of the protocol. Two other patients had hemorrhagic conversion without neurological worsening. Baseline and follow-up SPECT scans were performed in 12 patients. Ten of the 12 patients had improved blood flow at 24 h compared to baseline and had more neurological improvement, both early and late, than the 2 patients with persistently impaired perfusion.

INTRAVENOUS ADMINISTRATION: CONTROLLED TRIALS

The results of three small randomized, placebo-controlled trials of thrombolytic therapy were reported (Table 3). Two trials used rt-PA, whereas one employed ancrod.

Mori and colleagues *(21)* recruited 31 patients with acute carotid territory ischemia and randomly assigned them to receive either placebo (12 patients), 20 megaunits duteplase (approx 50 mg, 9 patients), or 30 megaunits (approx 80 mg, 10 patients) intravenously over 60 min *(21)*. Patients were eligible for treatment within 6 h of stroke onset, and all had pre- and posttreatment angiography. Despite the small sample sizes, there was a rough balance in baseline neurological deficits, as determined by the Hemispheric Stroke Scale. The clinical results were reported as average difference scores from baseline. In the overall analysis, in which patients who died were assigned the maximum score, there were no apparent differences between the groups at 24 h; but by d 2, the 80 mg rt-PA group had improved from baseline compared to the placebo group. By d 30, all three groups had improved from baseline, but the group receiving 80 mg rt-PA had improved statistically significantly more than the placebo group. If the two deaths in the placebo group were excluded from this analysis (none died in the 80 mg rt-PA group), then the difference in scores on the survivors between the groups were not significantly different at 30 d, but remained different up to d 7.

Parenchymal hematomas were reported in one patient in each of the treatment groups, including the placebo group. Hemorrhagic infarction was reported in 30% of the 80 mg group, 56% of the 50 mg group, and 33% of the placebo group. None of the differences were statistically significant. The incidence of neurological deterioration with hemorrhagic transformation was not reported.

Table 3
Randomized Trials of Intravenous Therapy

Study	Agent	# Patients	Treatment window	Results
Mori (1992)	rt-PA (duteplase)	12-control 9–20 MIU 10–30 MIU	0–6 h	Improved arterial recanalization and neurological scale difference scores in treated groups.
Bridging Study (1992)	rt-PA (alteplase)	10-control 10–0.85 mg/kg 3-control 4–0.85 mg/kg	0–90 min 91–180 min	60% early improvement in treated groups; 10% in controls. 1 fatal hemorrhage in control group, 2 with early improvement in each group.
Ancrod Group (1992)	Ancrod	68-control 64 Ancrod	0–6 h	No difference in neurological scale scores. Trends for improved mortality and functional outcome in treated groups.

Intended as a pilot feasibility study for a larger NINDS-sponsored trial, 27 patients were examined in the TPA Bridging Study, a randomized, double-blind, placebo-controlled trial of intravenous alteplase, 0.85 mg/kg given over 1 h with 10% of the total dose administered as an initial bolus *(22)*. Twenty patients (10 rt-PA and 10 placebo) were treated within 90 min from stroke onset, while 7 patients (4 rt-PA and 3 placebo) were treated from 91 to 180 min from onset. The primary end point was the proportion of patients who improved by 4 or more points on the NIH Stroke Scale as determined by a blinded evaluator at 24 h. Randomization produced approximate balance in the baseline stroke scale scores in the 0 to 90 min group. However, at 24 h, 60% of rt-PA-treated patients had improved by 4 or more points compared to 10% of the placebo-treated patients, a statistically significant difference ($p < 0.05$). There was no statistically significant difference in the group mean stroke scale scores at any of the follow-up time points, though, and the proportion of improvers was not statistically different at 1 wk or 3 mo. The numbers of patients in the 91–180 min group were too small to draw any meaningful conclusions, although the investigators reported the development of a fatal spontaneous hematoma in the placebo group. The investigators concluded that although the results were promising, larger studies were clearly needed.

Encouraged by results from a small pilot study performed in the late 1980s *(23)*, Olinger and colleagues *(24)* reported preliminary results from a larger randomized, controlled trial of ancrod in 132 patients treated within 6 hours of stroke onset. Ancrod, derived from the venom of the Malaysian pit viper, is a defibrinogenating agent that activates the thrombolytic system indirectly. The mean time to treatment was 4.6 h. While there was no statistically significant difference in the prospectively determined primary end point (Scandinavian Stroke Scale scores at 3 mo), post hoc analyses suggested trends in improvement in early mortality and functional outcome at 3 mo. Further studies of ancrod in acute ischemic stroke have recently been completed (*see* Chapter 8).

In 1992, Wardlaw and Warlow provided an overview analysis of the world's published experience, to date, which included experience with over 2500 patients *(25)*. They called for an end to further nonrandomized, uncontrolled trials of thrombolytic therapy in ischemic stroke and applauded the ongoing randomized trials being conducted worldwide at that time.

SUMMARY

The Phase 2 studies of intravenous thrombolytic therapy set the stage for the Phase 3 trials to come. The feasibility of rapid diagnosis and treatment of acute stroke was established. Patients could be treated as quickly as within 90 min of the onset of symptoms if angiography was not required, and within 6 h even if pretreatment angiography was thought to be necessary. A range of doses of rt-PA given early after the onset of symptoms was shown to be reasonably safe. As suggested by prior animal experience, the risk of symptomatic intracranial hemorrhage increased with increasing rt-PA dose, and with delay in treatment beyond 6 h.

Hemorrhages occurred in both ischemic and, less often, in uninvolved vascular territories, and also occurred in the absence of arterial recanalization. Occlusions of smaller arterial branches were more easily lysed than larger arteries, and neurological improvement correlated, though not exactly, with recanalization. Finally, a low, but clinically important incidence of symptomatic intracranial hemorrhage was observed in patients who were treated with neither thrombolytic drugs nor anticoagulants, further emphasizing the necessity of placebo-controlled trials to test not only the efficacy, but the safety of thrombolytic therapy for stroke.

Perhaps most importantly, these pilot studies demonstrated conclusively that ultra-rapid triage, diagnosis, and treatment of stroke patients was feasible. The significance of this demonstration in the face of nearly ubiquitois nihilism, cannot be over stated.

REFERENCES

1. Sussman BJ, Fitch TSP. Thrombolysis with fibrinolysin in cerebral arterial occlusion. *JAMA* 1958;167:1705–1709.
2. The National Institute of Neurological Disorders and Stroke rt-PA Stroke Study Group. Tissue plasminogen activator for acute ischemic stroke. *N Engl J Med* 1995;333:1581–1587.
3. Sloan MA. Thrombolysis and stroke. *Arch Neurol* 1987;44:748–768.
4. Levine SR, Brott TG. Thrombolytic therapy in cerebrovascular disorders. *Prog in Cardiovasc Dis* 1992;34:235–262.
5. Del Zoppo GJ, Pessin MS, Mori E, Hacke W. Thrombolytic intervention in acute thrombotic and embolic stroke. *Seminars in Neurology* 1991;11:368–384.
6. Sharma GVRK, Cella G, Parisi AF, Sasahara AA. Thrombolytic therapy. *N Engl J Med* 1982;306:1268–1276.
7. Del Zoppo GJ, Ferbert A, Otis S, et al. Local intra-arterial fibrinolytic therapy in acute carotid territory stroke. A pilot study. *Stroke* 1988;19:307–313.
8. Mori E, Tabuchi M, Yoshida T, Yamadori A. Intracarotid urokinase with thromboembolic occlusion of the middle cerebral artery. *Stroke* 1988;19:802–812.
9. Theron J, Courtheoux P, Casaseo A. Local intra-arterial fibrinolysis in the carotid territory. *AJNR* 1989;10:753–765.
10. Hacke W, Zeumer H, Ferbert A, Bruckmann H, del Zoppo GJ. Intra-arterial thrombolytic therapy improves outcome in patients with acute vertebrobasilar occlusive disease. *Stroke* 1988;19:1216–1222.
11. Matsumoto K, Satoh K. Topical intraarterial urokinase infusion for acute stroke. In: *Thrombolytic Therapy in Acute Ischemic Stroke*, Hacke W, del Zoppo GJ, Hirshberg M, eds. Springer-Verlag: Berlin. 1991; pp. 207–212.
12. Mobius E, Berg-Dammer E, Kuhne D, Ahser HC. Local thrombolytic therapy in acute basilar artery occlusion: experience with 18 patients. In: *Thrombolytic Therapy in Acute Ischemic Stroke*, Hacke W, del Zoppo GJ, Hirshberg M, eds. Springer-Verlag: Berlin. 1991; pp. 213–215.

13. Del Zoppo GJ, Poeck K, Pessin MS, et al. Recombinant tissue plasminogen activator in acute thrombotic and embolic stroke. *Ann Neurol* 1992;32:78–86.
14. Yamaguchi T, Hayakawa T, Kikuchi H, Abe T. Intravenous rt-PA in embolic and thrombotic cerebral infarction: A cooperative study. In: *Thrombolytic Therapy in Acute Ischemic Stroke*, Hacke W, del Zoppo GJ, Hirshberg M, eds. Springer-Verlag: Berlin. 1991; pp. 168–174.
15. Brott TG, Haley EC, Levy DE, et al. Urgent therapy for stroke. Part I. Pilot study of tissue plasminogen activator administered within 90 minutes. *Stroke* 1992;23:632–640.
16. Haley EC, Levy DE, Brott TG, et al. Urgent therapy for stroke. Part II. Pilot study of tissue plasminogen activator administered 91-180 minutes from onset. *Stroke* 1992;23:641–645.
17. Haley EC Jr, Lewandowski C, Tilley BC, and the NINDS rt-PA Stroke Study Group. Myths regarding the NINDS rt-PA Stroke Trial: Setting the record straight. *Ann Emerg Med* 1997;30:676–682.
18. Hennerici M, Hacke W, von Kummer R, Hornig C, Zangemeister W. Intravenous tissue plasminogen activator for the treatment of acute thromboembolic ischemia. *Cerebrovasc Dis* 1991;1(Suppl 1):124–128.
19. Von Kummer R, Hacke W. Safety and efficacy of intravenous tissue plasminogen activator and heparin in acute middle cerebral artery stroke. *Stroke* 1992;23:646–652.
20. Overgaard K, Sperling B, Boysen G, Pedersen H, Gam J, Ellemann K, Karle A, Arlien-Soborg P, Olsen TS, Videbaek C, Knudsen JB: Thrombolytic therapy in acute ischemic stroke. A Danish pilot study. *Stroke* 1993;24:1439–1446.
21. Mori E, Yoneda Y, Tabuchi M, et al. Intravenous recombinant tissue plasminogen activator in acute carotid artery territory stroke. *Neurology* 1992;42:976–982.
22. Haley EC, Broth TC, Sheppard GL, Barsan W, Brodeick J, Marler JR, Kongable GL, Spilker J, Massey S, Hansen CA, et al. Pilot Randomized Trial of Tissue Plasminogen Activator in Acute Ischemic Stroke. The t-PA Bridging Study. *Stroke* 1993;24:1000–1004.
23. Olinger CP, Brott TG, Barsan WG, et al. Use of ancrod in acute or progressing ischemic cerebral infarction. *Ann Emerg Med* 1988;17:1208–1209.
24. The Ancrod in Stroke Investigators. Ancrod in acute ischemic stroke. (Abst.) *Stroke* 1992;23:162.
25. Wardlaw JM, Warlow CP. Thrombolysis in acute ischemic stroke: does it work? *Stroke* 1992;23:1826–1839.

8

Intravenous Thrombolytic Therapy for Acute Ischemic Stroke

Results of Large, Randomized Clinical Trials

Rashmi U. Kothari, MD
and Joseph P. Broderick, MD

CONTENTS

INTRODUCTION
EFFICACY AND SAFETY OF TISSUE PLASMINOGEN ACTIVATOR
    IN STROKE
EFFICACY AND SAFETY OF STREPTOKINASE IN STROKE
CONCLUSION
REFERENCES

INTRODUCTION

Prior to the availability of computed tomography (CT) imaging, seven case series had reported the use of various thrombolytic agents for 249 patients who had ischemic strokes *(1–7)*. Mortality rates ranged from 20 to 50% and intracranial hemorrhage rates from 11 to 35% in these studies (*see* Chapter 6). These discouraging results reflect the fact that patients were treated days to weeks after symptom onset, and CT scanning was not yet available to appropriately exclude patients with hemorrhage.

During the 1980s, thrombolytic therapy was investigated in the setting of acute myocardial infarction (AMI), acute pulmonary embolism, and peripheral arterial disease. Subsequently, large clinical trials demonstrated that streptokinase and tissue-plasminogen activator (t-PA) improves cardiac function as well as survival in patients with AMI. Parallel with the successful treatment of AMI with thrombolytic therapy was the wide spread availability of CT in the United

From: *Thrombolytic Therapy for Stroke*
Edited by: P. D. Lyden © Humana Press Inc., Totowa, NJ

States. By the late 1980s, there were multiple encouraging case series of thrombolytic therapy for stroke reported in the medical literature *(15–18)*. Data from laboratory studies evaluating the use of thrombolytic agents in acute ischemic stroke suggested that time was an important factor in determining outcome and hemorrhage rate *(see* Chapters 4 and 7). Zivin et al. *(16)* reported reduced recovery rates as the delay between onset of ischemia and start of thrombolytic therapy progressed. In the early 1990s several pilot clinical protocols, preludes to larger randomized trials, reported similar results to the animal studies in regards to efficacy, safety, and time to treatment, discussed at length in the previous chapter.

Recently, the completion of several large, randomized, controlled trials of t-PA and streptokinase have given us important information regarding the safety of various thrombolytic agents, the importance of patient selection, and the time frame in which thrombolytic agents should be used. This chapter will review the findings of these large randomized trials.

EFFICACY AND SAFETY
OF TISSUE PLASMINOGEN ACTIVATOR IN STROKE

Randomized Trials of rt-PA Given Within 0–180 min of Stroke Onset

The National Institute of Neurological Disorders and Stroke (NINDS) recombinant tissue-plasminogen activator (rt-PA) Stroke Study was the first large randomized trial to demonstrate a benefit for a thrombolytic agent in acute stroke *(17)*. This two-part study was a randomized, double-blind trial of intravenous recombinant rt-PA versus placebo in patients with acute ischemic stroke treated within 3 h of stroke onset. The study was based on pilot studies and dose-escalation data that suggested that rt-PA in a dose of 0.9 mg/kg given intravenously within 3 h of stoke onset would prove beneficial while minimizing the risk of hemorrhage *(18,19)*.

The study had two parts. Part 1 enrolled 291 patients and tested whether rt-PA had early clinical activity, which was defined as a 4 point improvement over baseline on the National Institute of Health Stroke Scale (NIHSS) or complete resolution of neurologic deficit within 24 h of symptom onset. Part 2 enrolled 333 patients and used four outcome measures and a combined global test statistic (Table 1) to assess whether treatment with rt-PA conveyed clinical benefit at 3 mo after treatment.

Patients were randomized if they had an ischemic stroke with a clearly defined time of onset, a deficit measurable on the NIHSS, and a baseline CT that showed no evidence of intracranial hemorrhage. There were no exclusions based CT findings of ischemia. Half of all patients were treated within 90 min of symptom onset and the other half within 91–180 min of symptom onset. The investigators emphasized careful patient selection and strict adherence to the treatment protocol. Strict

Table 1

Percentage of Patients with Favorable Outcome* in Part 2 of the National Institute
of Neurological Disorders and Stroke rt-PA Stroke Study *(17)*

	rt-PA	Placebo	Odds ratio (95% CI)	p-value
Global test			1.7 (1.2–2.6)	0.008
Barthel Index	50%	38%	1.6 (1.1–2.5)	0.026
Modified Rankin Scale	39%	26%	1.7 (1.1–2.5)	0.019
Glasgow Outcome Scale	44%	32%	1.6 (1.1–2.5)	0.025
NIH Stroke Scale	31%	20%	1.7 (1.0–2.8)	0.033

*Scores of 95–100 on the Barthel Index, ≤1 on the Modified Rankin Scale and NIH Stroke Scale, and 1 1 on the Glasgow Outcome Scale were considered favorable outcomes by the investigators.

guidelines for blood pressure management were followed and the use of other anticoagulants or antiplatelet agents was prohibited for the first 24 h (*see* Chapter 17).

Outcomes for the study were as follows. In Part 1, no statistically significant difference was detected at 24 h between groups in the primary end point (a 4 point improvement on the NIHSS or complete resolution of neurologic deficit at 24 h). However, there was a 4 point difference in the median NIHSS at 24 h between the rt-PA and placebo group (8 vs 12, respectively, $p < 0.02$) *(20)*. In Part 2, patients who received rt-PA were 30% more likely to have little or no disability after 3 mo when compared to controls. This was also true for Part 1 and a combined analysis of both Parts 1 and 2. The benefit for t-PA was highly significant and was true for all four measures of outcome (Table 1). Using the global test statistic (a statistical tool that simultaneously evaluates all four outcome measures), the odds ratio for a favorable outcome in the rt-PA group was 1.7 (95% confidence interval, 1.2 to 2.6; $p = 0.008$). Treatment with rt-PA produced a favorable outcome regardless of the subtype of ischemic stroke (i.e., lacunar stroke, cardioembolic stroke, and so on).

Symptomatic intracerebral hemorrhage within 36 h after the onset of stroke occurred in 6.4% of patients given t-PA but only 0.6% of the placebo group ($p < 0.001$), Table 2. No significant difference in mortality was seen between t-PA (17%) and placebo groups (21%, $p = 0.30$). In a multivariable analysis, only stroke severity as measured by the NIHSS (five categories; OR = 1.8; 95% CI, 1.2 to 2.9) and brain edema (defined as acute hypodensity) or mass effect on baseline CT (OR, 7.8; 95% CI, 2.2 to 27.1) were independently associated with an increased risk of symptomatic intracerebral hemorrhage *(21)*. However, in either subgroup (patients with severe neurological deficit or CT findings of edema or mass effect) t-PA-treated patients were more likely than placebo-treated patients to have a favorable 3-mo outcome. These authors concluded that

Table 2
Randomized Trials of Tissue Plasminogen Activator

Study	Time to treatment	No. of patients	Dose and treatment group	3-mo mortality	Intracerebral hematoma[a]
NINDS rt-PA Acute Stroke Study (Part I) (17)	≤3 h	291	0.9 mg/kg rt-PA placebo	N/A N/A	6%[b] 0%[b]
NINDS rt-PA Acute Stroke Study (Part II) (17)	≤3 h	333	0.9 mg/kg rt-PA placebo	N/A N/A	7%[b] 1%[b]
NINDS rt-PA Acute Stroke Study (Part I & Part II combined) (17)	≤3 h	624	0.9 mg/kg rt-PA placebo	17% 21%	6.4%[b] 0.6%[b]
Alantis (22,23)	3–5 h[d]	579	0.9 mg/kg rt-PA placebo	N/A N/A	7.2%[b] 0.7%[b]
European Cooperative Acute Stroke Study (ECASS-I) (24)	≤6 h	620	1.1 mg/kg t-PA placebo	22.4%[b] 15.8%[b]	19.8%[b,c] 6.8%[b,c]
European Cooperative Acute Stroke Study-II (ECASS-II) (25)	≤6 h	800	0.9 mg/kg t-PA placebo	10.5% 10.7%	8.8%[b] 3.4%[b]

[a]Symptomatic intracerebral hemorrhage within 36 h.
[b]$p \leq 0.001$.
[c]Only rate of parenchymal intracerebral hemorrhage is available; no information regarding clinical deterioration is available.
[d]Initially 0–5 h study; however, protocol amended to 3–5 h following FDA approval of rt-PA under 3 h.
NA = not available.

despite a higher rate of intracerebral hemorrhage, patients with severe strokes or edema or mass effect on the baseline CT are reasonable candidates for t-PA if administered within 3 h of stroke onset. In June of 1996, the FDA approved the use of rt-PA given within 3 h of stroke onset in patients with acute ischemic stroke, based primarily on the data from Parts I and II of the NINDS rt-PA trial.

Randomized Trial of rt-PA Given Within 3–5 h of Stroke Onset

Because of the narrow therapeutic window and the small percentage of patients presenting within this narrow time frame, efforts were made to evaluate the use of rt-PA beyond the 3-h time window. The Alteplase Thrombolysis for Acute Noninterventional Therapy in Ischemic Stroke (Alantis) study was a double-blind, randomized trial evaluating the safety and efficacy of 0.9 mg/kg of intra-venous t-PA in patients with acute ischemic stroke *(22)*. It was initially designed to evaluate patients treated within 0–6 h (Part A). In December of 1993, after enrollment of 142 patients, the time window was changed (Part B) to 0–5 h owing to the Safety Committee (DMSB) concerns in the 5–6 h group. Time from onset to treatment in Part B was further modified following FDA approval of t-PA for patients with acute ischemic stroke treated within 3 h. The protocol was amended to evaluate patients treated within 3–5 h. For Part B, a total of 619 patients were enrolled of which 613 were randomized. The trial ended prematurely in July 1998 based on the DSMB analysis indicating that "treatment was unlikely to prove beneficial" *(22)*. In the final analysis of Part B data, the median time to treatment was 4.5 h with only 31 patients treated within 3 h. There was no difference in the primary end point (the percentage of patients with a NIHSS ≤ 1 at 90 d) between placebo and t-PA treated patients (34% for both groups, p = ns), however the symptomatic ICH rate was greater in the t-PA treated patients (1.3% vs 6.7%) *(23)*.

Tissue-Plasminogen Activator Within 0–6 h

There have been two, large randomized trials evaluating the safety and effi-cacy of t-PA in stroke patients treated within 0–6 h (European Cooperative Acute Stroke Study) ECASS and ECASS II *(24,25)*. ECASS was the first large, pub-lished, randomized trial of intravenous rt-PA in patients with acute ischemic stroke *(24)*. It was published 2 mo prior to the publication of the NINDS trial and 7 mo prior to the FDA approval of rt-PA given within 3 h. ECASS was a multi-center, double-blind, randomized trial of 1.1 mg/kg of intravenous rt-PA vs placebo in patients with acute ischemic stroke, treated within 6 h of symptom onset. Patients were eligible if they were 18 yr or older and had a clinical diag-nosis of moderate to severe hemispheric stroke. Patients with coma, hemiplegia plus fixed eye deviation, global aphasia, vertebrobasilar stroke, or those with a CT scan showing hypodensity in more than one-third of the middle cerebral artery territory were to be excluded. The primary end points were the 90-d Barthel

Index and the Modified Rankin Scale. Secondary end points included 30-d mortality.

A total of 620 patients were entered in the trial (the intent-to-treat population). In this intent-to-treat population, there was no difference in 3 mo neurological outcome or 30-d mortality in patients treated with rt-PA and placebo (*see* Table 2) *(24)*. Hemorrhagic infarction was more frequent in the placebo-treated group (30.3% vs 23%, $p < 0.001$), but parenchymal hematoma was more frequent in the rt-PA treated group (19.8% vs 6.5%, $p < 0.001$). Death associated with hemorrhage occurred in 19 of the rt-PA treated patients and in 7 of the placebo patients.

In a subset of patients, there was evidence of neurological improvement in the rt-PA treated group. Before enrolling patients, the ECASS investigators had anticipated that up to 20% of the patients would have major protocol violations, but would be inadvertently randomized and, indeed, a total of 109 patients treated in the study had major protocol violations. The protocol violations included 66 with abnormalities on the CT scans (mainly major early infarct signs), unapproved therapy in 12 patients (e.g., heparin in less than 24 h), deviation from the 90 ± 14-d time window for follow-up or lost follow-up in 20 patients, and 11 others (e.g., randomized but not treated). Prospectively, the remaining 511 patients were defined as the "target population" (the population that strictly met the inclusion and exclusion criteria). In the target population, the t-PA treated patients had a better outcome on two primary end points. First, the neurological outcome was improved in the rt-PA treated group vs placebo as measured by the median modified Rankin Scale (2 vs 3 respectively, $p = .035$). Second, of the rt-PA patients in the target population, 41% had a 3-mo modified Rankin Scale of 1 or 0 compared to 29% of the placebo-treated patients ($p < 0.01$) (Table 3). Mortality was not different in the two target population groups. Death associated with hemorrhage occurred in 10 patients treated with rt-PA as compared to 7 treated with placebo ($p =$ ns). Overall, the total parenchymal hematoma rate in the target population was 19.4% for rt-PA and 6.8% for placebo.

ECASS results sparked controversy. Skeptics pointed out that the real world population is the intent-to-treat population. For that group, no efficacy or suggestion of efficacy was identified. Optimists pointed out that proper patient selection is necessary for adequate evaluation of a given therapy. In the target population, there was evidence of benefit for patients treated with rt-PA. They argue that 66 of the 109 patients excluded from the target population had CT evidence of an already established major cerebral infarction. Such patients would not be expected to benefit from thrombolysis and should be excluded in future trials. The failure to show benefit in the rt-PA treated group may result from delaying treatment to greater than 4 h after symptom onset for the majority of the ECASS patients. Only 87 (14%) of the 620 patients were treated within 3 h of symptom onset. If all patients had been treated within 3 h, perhaps outcomes for the rt-PA treated patients would have been similar to that seen in the NINDS trial.

Table 3
Results of Europe Cooperative Acute Stroke Study (24)

	Intent-to-treat population (n = 620)		Target population (n = 511)	
	t-PA	*Placebo*	*t-PA*	*Placebo*
30-d mortality	18%*	13%*	15%	12%
Parenchymal hematoma	20%*	7%*	19%*	7%*
Modified Rankin Scale score 0–1 at 3 mo	36%	29%	41%*	29%*

*Significant ($p < 0.05$).

ECASS-II was designed to address the controversy raised by ECASS. ECASS-II was a multicenter, double-blind, randomized trial evaluating the safety and efficacy of intravenous rt-PA vs placebo within 6 h of stroke onset (25). A dose of 0.9 mg/kg of intravenous t-PA was used and strict blood pressure guidelines based upon the NINDS trial were followed. Similar to ECASS-I, but in contrast to the NINDS trial, patients with major signs of infarction on CT (>1/3 the MCA distribution), patients with coma or stupor, or patients with hemiplegia plus fixed eye deviation were excluded. The primary end point was the modified Rankin scale at 90 d, dichotomized for favorable (score 0–1) and unfavorable (score 2–6) outcome.

There were 800 patients randomized over the 14-mo study period. Despite implementation of a training course to improve CT assessment by investigators prior to and during the trial, there were 72 protocol violations; the majority of violations were resulting from CT criteria. There was no significant difference in the proportion of favorable outcome between the t-PA treated patients (40.3% [95% CI 35.6–45.4]) and the placebo-treated patients (36.6% [31.8–41.6]), $p = 0.277$. However, a *post-hoc* analysis of the modified Rankin Score at 90 d, dichotomized as independent (mRS=0-2) or not independent (mRS=3-6) found an absolute difference of 8.3% in favor of the t-PA treated patients (t-PA=54.3% [49.5–59.1] vs placebo=46.0% [41.1–50.9], $p = 0.024$). Though the incidence of symptomatic intracranial hemorrhage was significantly higher in the t-PA treated patients (8.8%) as compared to the placebo-treated group (3.4%), there was no significant difference in 30 or 90 d mortality between the two groups. The rate of symptomatic parenchymal hemorrhage within 36 h in the t-PA treated group was similar to that reported noted in the NINDS trial (*see* Table 2).

Summary

There have been two large randomized trials (NINDS Part 1 and 2) evaluating the use of t-PA within 3 h of stroke onset. These data show that patients treated with rt-PA within 3 h of symptom onset are at least 30% more likely to have no or min. deficits at 90 d as compared to those who receive placebo. The rate of symptomatic intracranial hemorrhage within 36 h was 6.4%, and there was no significant difference in 90 d mortality between treated and placebo groups.

There have been three large randomized trials evaluating the safety and efficacy of intravenous t-PA beyond this 3-h window. The majority of the patients in these trials have been treated greater than 3 h after stroke onset. None have found a significant improvement in outcome between the t-PA and placebo-treated patients in regards to their primary end points and also found significantly higher intracranial hemorrhage rates in the t-PA treated group. *Post-hoc* analysis from ECASS-I and ECASS-II suggests that there may be a subset of patients in this later time window who may benefit from intravenous t-PA, especially those with minimal or no CT evidence of infarction, however, further prospective trials are needed to verify this hypothesis.

EFFICACY AND SAFETY OF STREPTOKINASE IN STROKE

There have been three large randomized trials of streptokinase in the treatment of acute ischemic stroke *(26–28)*. Unfortunately, all three trials were halted because of increased rate of intracranial hemorrhage and higher mortality in the streptokinase-treated patients.

Randomized Trial of Streptokinase Given Within 0–4 h of Stroke Onset

The Australian Streptokinase Trial (ASK) is a double-blind randomized placebo controlled trial of patients with ischemic stroke who could be randomized and treated within 4 h of symptom onset *(26,29)*. Patients were treated with 1.5 million units of streptokinase plus 325 mg aspirin or intravenous placebo and aspirin over 60 min. ASK was suspended upon recommendation by the Safety and Monitoring Committee following analysis of the first 228 patients who had been treated between 3 and 4 h following stroke onset *(26)*. The recommendation was made because of increased mortality and symptomatic hemorrhage in the streptokinase patients treated within 3–4 h (Table 4). A specific *a priori* hypothesis was that outcomes would differ between those patients treated within 0–3 h and those treated after 3 h. Subsequent analysis of the 70 patients treated within 3 h as compared to the 270 that were treated after 3 h found that earlier treatment was safer and associated with significantly better outcomes than later treatment $(p = 0.04)$ *(29)*.

Randomized Trials of Streptokinase Given Within 0–6 h of Stroke Onset

There have been two large randomized trials of streptokinase given within 6 h of stroke onset *(27,28)*. The Multicenter Acute Stroke Trial - Europe (MAST-E)

Table 4
Randomized Trials of Streptokinase

Study	Time to treatment	No. of patients	Treatment group	Mortality	Intracerebral hematoma
Australian Streptokinase Study (ASK) (29)[b]	≤4 h	340	SK + 100 mg ASA vs 100 mg ASA	36.2%[a] 20.5%[a]	13.2%[a] 3.0%[a]
Multicenter Acute Stroke Trial—Europe (MAST-E) (27,62)[b]	≤6 h	310	SK vs Placebo	34% 18%	21.2%[a,c] 2.6%[a,c]
Multicenter Acute Stroke Trials—Italy (MAST-I) (28)[b]	≤6 h	622	SK + 300 mg ASA vs SK vs 300 mg ASA vs standard therapy	34%[a] 19% 10% 13%[a]	10%[c] 6%[c] 2%[c] 0.6%[c]

[a] $p \leq 0.001$.
[b] All studies terminated prior to completion due to increased mortality in treatment group.
[c] Symptomatic hemorrhage in hospital.
NA = not available.

was a multi-center double-blind randomized study of streptokinase compared to placebo in patients with hemispheric stroke who could be randomized and treated within 6 h from stroke onset (27). Patients were treated intravenously with 1.5 million units of streptokinase or placebo given over 60 min. The study was terminated upon recommendation from the Data Monitoring and Safety Committee following the analysis of data from 270 patients (310 enrolled) (30). The 10-d mortality in patients receiving streptokinase was 34% compared to 18% in the patients treated with placebo (p = 0.002) (Table 4) (27). The symptomatic hemorrhage rate was 21% in the streptokinase patients and 3% in the placebo patients (p < 0.001) (27).

The Multicenter Acute Stroke Trial - Italy (MAST-I) was a multicenter randomized trial comparing treatment among four groups (28). Patients within 6 h of symptom onset were randomized to receive either 1.5 million units of streptokinase intravenously over 60 min, aspirin 300 mg per day for 10 d, intravenous streptokinase and aspirin, or control (standard treatment—no placebo). MAST-I was also suspended after 40% of planned recruitment (28). Patients receiving both streptokinase and aspirin had significantly greater 10-d mortality than those given neither (34% vs 13%, p < 0.001, see Table 4). There was no significant difference in mortality for those patients treated with streptokinase alone (19% vs 13%, p = 0.12) (28). Symptomatic cerebral hemorrhage rates were more frequent in the streptokinase-alone and streptokinase-plus-aspirin groups than in the group given neither (6% and 10%, respectively, vs 0.6%).

Summary

All three studies of streptokinase were suspended owing to increased rates of hemorrhage and mortality in the streptokinase treated group. Although pilot safety studies for streptokinase were carried out prior to beginning the randomized trials, dose-escalation safety studies were not performed. The 1.5 million unit dose is identical to the dose used for myocardial infarction. In contrast, two dose-finding, dose-escalation trials of intravenous rt-PA preceded the larger randomized trials of rt-PA. The doses selected for the subsequent randomized trials of rt-PA were approx 60–75% of the doses used for AMI. A lower dose of streptokinase (e.g., 0.9–1.2 million units) may have been better tolerated by stroke patients without sacrificing efficacy. Safety in the streptokinase trials may also have been significantly better if earlier treatment had been required. The two dose-finding, dose-escalation trials of intravenous rt-PA indicated a statistically significant relationship of later treatment to the occurrence of thrombolysis-related intracerebral bleeding. Further development of streptokinase as intravenous therapy for acute ischemic stroke is unlikely because of the negative findings from these studies.

CONCLUSION

Intravenous tissue plasminogen activator improves 3-mo neurologic outcome if given within 3 h of symptom onset in patients with acute ischemic stroke. Administration of intravenous rt-PA beyond the 3-h window or in doses greater than 0.9 mg has not been shown to be efficacious. The use of streptokinase at a dose of 1.5 million units has not been shown to be efficacious or safe in patients with acute ischemic stroke

REFERENCES

1. Clarke RL, Clifton E. The treatment of cerebrovascular thromboses and embolism with fibrinolytic agents. *Am J Cardiology* 1960;6:546–551.
2. Herndon RM, Meyer JS, Johnson JF. Fibrinolysin therapy in thrombotic diseases of the nervous system. *J Mich St Med Soc* 1960;59:1684–1692.
3. Meyer JS, Gilroy J, Barnhart MI, Johnson JF. Anticoagulants plus streptokinase therapy in progressive stroke. *JAMA* 1964;189:373.
4. Meyer JS, Gilroy J, Barnhart MI, Johnson JF. Therapeutic thrombolysis in cerebral thromboembolism. *Neurology* 1963;13:927–937.
5. Fletcher AP, Alkjersig N, Lewis M, Tulevski V, Davies A, Brooks JE, Hardin WB, Landau WM, Raichle ME. A pilot study of urokinase therapy in cerebral infarction. *Stroke* 1976;7:135–142.
6. Fears R. Biochemical pharmacology and therapeutic aspects of thrombolytic agents. *Pharmacol Rev* 1990;42:202–222.
7. Larcan A, Laprevote-Heully MC, Lambert H, et al. Indications des thrombolytiques au cours des accidents vasculaires cerebraux thrombosants traites par ailleurs par O.H.B. (2ATA). *Therapie* 1977;32:259–270.
8. Zeumer H, Freitag HJ, Grzyska V, et al. Interventional neuroradiology: Local intr-arterial fibrinolysis in acute vertebrobasilar thromboembolic disease. *Am J Neuroradiol* 1983;4:401–404.
9. Henze T, Boerr A, Tebbe U, et al. Lysis of basilar artery occlusion with tissue plasminogen activator. *Lancet* 1987 (letter)2:1391.
10. Jafar JJ, Tan WS, Crowell RM. Tissue plasminogen activator thrombolysis of a middle cerebral artery embolus in a patient with an arteriovenous malformation. *J Neurosurg* 1991;74:808–812.
11. Kaufman HH, Lind TA, Clark DS. Non penetrating trauma to the carotid artery with secondary thrombosis and embolism: Treatment by thrombolysin. *Acta Neurochirurgica* 1977;37:219–244.
12. Nenci GG, Gresele P, Taramelli M, Agnelli G Signorini E. Thrombolytic therapy for thromboembolism of vertebrobasilar artery. *Angiology* 1983;34:361–371.
13. Zeumer H, Hacke W, Kolmann HL, Poeck K. Lokale fibrinolysetherapie bei basilaris-thrombose. *Dtsch Med Wochenschr* 1982;107:728–731.
14. Zeumer H, Ferbert A, Ringelstein EB. Local intra-arterial fibrinolytic therapy in inaccessible internal carotid occlusion. *Neuroradiology* 1984;26:315–317.
15. Jungreis CA, Wechsler LR, Horton JA. Intracranial thrombolysis via a catheter embedded in the clot. *Stroke* 1989;20:1578–1580.
16. Zivin JA, Lyden PD, DeGirolami U, Kochhar A, Mazzarella V, Hemenway CC, Johnston: Tissue Plasminogen Activator: Reduction of Neurologic Damage After Experimental Embolic Stroke. Arch Neurol 1988;45:387–391.

17. The NINDS rt-PA Stroke Study Group. Tissue plasminogen activator for acute ischemic stroke. *N Engl J Med* 1995;333:1581–1587.
18. Haley Jr EC, Levy DE, Brott TG, Sheppard GL, Wong MCW, Kongable GL, Torner JC, Marler JR. Urgent therapy for stroke. Part II. Pilot study of tissue plasminogen activator administered 91–180 minutes from onset. *Stroke* 1992;23:641–645.
19. Brott TG, Haley Jr EC, Levy DE, Barsan W, Broderick J, Sheppard GL, Spilker J, Kongable GL, Massey S, Reed R, Marler JR. Urgent therapy for stroke. Part I. Pilot study of tissue plasminogen activator administered within 90 minutes. *Stroke* 1992;23:632–640.
20. Haley, EC jr, Lewandowski C, Tilley BC, NINDS rt-PA Stroke Study Group: Myths regarding the NINDS rt-PA Stroke Trial: Setting the record straight. Ann Emerg Med November 1997;30:676–682.
21. The NINDS t-PA Stroke Study Group: Intracerebral Hemorrhage after intravenous t-PA therapy for ischemic stroke. Stroke. 1997;2109–2118.
22. Clark W, Albers GW, for the ATLANTIS Stroke Study Investigators: The ALANTIS rt-PA (ALTEPLASE) Acute Stroke Trial: Final Results. (Abstract) Stroke 1999;30:234.
23. Clark W, Wissman, S, Albers, G, Jhamandas, J, Madden, K, Hamilton, S, for the ATLANTIS Study Investigators: Recombinant Tissue-Type Plasminogen Activator (Alteplase) for Ischemic Stroke 3 to 5 Hours After Symptom Onset. JAMA 1999;282:2019–2026.
24. Hacke W, Kaste M, Fieschi, C, von Kummer R, Davalos A, Meier D, et al., for the ECASS Study Group. Intravenous Thrombolysis with recombinant tissue plasminogen: Activator for Acute Hemispheric Stroke. The European Cooperative Acute Stroke Study. *JAMA* 1995; vol. 274,13:1–17.
25. Hacke W, Kaste M, Fieschi C, von Kummer R, Davalos A, Meier D, et al., for the Second European-Australiasian Acute Stroke Study Investigators: Randomized double-blind placebo-controlled trial of thrombolytic therapy with intravenous alteplase in acute ischaemic stroke (ECASS II). Lancet 1998; 352:1245–1251.
26. Donnan GA, Davis SM, Chambers BR, Gates PC, Hankey GJ, Stewart-Wynne EG, et al. Trials of streptokinase in severe acute ischaemic stroke. *Lancet* 1995;345:578–579.
27. The Multicenter Acute Stroke Trial-Europe Study Group: Thrombolytic therapy with streptokinase in acute ischemic stroke. N Engl J Med 1996;335:145–150.
28. Multicentre Acute Stroke Trial—Italy (MAST-I) Group. Randomized controlled trial of streptokinase, aspirin, and combination of both in treatment of acute ischaemic stroke. *Lancet* 1995:346:1509–1514.
29. Donnan GA, Davis SM, Chambers BR, Gates PC, Hankey GJ, McNeil JJ, et al., for the Australian Streptokinase (ASK) Trial Study Group. Streptokinase for acute ischemic stroke with relationship to time of administration. JAMA 1996;276:961–966.
30. Hommel M, Boissel JP, Comu C, Boutitie F, Lees KR, Sasson G, et al., for the MAST Study Group. Termination of trial of streptokinase in severe acute ischaemic stroke. *Lancet* 1994;315:57.

9

Further Analysis of NINDS Study
Long-Term Outcome, Subgroups and Cost Effectiveness*

Susan C. Fagan, PharmD,
Thomas Kwiatkowski, MD,
and Patrick Lyden, MD

CONTENTS

INTRODUCTION
COST EFFECTIVENESS
SUB-GROUP ANALYSIS
LONG-TERM OUTCOME
REFERENCES

INTRODUCTION

Following the initial publication of the National Institute of Neurological Disorders and Stroke (NINDS) tissue-plasminogen activator (t-PA) Stroke Trial results, the NINDS investigators published a series of additional data and analyses. These analyses were necessary because not all the relevant data could be included in the primary report, and to answer criticisms of the original article. Some of these analyses are summarized in other chapters, including 12 and 17. In this chapter, we will focus on three important issues: cost effectiveness, subgroup selection, and long-term follow-up. The cost effectiveness issue is critical because thrombolytic drugs are expensive. To show that the drug cost is worthwhile, we examined the costs of stroke care absent treatment, including how

Portions of the text, data, and figures in this chapter are adapted from three separate publications, with permission (1–3).

From: *Thrombolytic Therapy for Stroke*
Edited by: P. D. Lyden © Humana Press Inc., Totowa, NJ

costs might increase or decrease with successful treatment. Subgroup selection is addressed because some have advocated such analysis to help select patients at particular risk or susceptibility of benefit. We used regression modeling to rigorously identify any subgroups that could be preferred for treatment. To ensure that the benefits of thrombolysis were sustained over the long term, we followed the original cohort of patients up to 1 yr after their stroke. The essentials of these three follow-up analyses, cost effectiveness, subgroup selection, and long-term follow-up, have been published, so only brief descriptions of the methods will be given (1–3). We will try to put the results of these analyses into perspective for the practicing clinician.

COST EFFECTIVENESS

The cost effectiveness of t-PA was demonstrated in 1998 (1). We used a rigorous methodology to estimate the cost savings and any additional costs associated with thrombolytic stroke therapy. Certain assumptions about stroke costs and outcomes were based on data from the literature and from the original study (see Table 1). Then, to account for possible errors in the assumptions, a simulation method was used to vary the values of those assumptions. For example, we estimated that the cost of in-patient rehabilitation might be $21,233, but in the simulation, this assumption was varied from $10,000 to $40,000. Using these simulations, it was possible to estimate not only the costs of thrombolytic therapy, but also the likelihood of that estimate being correct.

Methods

Health and economic outcomes from the NINDS rt-PA Stroke trial, comparing t-PA and placebo, were estimated using a Markov modeling approach. A Markov model allows decision analysis of problems that are ongoing. Over time a patient can be in any one of a set of states and can transition between states based on probabilities defined by empiric data or assumptions. To illustrate, a patient may transition from no disability to moderate disability because of a recurrent stroke, the rate of which may be predicted to be 5% per year. For our purpose, a Markov model was particularly appropriate because it allowed us to focus on the impact of stroke over the lifetime of the patient.

We used sensitivity analyses to assess the probability that the model accurately estimated costs and outcomes. First, a one-way sensitivity analysis was performed for each assumption by varying it from minimum to maximum values although all others were held at their baseline values. This process determined which assumptions had the greatest impact on the findings. Next, the overall certainty of the findings was estimated using a Monte Carlo multi-way sensitivity analysis and spreadsheet forecasting software (Crystal Ball®, Decisioneering Inc., Boulder, CO). The Monte Carlo simulation allowed each assumption to vary randomly across their range of values over 10,000 iterations.

Table 1

Assumptions used to Estimate Cost Effectiveness of Thrombolytic Therapy for Stroke

Epidemiological Assumptions	Low	Best	High
Stroke recurrence rate per year	0.03	0.052	0.08
Recurrent stroke mortality	0.1	0.19	0.3
Multiplier for age specific mortality**	1.25	2.67	4
Discharge to NH from rehab - age 65 to 75	0.13	0.18	0.21
Discharge to NH from rehab - age > 75	0.24	0.32	0.34
Disability Distribution (Utilities)			
Rankin 0 - No Symptoms	0.85	0.90	0.95
Rankin 1 - No Disability Despite Symptoms	0.70	0.80	0.9
Rankin 2 - Slight Disability	0.35	0.46	0.65
Rankin 3 - Moderate Disability	0.20	0.34	0.5
Rankin 4 - Moderate/Severe Disability	0.12	0.30	0.45
Rankin 5 - Severe Disability	–0.20	–0.02	0.2
Dead	0.00	0.00	0.00
Cost Assumptions			
Cost/day of hosp	$1000	$1200	$1400
Average t-PA acquisition cost	$2100	$2230	$2400
Preparation and administration of t-PA	$10	$20	$30
Physician cost for administration of t-PA	$200	$300	$400
ICU additional cost for t-PA patients	$600	$775	$1000
ICH additional cost	$3000	$4500	$6000
Inpatient Rehabilitation	$10,000	$21,233	$40,000
Outpatient Rehabilitation	$1200	$2236	$2500
Nursing home cost per year	$20,000	$39,996	$50,000

NH = nursing home; ICU = intensive care unit; ICH = intracerebral hemorrhage.

** = Inflates U.S. age-specific mortality rate to account for the increase in mortality observed in patients who have had a stroke.

We used the number of quality-adjusted-life-years (QALYs) saved as the health outcome summary measure. This measure is standard for these sorts of studies, in which no effect on mortality is expected. We therefore predicted that the main impact of t-PA would be an increase in the quality of the patients' life (through decreased disability) rather than the "quantity" of life (no decreased mortality). The economic outcome summary measure of the model is the difference in estimated health care costs between the two treatment alternatives. We used the modified Rankin disability scale *(2)* as a disability measure because of its relative simplicity compared to the Barthel Index (scale of 0–5 vs 0–100) and its potential for translation into utilities (mild, moderate, severe) *(3)*. The Rankin scale divides disability into one of six states: 0: perfect health/no symptoms; 1: symptoms but no disability; 2: minor disability; 3: moderate disability, 4: severe disability, and 5: death *(2,4)*. The scale has been modified for use in clinical trials by the addition of the death rating, which was not present in the original scale. The modified Rankin scale is considered to have reasonable reliability and validity and is one of the most widely used scales in stroke research.

ASSUMPTIONS

Since we desired to model outcome for 30 yr following stroke, and since data from the NINDS rt-PA Stroke Study was only available for 1 yr, certain assumptions had to be made, as listed in Table 1. Stroke recurrence rate and age-adjusted mortality could be estimated from natural history studies available in the literature. We assumed that among survivors after a recurrent stroke there was an equal chance of Rankin categories of equal or greater disability. Each of the Rankin categories was assigned a utility value based on the results of a published patient preference survey for stroke outcomes *(5)*. A score of 100 was assigned for perfect health, 51 for minor disability, 40 for moderate disability, 9.8 for death, and 8 for severe disability. Since patients were unlikely to have been in "perfect health" prior to their index stroke, a utility of 90 was assigned to a Rankin rating of 0 or no symptoms. For cost assumptions, no published accepted estimate existed and wide extrapolations were required in many situations. For instance, the mode and utility of outpatient rehabilitation vs inpatient rehabilitation varied markedly from region to region in the United States. Also, in foreign countries, inpatient rehabilitation is often part of the acute hospital stay. In assumptions with greater uncertainty, the ranges of values used in the sensitivity analyses were broadened.

Results

NINDS rt-PA STROKE TRIAL DATA

The initial hospital stay was 12.4 ± 11 days for t-PA treated patients, compared to 10.9 ± 10 days for placebo treated patients in the trial ($p = 0.02$–Wilcoxon Rank Sum Test). The difference was attributable to the treatment, and not to other confounding factors such as stroke subtype. Disability status over the first year after a stroke is listed in Table 2. Discharge disposition data for 535 of the 572 patients alive at discharge are summarized in Table 3. More patients treated with t-PA were discharged to their own (or a relative or friend's) home and fewer required inpatient rehabilitation and nursing home care (Table 3, $p = 0.002$–chi-squared).

SENSITIVITY ANALYSES

The health and economic outcomes, calculated per 1000 patients potentially eligible for early thrombolytic therapy, are shown in Table 4. Assuming that 1000 patients are treated, the table lists the number of resulting "life-years" in each category. The column marked "Difference" shows the net increase or decrease in life-years in each category owing to treatment. For example, an additional 694

Table 2
Actual Distribution of Patients by Modified Rankin Disability Scores
and Deaths by Time from Randomization

Disability category	10 D		3 Mo		6 Mo		1 Yr	
	PLA	t-PA	PLA	t-PA	PLA	t-PA	PLA	t-PA
Rankin 0	23	49	33	57	33	59	32	61
Rankin 1	31	52	50	74	56	68	50	66
Rankin 2	29	26	36	23	32	25	36	23
Rankin 3	29	29	44	40	50	42	38	39
Rankin 4	87	68	60	42	42	30	34	19
Rankin 5	77	63	20	19	18	14	17	14
Dead	31	23	64	54	72	65	87	76
Total Patients with Data	307	310	307	309	303	303	294	298

Data are from patients in the NINDS rt-PA Stroke Trial. Total n = 312 per t-PA and placebo groups. Patients with missing values were excluded.
PLA = placebo.

Table 3
Disposition Results from the NINDS rt-PA Stroke Trial

Discharge destination	Number (%) t-PA	Number (%) placebo
Home	151 (48)	112 (36)
Rehabilitation Unit	91 (29)	115 (37)
Nursing Home	22 (7)	39 (13)
Dead	35 (11)	40 (13)
Other Facility	13 (4)	6 (2)

Compared home to all other dispositions, chi-square test $p < 0.01$.

life-years will accrue into the best outcome, Rankin = 0, per 1000 patients treated. The results of the Monte Carlo simulation are shown in the last column as 90% certainty ranges for each outcome. These ranges represent the forecasts for each outcome that lie between 5th and 95th percentile of the 10,000 predicted values for each outcome. An outcome in which the range of values significantly straddles zero would have a low probability of occurring, whereas an outcome in which more than 90% of the predicted values are on one side of zero would be more likely. Inspection of this column shows that thrombolytic treatment is associated with an increase in the number of life-years in the Rankin = 0 category, and a decrease in the number of life years in the moderate/severe category.

For every 1000 patients treated with t-PA, the model predicts 55 more intracerebral hemorrhages and 116 more patients discharged home, compared to pla-

Table 4
One-way Sensitivity Analysis of Health and Economic Outcomes per 1000 Patients Eligible to be Treated with t-PA

Health outcomes	Placebo	TPA	Difference	5th and 95th percentiles*
Life Years by Rankin Category				
Rankin 0 - No Symptoms	826	1520	694	257 to 1072
Rankin 1 - No Disability Despite Symptoms	1394	1866	472	-244 to 1017
Rankin 2 - Slight Disability	1101	776	-325	-719 to -59
Rankin 3 - Moderate Disability	1268	1322	54	-357 to 393
Rankin 4 - Moderate/Severe Disability	1366	959	-407	-863 to -133
Rankin 5 - Severe Disability	1179	1054	-125	-514 to 147
Total Life Years (30 yr)	7135	7498	363	-985 to 982
QALYs	3183	3934	751	-15 to 1142
*Economic outcomes (discounted**, $ thousands)*				
t-PA acquisition cost	0	2250	2250	2135 to 2406
Physician cost for t-PA administration	0	300	300	206 to 389
Initial hospitalization	14,923	14,121	(803)	-2282 to 1236
Future hospitalization for stroke	5222	5493	271	-861 to 813
Nursing Home	32,975	28,157	(4818)	-12,195 to -1002
Rehabilitation	11,146	9768	(1378)	-3970 to -398
Total cost (acute plus long-term care)	62,716	58,461	(4255)	-13,022 to 531
Cost at 1 yr	29,810	29,207	(604)	-3481 to 2004
Cost-Effectiveness ($1000)				
Hospitalization cost per additional patient discharged home			15	1.9 to 80
Cost per QALY gained			(8)	-76 to 17

*Represents the estimated 5th and 95th percentiles for the distribution of possible values of the difference based on the Monte Carlo one-way sensitivity analysis using the ranges specified and 10,000 iterations.
**Discounted at 5% per year.
QALYs = Quality adjusted life years.

cebo. Discounted costs for hospitalization are about $1.7 million greater owing to treatment. However, costs for nursing home care and rehabilitation, are significantly reduced by t-PA treatment by about $4.8 and $1.3 million, respectively. The increase in acute care costs represents an incremental cost of $15,000 for each additional patient discharged home rather than a rehabilitation facility or nursing home. The overall impact on both acute and long-term costs (90% certainty) is a net decrease of over $4 million (–13 million to 531 thousand) to the health care system for every 1000 patients treated. The estimated impact on long-term health outcomes is 751 QALYs saved over 30 yr for 1000 patients. The results of the multi-way sensitivity analysis showed the probabilities are 93% and 94% that treatment with t-PA results in decreased cost and increased QALYs, respectively. The one-way sensitivity analysis showed that variation of each of the assumptions from their minimum to maximum values still resulted in positive QALYs and cost savings. The variables with the largest impact on health outcome were the t-PA hemorrhage rate and the overall mortality factor. As the hemorrhage rate was varied from 6% to 20%, the number of QALYs saved decreased from 765 to 335. As the overall mortality factor was varied from 1.25 to 4, the number of QALYs saved decreased from 1129 to 575. The variables with the largest impact on cost were initial length of stay and annual nursing home cost. In order to eliminate the overall cost savings, the t-PA group length of stay would have to exceed the placebo group by 2.1 d or the annual nursing home cost would have to be less than $4700 per year. The t-PA drug cost had minimal impact.

Implications for Clinicians

The decision to administer t-PA to an eligible patient should be based on the proven health benefits alone, as detailed in Chapters 7 and 17. The cost-effectiveness analysis becomes important only when forecasting budget costs at a macro level for a health care system. Also, the costs of interventions designed to increase the number of eligible patients could be compared to the predicted cost savings. Our analysis has been criticized for excluding the costs of developing acute stroke teams and improving prehospital care, but we believe strongly that these costs do not belong to t-PA, but rather to good stroke management. For example, the emergency department assessment for t-PA eligibility should be identical to that used to distinguish ischemia from hemorrhage and triage appropriately. Additionally, protocol changes required to manage acute stroke urgently generally don't require costly, new technology, but rather expeditious use of existing resources (6).

Hospitalization costs were decreased since t-PA shortened the length of hospital stay. Considering all hospitalization costs, however, including cost of the drug and management of symptomatic hemorrhages in some cases, t-PA use was estimated to increase hospitalization costs by approx $15,000 for each additional patient discharged home rather than to a nursing home or inpatient rehabilitation.

The 1-yr cost savings of $600,000 dollars per 1000 treated patients indicates that the additional hospitalization costs are probably recovered within a year.

The sensitivity analysis strongly supports the reality of the cost savings we report, with probabilities greater than 90% that t-PA increases quality of life and decreases health care costs. The analysis beyond 1 yr required many assumptions, so we analyzed a pessimistic scenario that assumed no differences between treatment and placebo beyond 1 yr. Even with this highly unrealistic scenario, treatment with t-PA remained cost effective. Thus, thrombolytic stroke therapy joins a very small number of therapies that not only saves disability, but also saves dollars. To put these results in perspective, note that few other therapies result in net cost savings to the health care system; two traditional examples are prenatal care and early childhood vaccinations (7–11). These therapies cost money to administer, but overall there is a net cost reduction owing to lower disease incidence. Actual cost savings are realized to the health system when reduced disability at discharge translates into a significant reduction in the utilization of subacute and long-term care facilities. In this analysis, t-PA for eligible stroke patients appears to represent a "win-win" situation: improved patient outcomes are associated with a net cost savings to the health care system. Truly integrated health systems that cover both acute and long-term care facilities are rare, however. The payer responsible for the increased hospitalization costs may not be the one to benefit from reduced long-term costs. To rationalize this inequity may necessitate increased reimbursement or adjusted capitation rates for acute stroke admissions.

SUB-GROUP ANALYSIS

The inclusion and exclusion criteria used in the original study are now used to select eligible patients for thrombolytic therapy. In applying the selection criteria to individual patients (see Chapter 17), it would be useful to know if there are any particular subgroups of patients with increased likelihood to benefit or suffer harm from t-PA. Indeed, some critics of the original work have noted the lack of such subgroup data in the literature (12). To address these concerns, we compared outcome in t-PA and placebo-treated patients with pretreatment information to identify subgroups that may or may not particularly benefit from t-PA treatment (13).

Methods

In the original report, we found that odds of a good outcome were associated with age, race, gender, smoking, problem drinking, diabetes, hypertension, atherosclerosis, atrial fibrillation, other cardiac disease, stroke subtype, baseline NIHSS, presence of thrombus or early signs of infarction (hypodensity or midline shift) on baseline CT scan, admission and baseline blood pressure (14) (see

Table 5). None of the findings, however, could be used to subselect patients, since the odds ratios were calculated using univariate models. That is, we did not correct for the fact that some of these variables interact with each other; such an interaction could erroneously indicate a subgroup of patients susceptible to increased benefit or harm. To account for such interactions, we used a multivariable modeling method. In a rigorous and stepwise manner, we sequentially tested each variable, and each interaction between variables, for possible influence on response to treatment. In this analysis we found that race, diabetes, hypertension, baseline mean arterial pressure, and baseline systolic blood pressure showed a significant interaction with t-PA treatment. The selected variables and interactions were then included in a multivariable model, and interactions among confounding variables were identified.

Results

To illustrate the preliminary univariate results, the effect of age on outcome is shown in Fig. 1. In each decile the proportion of responders was greater in the t-PA group. Similarly, the effect of stroke subtype is illustrated in Fig. 2. Again, the benefit of thrombolysis was apparent in each subtype of ischemic stroke. During the multivariable analysis, however, we found significant confounding interactions among several variables. Age-by-baseline NIHSS and age-by-mean arterial pressure interactions were significant (i.e., patients with older age and higher baseline stroke scale scores or older age and higher admission mean arterial blood pressure were less likely to have a favorable outcome). None of the two-way interactions significantly interacted with treatment, however, suggesting that none of these confounds influenced patient responsiveness to treatment. This concept is illustrated in Fig. 3. The proportion of patients who achieve a favorable outcome declines markedly with increasing levels of severity. In each severity quartile, however, the proportion of favorable responders is always greater in the thrombolysis group, and the relative benefit is always positive, ranging from 20 to 40%. Thus, although many variables adversely affect outcome, none reduce the chances of favorable response to thrombolysis.

Table 6 shows the final results of the multivariable model process. Treatment with t-PA remained strongly and independently associated with favorable outcome (global odds ratio 1.96, $p < 0.0001$). The only terms that remained important predictors of outcome, after correcting for the influences of all other confounding variables, were the age-by-NIH Stroke Scale interaction term, diabetes, admission mean arterial pressure-by-age interaction, and thrombus or hypodensity/mass effect on baseline CT scan (i.e., for all randomized patients, global odds ratios <1). None of these terms, however, had a significant interaction with t-PA treatment. That is, each of the variables and interactions in Table 6 significantly influenced outcome, but none of them influenced the likelihood of differential response to t-PA. In nearly all subgroups, the proportion of

Table 5

Relationship between Baseline Covariates and Outcome (Global Odds Ratio): Univariate Analyses and Treatment Interactions

Variable	Global odds ratio	95% confidence limits	p-value*	Treatment interaction p-value**
t-PA Treatment	1.86	1.38–2.5	<0.001	
Age	0.97	0.95–0.98	<0.001	0.49
Race				
Hispanic vs Black	1.05	0.49–2.21	0.31	0.13
Hispanic vs White	1.34	0.65	0.10	0.83
Gender	1.29	0.95–1.75	0.007	0.78
Cigarette Smoking in Previous Year	1.54	1.13–2.10	0.01	0.98
Drinking Problems	1.48	1.10–2.00	0.004	0.05
History of Diabetes	0.57	0.39–0.84	<0.001	0.19
History of Hypertension	0.55	0.41–0.75	0.04	0.34
History of Atherosclerosis	0.69	0.49–0.98	0.008	0.96
History of Atrial Fibrillation	0.57	0.38–0.86	0.18	0.66
History of Other Cardiac Disease	0.82	0.61–1.10	0.79	0.99
Prior Stroke	0.96	0.70–1.31	0.78	0.68
Aspirin (NSAID)	0.96	0.70–1.31	0.008	0.78
Baseline Stroke Sub-types***				
Small vs Cardioembolic	0.44	0.28–0.69		
Small vs Large	0.45	0.29–0.71		
Small vs Other	0.69	0.27–1.71		
Baseline NIH Stoke Scale	0.86	0.84–0.88	0.0001	0.78
Early CT Findings With Thrombus	0.43	0.28–0.66	0.0001	0.53
Early CT Findings Without Thrombus	0.65	0.33–1.26	0.20	0.42
Weight (actual, ranked)	1.00	1.00–1.00	0.87	0.69
Percent of Correct Dose (ranked)	1.00	1.00–1.00	0.30	0.80

Admission Blood Pressure (MAP)	0.99	0.99–1.00	0.12	0.18
Admission Systolic Blood Pressure	1.00	0.99–1.00	0.14	0.53
Admission Diastolic Blood Pressure	0.99	0.99–1.00	0.22	0.89
Baseline Blood Pressure (MAP)	0.99	0.98–1.00	0.22	0.64
Baseline Systolic Blood Pressure	0.99	0.99–1.00	0.13	0.14
Baseline Diastolic Blood Pressure	0.99	0.98	0.27	0.33
Centers	1.01	0.94–1.08	0.82	0.23
Time From Stroke Onset to Treatment	1.00	1.00–1.01	0.62	0.28
Admission Temperature	1.15	1.003–1.33	0.046	0.83

*Association of specified variable with outcome (global) including treatment effect.

**Association of specified treatment interaction with outcome (global) in model including the interaction and effects for treatment and the other variable in the interaction.

***Stroke Subtype was diagnosed based on all information available to the treating physician prior to starting t-PA therapy. Small = small vessel (lacunar), large = large vessel.

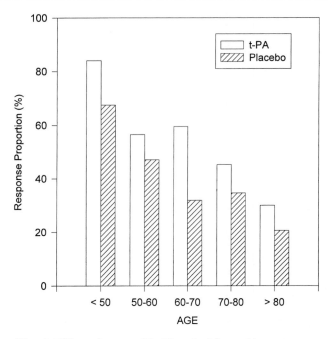

Fig. 1. Effect of age on likelihood of favorable response.

patients with favorable outcome is greater in the t-PA treated group. Further-more, in the 49 patients with age > 75 and admission NIHSS > 20 there appeared to be no favorable response to treatment. However, closer evaluation of this subgroup, including analysis of outcome categories such as mild or moderate, suggested a treatment benefit, as shown in Fig. 4. The proportion of patients who achieved a nearly normal score on the NIHSS was zero, suggesting no benefit. In the mild category, though, with NIHSS scores between 2 and 8, there was a significant benefit in the treated group *(13)*. Similarly in this most severe patient cohort, the treated group was significantly more likely to show independence in Activities of Daily Living, as shown in Fig. 4 by the proportion with Barthel Index scores greater than 50.

Implications for Clinicians

Despite rigorous procedures, and a liberal p-value cut-off of 0.1, we could identify no pretreatment information that predicted a differential response to t-PA treatment. Thrombolytic treatment was independently and strongly associated with increased likelihood of favorable outcome 3 mo after stroke *(14)*. After other confounding variables were included in the multivariable model, the absence of any interactions with treatment suggests a persistent beneficial effect of t-PA treatment across all subgroups tested. Although tempting, it is fallacious

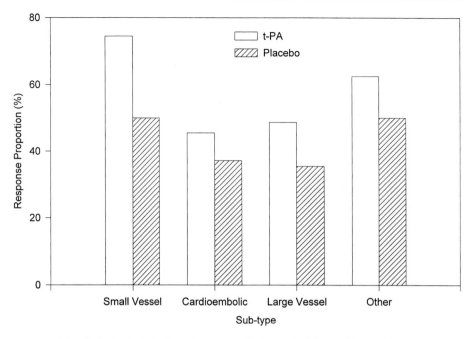

Fig. 2. Effect of stroke subtype on likelihood of favorable response.

to select a subgroup from univariate data, such as Table 5, and conclude that t-PA is not beneficial for that subgroup *(15)*. The broader trend of t-PA benefit demonstrable across all subgroups, using rigorous statistical methods, makes the single isolated subgroup aberration more likely to be a random occurrence related to small sample size in the subgroup than a clinically meaningful, biological trend *(15)*. That is, we found no evidence to justify withholding t-PA from any of the subgroups we studied.

There are a few limitations to the analysis presented here. The original trial included enough patients to address the primary hypothesis, not the subgroup analyses. Nevertheless, power analyses showed that we could have detected significant treatment interactions with a power greater than 90%: if an important interaction was present, there is a greater than 90% probability that we would have found it. Another limitation is the selection of variables for the analysis. We chose 27 baseline data items that were likely to be related to either outcome or differential treatment response. There could be other variables but we found no literature supporting inclusion of such. In prior studies, the variables usually associated with long-term stroke outcome included age, severity, smoking, diabetes, heart disease and hypertension *(16–18)*. These same variables appeared in our analyses, suggesting that there are probably not other important variables missing.

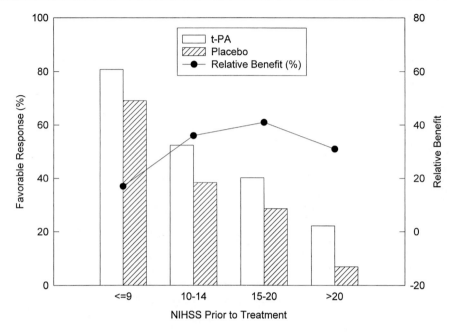

Fig. 3. Effect of stroke severity (NIHSS) on likelihood of a favorable response.

Some of the predictor variables show important effects on long-term outcome. Patients with more severe baseline deficits, or who are older, do poorly over the long term, but t-PA was effective in such patients (Figs. 1 and 3). There was no threshold value for age, NIHSS score, or any particular stroke subtype that precluded t-PA treatment. Thus, t-PA offers some benefit for older, sicker patients, even if the overall likelihood of a good outcome is less (Fig. 4). The careful clinician will note, however, that the t-PA package insert cautions that use in patients with an NIHSS score greater than 22 may be hazardous. The analyses reported here were not available to the US Food and Drug Administration at the time the drug was approved for stroke. Since then, it has become clear that no single value of the NIHSS can be used rigidly for selecting patients; the clinician must exercise judgment in each case.

LONG-TERM OUTCOME

In the original report, benefit of thrombolysis was demonstrated using follow-up data obtained 3 mo after stroke. Although the 3-mo outcome of patients treated with t-PA for acute ischemic stroke is compelling, showing a long-term benefit would solidify the case for the use of t-PA in similar patients. Any short-term risk would be offset by a long period of disease-free survival, long-term independence, and reduced long-term supportive care costs. If a long-term ben-

Table 6
Final Multivariate Model Comparing Possible Predictor Variables to Outcome Using 3-Mo Outcome Data

Variable	Global odds ratio	95% confidence limits	p-value
t-PA Treatment	2.02	1.45, 2.81	0.0001
Age X NIHSS*	0.993	0.993,0.998	0.0001
History of Diabetes	0.47	0.31, 0.72	0.0004
Age X Admission Map	*1.0009	1.000, 1.0016	0.026
Early CT Findings With Thrombus	0.49	0.29, 0.80	0.0046

*Age, NIH Stroke Scale and admission Mean Arterial Pressure are also included individually in the model. Their odds ratios are not shown, as they cannot be interpreted directly in the presence of the interaction.

NIHSS

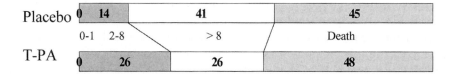

Barthel

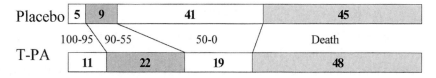

Fig. 4. Effect of tPA on outcome (Barthel and NIHSS) in 49 patients with age older than 75 and baseline severity greater than 20. Note the beneficial effect in mild and moderate categories. See text for explanation.

efit could not be demonstrated, however, the argument in favor of thrombolytic stroke therapy weakens. The decision to use thrombolysis for stroke would depend on the short-term benefits and risks only.

To address these important issues, the 1-yr outcome data for patients enrolled in the NINDS t-PA stroke study will be presented *(19)*. These data may allow clinicians to understand the true benefit of t-PA for patients with acute ischemic stroke, especially with regard to long-term quality of life issues.

Methods

All patients enrolled in the original trial were followed for 1 yr and outcome data were collected at 24 h and 3, 6, and 12 mo following stroke. Telephone contact was made at 6 and 12 mo to determine the patient's status (alive or dead); their ability to perform daily activities (Barthel Index) (20) and assessment of functional disability (Modified Rankin) (2) and Glasgow Outcome Scales (4). Data were also collected for serious medical events including intracerebral hemorrhage and recurrent stroke. During the entire follow-up period, telephone evaluators (certified nurse coordinators or study physicians), patients, and their caregivers remained blinded to treatment allocation. Several studies have validated telephone assessment of stroke outcome (20–22). Using an intention-to-treat analysis, patients who died before follow-up or those for whom follow-up was unavailable, were assigned the most unfavorable scores for all outcome measures.

A total of 624 patients were randomized into the NINDS t-PA Stroke Trial: 291 in Part 1 and 333 in Part 2. Only 15 patients (2.4% : 7 t-PA, 8 placebo) were not available for 6-mo follow-up and 26 patients (4.1% : 14 t-PA, 8 placebo) were unavailable for follow-up at 1 yr for all the three scales. Under the intent-to-treat analysis, these patients were considered to have an unfavorable outcome in each scale. By assigning an unfavorable outcome to these patients, a worst-case scenario for treatment with t-PA is created; i.e., all of these patients are assumed to have done poorly, therefore, biasing the results against treatment. If any of these patients had a good outcome, the actual benefit of t-PA will be underestimated in the analyses.

Results

A favorable outcome at 6 and 12 mo occurred more often in t-PA compared to placebo-treated patients. The odds ratio (95% confidence intervals) for favorable outcome at 6 mo was 1.7 (1.3, 2.3) and for 1 yr 1.7 (1.2, 2.3). A similar pattern is seen in the univariate tests for Barthel Index, Modified Rankin, and Glasgow Outcome Scales. The distributions of outcome scores for the three scales are summarized in Fig. 5. For each scale, the proportion of patients improved to minimal or no disability was greater in the t-PA group. The proportions of patients suffering moderate or severe disability, or death, were reduced by t-PA on all three scales. At 1 yr, the range of absolute improvement was 11 to 13% and relative improvement 32 to 46% for the three outcome scales. The distributions are summarized in Fig. 6. These results are very similar to those seen at 3 mo: t-PA treated patients were at least 30% more likely to be independent of their stroke symptoms at 1 yr compared to placebo patients; (relative risk 1.3–1.5 for the individual scales at 1 yr). Importantly, the favorable outcomes were not accompanied by an increase in severe disability or mortality.

Barthel Index

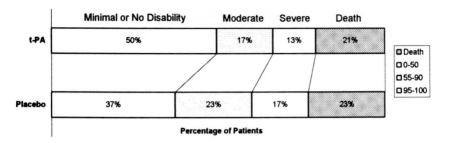

Modified Rankin Scale

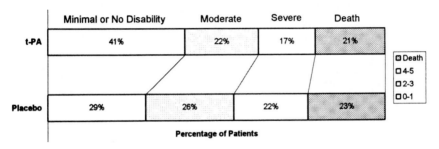

Glasgow Outcome Scale

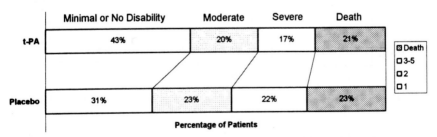

Fig. 5. Effect of tPA on outcome 6 mo following stroke. See text for explanation.

In the treatment group, there were 23 symptomatic hemorrhages during the first 3 mo of which 20 occurred within the first 36 h. Six (26%) of these patients were alive at 1 yr. In the placebo group, 4 symptomatic hemorrhages occurred within 3 mo, 2 of which occurred within 36 h. One (25%) of these four patients was alive at 12 mo. Between 3 mo and 1 yr there were 2 additional symptomatic

Barthel Index

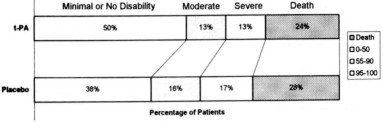

Modified Rankin Scale

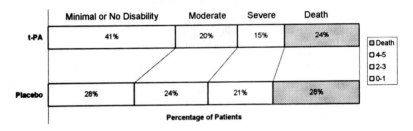

Glasgow Outcome Scale

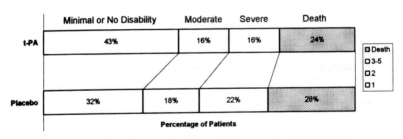

Fig. 6. Effect of tPA on outcome 1 yr following stroke. See text for explanation.

hemorrhages in the treatment group, of which one survived to 1 yr. In the placebo group, there was one additional symptomatic hemorrhage between 3 mo and 1 yr, and this patient did not survive.

The proportion of patients surviving between 3 and 12 mo after stroke was consistently higher in the t-PA group compared to placebo, illustrated in Fig. 7. However, there were no statistically significant differences in mortality between the two groups at 6 mo ($p = 0.31$) and 1 yr ($p = 0.29$). Recurrent stroke in 1 yr occurred in 34/624 patients, including two patients with two recurrences. Recur-

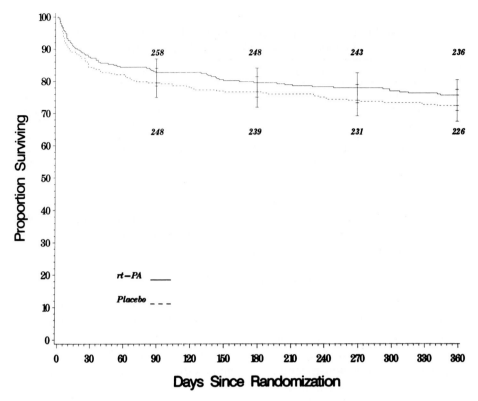

Fig. 7. One-year survival in the NINDS tPA Stroke Trial.

rent stroke in the first 3 mo occurred in 24 of these 34 patients (12 t-PA, 12 placebo). The recurrence rate difference between treatment groups was not significant, using the log-rank test ($p = 0.89$ at 6 mo and 0.96 at 1 yr).

Using the subgroup analysis methods described above, we also fit a multivariable model to identify baseline variables associated with a favorable outcome or death at 6 mo and 1 yr *(3)*. The final multivariable models are presented in Table 7 for the 12-mo outcomes. Variables included in the 6-mo final model were diabetes, age, NIHSS score at baseline, age by NIHSS score interaction, early CT findings including hyperdense artery sign, time (from stroke onset to treatment), and time by treatment interaction. The variables remaining in the final 12-mo model were diabetes, age, NIHSSS, and age by NIHSSS interaction. There was no interaction between treatment response and presumed stroke subtype at 6 and 12 mo, confirming that no particular subgroup was more likely to benefit from thrombolysis.

The baseline variables that were predictors of death at 12 mo were age, NIHSS score, diabetes, and diabetes by age interaction. After adjusting for these vari-

Table 7
Final Multivariate Model Comparing Possible Predictor Variables
To Outcome Using One-Year Outcome Data.

Variable	Global odds ratio	95% confidence limits	p-value
t-PA Treatment	1.81	1.27, 2.57	0.001
Age X NIHSS*	0.996	0.993,0.999	0.002
History of Diabetes	0.39	0.25, 0.62	0.001

*Age, NIH Stroke Scale and admission Mean Arterial Pressure are also included individually in the model. Their odds ratios are not shown, as they cannot be interpreted directly in the presence of the interaction.

ables identified as prognostic for death at 12 mo, treatment with t-PA remained significant. Patients with higher baseline NIHSS score have a lower chance of survival than patients with lower NIHSS scores.

Implications for Clinicians

Consistent benefit of t-PA at 3 mo, 6 mo, and 1 yr indicate that the beneficial effect of t-PA is durable over the long term. The data strongly argue in favor of the use of t-PA for acute ischemic stroke when patients can be treated within 3 h of symptom onset. The long-term follow-up of patients enrolled in the NINDS t-PA Stroke study demonstrates that the magnitude of benefit associated with t-PA 3 mo after stroke was sustained at 6 mo and 1 yr. Patients treated with t-PA were at least 30% more likely than placebo-treated patients to have minimal or no disability at 6 mo and 1 yr after treatment. In addition, t-PA treated patients at 1 yr were less likely to be severely disabled or to have died from their stroke. These figures demonstrate an overall improvement for t-PA treated patients. Treated patients were also more likely to have lesser degrees of disability with fewer moderately or severely disabled patients.

Multivariable analysis revealed similar results to that reported for the 3 mo favorable outcome *(see above)* where associated baseline characteristics included age interacting with baseline NIHSS, age interacting with admission blood pressure, early CT findings and diabetes. Consistent with the 3-mo model, age interacting with baseline NIHSSS and diabetes remained in both the 6 and 12 mo models. This data suggests that for any age, patients with a higher NIHSSS at baseline have less chance of having a favorable outcome compared to the patients with a lower NIHSS. As of 3 mo, however, none of the identified variables associated with 6 or 12 mo favorable outcome interacted with treatment: patients cannot be selected for treatment *a priori* based on the presence or absence of these features (as in Fig. 4). In addition, after adjusting for other baseline variables, an association between presumed stroke subtype and favorable outcome over the long term could not be detected. This suggests that patients should not be selected for or excluded from treatment with t-PA based solely on stroke mechanism.

SUMMARY

In this chapter we amplified on much of the data presented in the NINDS t-PA for stroke trial to show three points: thrombolytic therapy for stroke is cost effective; there are no particular subgroups to be preferred or avoided for treatment; and the benefits are sustained over the long term. These data could not be included in the original report, but the main points have now all been subjected to peer review and are published. Taken together with the initial report, these analyses show that in the NINDS trial, thrombolytic therapy was effective.

REFERENCES

1. Fagan SC, Morgenstern LB, Petitta A, Ward RE, Tilley B, Marler JR, et al. NINDS rt-PA Stroke Study Group. Cost-effectiveness of tissue plasminogen activator for acute ischemic stroke. *Neurology* 1998;50:883–890.
2. Rankin J. Cerebral vascular accidents in patients over the age of 60: Prognosis. *Scott Med J* 1957;2:200–215.
3. Mahoney FT, Barthel DW. Functional evaluation: Barthel Index. Md State Med J 1965;14:61–65.
4. Jennett B, Bond M. Assessment of outcome after severe brain damage. A practical scale. Lancet 1975;480–484.
5. Solomon NA, Russo CJ, Lee J, Schulman KA. Patient preferences for stroke outcome. Stroke 1994;25:1721–1725.
6. Tilley BC, Lyden PD, Brott TG, Lu M, Levine SR, Welch KMA. Total quality improvement method for reduction of delays between emergency department admission and treatment of acute ischemic stroke. *Arch Neurol* 1997;54:1466–1474.
7. Avruch S, Cackley AP. Savings achieved by giving WIC benefits to women prenatally. *Public Health Rep* 1995;110:27–34.
8. Schoenbaum SC, Hyde JN, Baroshesky L, Crampton K. Benefit-cost analysis of rubella vaccination policy. *N Engl J Med* 1976;294:306–310.
9. Koplan JP, Schoenbaum SC, Weinstein MC, Fraser DW. Pertussis vaccine—an analysis of benefits, risks and costs. *N Engl J Med* 1979;301:906–911.
10. Koplan JP, Preblud SR. A benefit-cost analysis of mumps vaccine. *Am J Dis Child* 1982;136:362–364.
11. Cutting WA. Cost-benefit evaluations of vaccination programmes. *Lancet* 1980;8195 part 1:634–635.
12. Furlan A, Kanoti G. When Is Thrombolysis Justified in Patients with Acute Ischemic Stroke? A Bioethical Perspective. *Stroke* 1997;214–218.
13. NINDS TPA Stroke Study Group. Generalized Efficacy of t-PA for Acute Stroke. *Stroke* 1997;28:2119–2125.
14. NINDS rt-PA Stroke Study Group. Tissue plasminogen activator for acute ischemic stroke. *N Engl J Med* 1995;333:1581–1587.
15. Yusuf S, Wittes J, Probstfield J, Tyroler H. Analysis and Interpretation of Treatment Effects in Subgroups of Patients in Randomized Clinical Trials. *JAMA* 1991;266:93–98.
16. Carlberg B, Asplund K, Hägg E. The prognostic value of admission blood pressure in patients with acute stroke. *Stroke* 1993;24:1372–1375.

17. Loewen SC, Anderson BA. Predictors of stroke outcome using objective measurement scales. *Stroke* 1990;21:78–81.
18. Katz S, Ford AB, Chinn AB, Newill VA. Prognosis after strokes: II. Long-course of 159 patients. *Medicine* 1966;454:236–246.
19. Kwiatkowski TG, Libman RB, Frankel M, Tilley BC, Morgenstern LB, Lu M, et al. Effects of tissue plasminogen activator for acute ischemic stroke at one year. The National Institute of Neurological Disorders and Stroke rt-PA Stroke Study Group. *N Engl J Med* 1999; 340:1781–1787.
20. Lyden P, Broderick J, Mascha E, NINDS rt-PA Stroke Study Group. Reliability of the Barthel Index Outcome Measure selected for the NINDS t-PA Stroke Trial. In: Thrombolytic Therapy in Acute Ischemic Stroke III, Yamaguchi T, Mori E, Minematsu K, del Zoppo G, eds. Springer-Verlag: Tokyo. 1995; pp. 327–333.
21. Shinar D, Gross CR, Bronstein KS, Licata-Gehr EE, Eden DT, Cabrara AR, Fishman IG, Roth AA, Barwick JA, Kunitz SC. Reliability of the activities of daily living scale and its use in the telephone interview. *Arch Phys Med Rehabil* 1987;68:723–728.
22. Candelise L, Pinardi G, Aritzu E, Musicco M. Telephone interview for stroke outcome assessment. *Cerebrovasc Dis* 1994;4:341–343.

10 Intra-Arterial Thrombolysis in Acute Ischemic Stroke

Anthony J. Furlan, MD,
Randall Higashida, MD,
Irene Katzan, MD, and Alex Abou-Chebl, MD

CONTENTS

INTRODUCTION
INITIAL PATIENT SELECTION
    FOR DIRECT INTRA-ARTERIAL THROMBOLYSIS
GENERAL TECHNIQUE OF IA THROMBOLYSIS
THROMBOLYTIC AGENT
ADJUNCTIVE THERAPY
RATIONALE FOR IA THROMBOLYSIS
SELECTED CASE SERIES OF IA THROMBOLYSIS:
    CAROTID TERRITORY
SELECTED CASE SERIES IA THROMBOLYSIS:
    VERTEBROBASILAR TERRITORY
THE PROLYSE IN ACUTE CEREBRAL THROMBOEMBOLISM TRIALS
    (PROACT I AND PROACT II)
BRAIN HEMORRHAGE AND IA THROMBOLYSIS
IV VS IA THROMBOLYSIS
LIMITATIONS OF IA THROMBOLYSIS
SPECIAL SETTINGS FOR IA THROMBOLYSIS
SUMMARY AND FUTURE DIRECTIONS
REFERENCES

INTRODUCTION

Intra-arterial (IA) thrombolysis provides an alternative to intravenous (IV) thrombolysis in selected patients with acute ischemic stroke. Recent advances in

From: *Thrombolytic Therapy for Stroke*
Edited by: P. D. Lyden © Humana Press Inc., Totowa, NJ

the field of neurointerventional radiology, with the development of extremely soft, compliant microcatheters and steerable microguidewires, along with high resolution fluoroscopy and digital imaging, and nonionic contrast agents, have made it feasible and safe to access the major intracranial blood vessels around the circle of Willis from a percutaneous transfemoral approach under local anesthesia. Rapid local delivery of fibrinolytic agents is now feasible using these techniques and is performed at many major medical centers in selected patients with acute cerebral ischemia.

INITIAL PATIENT SELECTION
FOR DIRECT INTRA-ARTERIAL THROMBOLYSIS

The initial clinical and computed tomography (CT) scan selection criteria for IA thrombolysis are similar to those for IV tissue-plasminogen activator (t-PA) *(1)*. IA thrombolysis has been used most successfully in patients with acute middle cerebral artery (MCA) occlusion. There is evidence that the treatment window for IA thrombolysis extends to at least 6 h from stroke onset in patients with MCA occlusion. Other potential candidates for IA thrombolysis include patients with extracranial internal carotid artery (ICA) occlusion, intracranial carotid artery "T" occlusion or basilar artery occlusion.

Patients who present with an acute stroke within 6 h of onset should initially be examined by a neurologist familiar with the IV t-PA selection criteria. The baseline National Institutes of Health Stroke Scale score (NIHSS) in most patients considered for IA thrombolysis is >10. Baseline laboratory evaluation should include a complete blood count with platelets and differential, coagulation studies, including thrombin time, activated partial thromboplastin time, and International normalization ratio (INR), activated clotting time (ACT), fibrinogen, plasminogen and alpha 2-antiplasmin levels, serum electrolytes, and an electrocardiogram.

A CT scan is performed to exclude hemorrhage and major early signs of infarction which would preclude thrombolytic therapy. The precise site of arterial occlusion in patients with acute ischemic stroke of <6 h duration cannot be determined solely on the basis of a neurological examination (NIHSS) and CT scan *(2)*. In about 33% of patients with acute stroke owing to occlusion of the MCA the CT scan will demonstrate an hyperdense MCA sign signifying thrombus in the MCA (Fig. 1) *(3)*. Patients with an appropriate clinical picture and a hyperdense MCA sign on CT should be considered for immediate angiography and IA thrombolysis. If quickly available, noninvasive testing with carotid duplex and transcranial doppler, CT angiography (CTA), or magnetic resonance angiography (MRA) can be used to screen for major vessel occlusions treatable with IA thrombolysis.

GENERAL TECHNIQUE OF IA THROMBOLYSIS

In patients with appropriate clinical and CT criteria, a complete four vessel cerebral angiogram, from a transfemoral approach, should be performed to evalu-

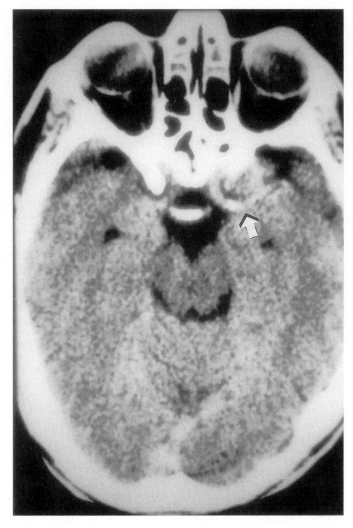

Fig. 1. Hyperdense MCA sign signifying thrombus in the proximal left MCA (arrow).

ate the site of vessel occlusion, extent of thrombus, number of territories involved, and collateral circulation. A diagnostic catheter is guided into the high cervical segment of the vascular territory to be treated, followed by the introduction of a 2.3 French coaxial Rapid Transit Microcatheter with an 0.016″ Instinct steerable microguidewire. (Cordis Endovascular Systems, Miami Lakes, Florida) Under direct fluoroscopic visualization, the microcatheter is gently navigated through the intracranial circulation until the tip is embedded within or through the central portion of the thrombus (Fig. 2).

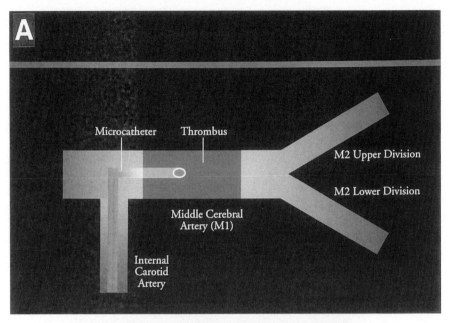

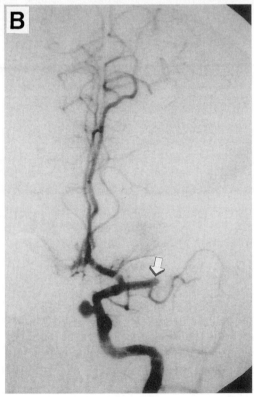

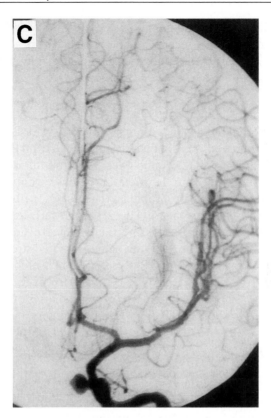

Fig. 2. *(opposite page)* **(A)** Illustration of microcatheter placement into an MCA clot; **(B)** Angiogram demonstrating acute occlusion of the M1 segment of the MCA (arrow); **(C)** Recanalized MCA after 600,000 U IA urokinase.

Many variations in catheter design and delivery technique have been described *(4)*. Two types of microcatheters are being used most often for local cerebral thrombolysis, depending upon the extent of clot formation. For the majority of intra-arterial cases, a single end hole microcatheter is used, whereas for longer segments of clot formation, multiple side hole infusion microcatheters are used. Superselective angiography through the microcatheter is performed at regular intervals to assess for degree of clot lysis and to adjust the dosage and volume of the thrombolytic agent.

A superselective angiogram is performed and if there is partial clot dissolution, the catheter is advanced into the remaining thrombus where additional thrombolysis is performed. As the thrombus is dissolved, the catheter is advanced into more distal branches of the intracranial circulation, so that the majority of the thrombolytic agent enters the occluded vessel and is not washed preferentially into adjacent open blood vessels. Recanalization can be achieved up to 2 h after the procedure begins, although a successful procedure is unlikely if the vessel is at least not partially recanalized before 1 h. The goal is to achieve rapid recanalization with as little thrombolytic agent as possible to limit the extent of brain infarction and to reduce the risk of hemorrhage.

THROMBOLYTIC AGENT

The agent preferred by most neurointerventionalists for IA thrombolysis has been urokinase (Abbokinase®; Abbott Laboratories, Abbott Park, Illinois), in the dose range of 25,000 to 50,000 units over 5–10 min intervals, at the rate of 250,000–500,000 units per hour. However, urokinase is currently not commercially available. Recombinant prourokinase (r-proUK) is a fibrin selective proenzyme which is converted to urokinase (UK) at the clot surface by fibrin associated plasmin. The recanalization efficacy, safety and clinical efficacy of recombinant prourokinase (r-proUK) in patients with acute ischemic stroke owing to MCA occlusion were demonstrated in the Prolyse in Acute Cerebral Thromboembolism Trials (PROACT I and PROACT II) (5,6). However, r-proUK is not yet FDA approved and is not available for general use. Doses of 20 mg to 50 mg of IA t-PA over 1 h have been used by various investigators, but there is considerable uncertainty about the effective dose range and safety of IA t-PA in the cerebral circulation.

ADJUNCTIVE THERAPY

Once a site of vascular occlusion is angiographically confirmed that corresponds to the patient's neurological deficit, IV heparin is given by most neurointerventionalists. Systemic anticoagulation with heparin reduces the risk of catheter related embolism. Also, the thrombolytic effect of some agents such as r-proUK is augmented by heparin. Another rationale for antithrombotic therapy is prevention of acute reocclusion which is more common with atherothrombosis than with cerebral embolism. These indications are counterbalanced by the potentially increased risk of brain hemorrhage when heparin is combined with a thrombolytic agent.

There is no standard heparin regimen established for IA thrombolysis in acute stroke. Some neurointerventionalists employ weight adjusted heparin keeping the ACT between 200–300. PROACT I (5) reported a 27% rate of symptomatic brain hemorrhage when a conventional heparin regimen (100 U/kg bolus, 1000 U per hour for 4 h) was employed with IA r-proUK. Subsequently a standard low dose heparin regimen was used (2000 U bolus, 500 U per hour for 4 h) which reduced the symptomatic brain hemorrhage rate with IA r-proUK to 7% in PROACT I and 10% in PROACT II. This dose of heparin does not prolong the Activated Partial Thromboplastin Time (APTT) in most patients. Based on the PROACT trials, many neurointerventionalists now employ the low dose heparin regimen during IA thrombolysis.

The potent IIb/IIIa platelet inhibitor abciximab (Reopro, Centocor) has been used successfully instead of heparin in patients undergoing acute or elective cerebrovascular interventions *(7)*. Coronary doses of abciximab appear to be safe in patients with acute ischemic stroke up to 24 h after onset *(8)*. IIb/IIIa agents may be most efficacious when the risk of acute reocclusion is great such as basilar artery atherothrombosis. The safety and efficacy of IIb/IIIa agents in patients with embolic occlusion of cerebral vessels, which is the usual cause of MCA occlusion, is less clear.

RATIONALE FOR IA THROMBOLYSIS

The recanalization efficacy of thrombolysis varies with the site of arterial occlusion *(9)*. Patients with ischemic stroke of <6 h duration have a wide variety of arterial occlusion sites, and 20% have no visible occlusion, despite similar neurological presentations *(2)*. In the IV thrombolysis stroke trials neither the sites of arterial occlusion nor the recanalization rates are known. IA thrombolysis permits documentation of both the site of arterial occlusion and recanalization rates.

Recanalization rates with IA thrombolysis are superior to IV thrombolysis for major cerebrovascular occlusions. Recanalization rates for major cerebrovascular occlusions average 70% for IA thrombolysis compared to 34% for IV thrombolysis *(9)*. The differences in recanalization rates are most apparent with large vessel occlusions such as the internal carotid artery (ICA), which is the most resistant vessel to any thrombolysis, the carotid T segment and the proximal (M1) segment of the MCA *(9,10)*. Recanalization has been linked with improved clinical outcome especially in patients with good collateral blood flow and no major early signs of infarction on CT.

The time window for IA thrombolysis appears to be at least 6 h for MCA occlusion, and may be even longer in the vertebrobasilar circulation with some reports of successful therapy up to 48 h after stroke onset *(11)*. The possibly longer time window in posterior circulation occlusions may be owing to greater collateral blood flow in that region *(12)*.

SELECTED CASE SERIES
OF IA THROMBOLYSIS: CAROTID TERRITORY

Early attempts at IA thrombolysis for carotid artery territory occlusions include the reports of Sussman et al. (1958) *(13)*, Atkin et al. (1964) *(14)*, and Labauge et al. (1978) *(15)*. Zeumer *(16)* is often credited with ushering in the modern era of IA stroke thrombolysis in 1983 with a series of case reports describing IA thrombolysis for internal carotid artery occlusion with UK or streptokinase (SK).

In 1988, del Zoppo et al. *(17)* reported 20 patients treated with either IA, SK or UK. Complete recanalization occurred in 15 cases (75%) and 10 patients

(50%) had improvement of neurological symptoms. There were 3 deaths (15%) and 3 patients (15%) with embolic strokes in his series.

Also in 1988, Mori et al. *(18)* reported a series of 22 patients treated for acute occlusion of the MCA with IA UK, in doses ranging between 80,000 to 1.32 million units. Recanalization occurred in 10 cases (45%), of which 4 were complete and 6 had residual stenosis. There was symptomatic improvement in 8 of the 10 (80%) cases with recanalization. In addition, there was a significant correlation between recanalization and improved clinical outcome in his series.

Theron et al. *(19)* reported 12 patients with carotid territory occlusions treated with local IA SK or UK. Most patients were treated within 10 h of stroke onset, although in one case symptoms had recurred over 5 wk. Theron et al. speculated that occlusions involving the lenticulostriate vessels carry the highest risk of hemorrhage since the two symptomatic brain hemorrhages in this series both occurred among the 5 patients with occlusions at this level.

Zeumer et al. (20) reported their experience with local IA UK (750,000 IU) or t-PA (20 mg) given over 2 h in 31 patients with acute carotid territory and 28 patients with acute vertebrobasilar occlusion. All patients received a bolus injection of 5000 IU heparin followed by a 1000 IU/h intravenous heparin infusion during the procedure. In carotid territory patients, treatment had to be finished by the 6th hour after stroke onset. Assuming a very bad prognosis, no time limit was placed on vertebrobasilar cases and the average delay to treatment was 8 h. In the carotid territory, recanalization was achieved in 94% of patients (complete 38%). Five types of carotid territory occlusions were identified: 1) carotid siphon C1/2 segment only; 2) MCA M1; 3) MCA M1 plus M2; 4) MCA M2 or M3; 5) multiple occlusions or multiple emboli beyond M1 and A1. Optimal recanalization and clinical results were obtained only in type 1 and type 4 occlusions. The neurological deficit was minimal or mild in 32%. In the vertebrobasilar territory, a 100% recanalization rate was achieved (complete 75%). The mortality rate was 65%; 7 patients (25%) had a minimal or mild deficit. There were no brain hemorrhages with clinical neurological deterioration, and no apparent difference in efficacy between IA UK and t-PA.

Higashida et al. *(21)* in 1994 also reported their results in 27 cases who were treated for an acute arterial occlusion in 45 vascular territories. Clinically there was neurological improvement in 18 (66.7%) cases. Complications directly related to therapy included symptomatic intracranial hemorrhage in three cases (11.1%). In 8 (29.6%) patients, there was no evidence of clinical improvement and in long-term follow-up there were 9 (33.3%) patient deaths.

In an attempt to speed the time to recanalization, Freitag et al. *(22)* compared 40 patients with carotid territory stroke treated with IA UK or IA t-PA to 15 patients treated with up to 30 mg IA t-PA plus lys-plasminogen (PG). Only 1 patient (2%) experienced brain hemorrhage with clinical neurological deterioration. 40% of the UK-t-PA patients had a Barthel index score >90 at 3 mo compared to 60%

in the lys-PG/t-PA group. For vertebrobasilar patients, long-term survival was 50% in the UK-t-PA group ($n = 20$), and 58% in the lys-PG/t-PA group ($n = 12$).

Matsumoto and Satoh *(23)* have studied IA thrombolysis in 93 patients (1995). This series is atypical in that a 24 h entry window was used. Fifty-seven patients received regional IA UK with a maximal dose of 1,200,000 IU. Nineteen patients received local IA UK, and 18 patients received local IA t-PA. Among the 36 patients with ICA occlusions, none completely recanalized with regional UK ($n = 21$), whereas 33% recanalized with local IA UK (3 of 8) or IA t-PA (2 of 7). Outcome was said to be good or excellent in 8 patients (22%); the mortality rate was 44% (16 of 36). Fourty-one patients had MCA occlusions. The MCA complete recanalization rates were: regional UK, 62% (13 of 21); local UK, 64% (7 of 11); local t-PA, 78% (7 of 9). Clinical outcome was good or excellent in 37% of all MCA patients, and 50% for patients treated with local thrombolysis. Overall MCA mortality was 22% (9 of 41). The parenchymal hematoma rate for ICA occlusion was 6% (2 of 36), and for MCA occlusion 10% (4 of 41). Fourteen of 16 patients with basilar artery occlusion received regional UK (2 local t-PA). Fourty-four percent of basilar artery cases had a 1/3 good or excellent outcome, although 31% died. There was one parenchymal hematoma (6%) in the basilar artery group. Gotoh and Ogata *(24)* reported a 93% recanalization rate in 14 patients (12 MCA) treated with local IA UK starting at the distal clot interface. There were no complications.

Gönner et al. *(25)* retrospectively analyzed a series of 43 consecutive patients treated with IA thrombolysis and found that there was a statistically significant improvement in the success of recanalization if therapy was initiated within 4 h of stroke onset compared to patients treated after 4 h. Lansberg and colleagues *(26)* reported a 73-yr-old patient who received IA t-PA into three occluded left hemispheric vessels. On diffusion-weighted magnetic resonance imaging (DWI) there was no abnormality in the region of the vessel successfully recanalized under 3 h from onset but there were DWI abnormalities in the region of the artery recanalized at 3.5 h and in the territory of the vessel that failed to reopen.

SELECTED CASE SERIES IA THROMBOLYSIS: VERTEBROBASILAR TERRITORY

The natural history of basilar artery occlusion is extremely poor with mortality ranging from 83% to 91% *(27)*. Because of this poor natural history, IA thrombolysis has been preferred in patients with acute basilar artery occlusion. Approximately 278 cases have been reported with an overall basilar artery recanalization rate of 60% *(28)*. Basilar artery occlusions are usually owing to atherothrombosis. There is a high incidence of residual stenosis after basilar artery recanalization which often requires adjuvant therapies including angioplasty, antithrombotic, and antiplatelet agents, and, recently, stenting *(28a)*.

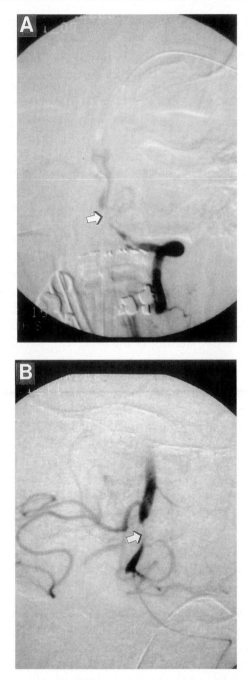

Fig. 3. (A) *(continued on opposite page)* Angiogram demonstrating acute thrombosis of the junction of the distal left vertebral and basilar artery (arrow); **(B)** Microcatheter placement within proximal basilar artery. Thrombus partially

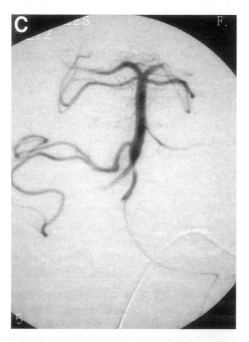

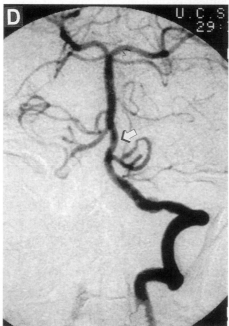

recanalized after 200,000 U IA urokinase (arrow); **(C)** Further recanalization of basilar artery thrombus; **(D)** Final basilar artery recanalization (arrow) after 600,000 U IA urokinase.

In a compilation of reported cases of vertebrobasilar IA thrombolysis, the mortality in patients failing recanalization was 90% compared to 31% mortality in patients achieving at least partial recanalization *(28)*. Good outcomes are strongly associated with recanalization after thrombolytic therapy (see Fig. 3). Hacke et al. *(29)* described 65 consecutive patients with vertebrobasilar occlusion treated either with local IA UK or IA SK plus heparin (*n* = 43) or conventional antiplatelet/anticoagulation therapy (*n* = 22). The recanalization rate among thrombolysis cases was 44% (19 of 43). All patients without recanalization died, whereas 14 of 19 with recanalization survived, 10 with a favorable outcome. The mortality rate with conventional therapy was 86% compared to 67% with thrombolysis. The rate of brain hemorrhage with clinical neurological deterioration was 7% in thrombolysis patients. Schumacher et al. *(30)* reported 29 patients with vertebrobasilar occlusion of <6 h duration treated with up to 1,500,000 IU local UK plus IV heparin. Recanalization was achieved in 66%. There was no or minimal deficit in 45%. The mortality rate was 45%.

Recanalization rates depend upon the location of the vertebrobasilar occlusion. Distal basilar occlusions have higher recanalization rates than proximal occlusions. Emboli often lodge in the distal basilar artery and are easier to lyse than atherosclerosis related thrombi, the usual cause of proximal basilar occlusions *(31)*. Short segment occlusions are easier to lyse than longer segment occlusions *(32)*. Younger patients have higher recanalization rates *(33)*, probably resulting from the increased incidence of embolic occlusions seen in this age group.

The timing of IA vertebrobasilar thrombolysis is often a difficult decision. The presence of coma or tetraparesis for several hours portends a poor prognosis, despite recanalization *(29,31,33)*. Such symptoms do not preclude survival, however, and recovery has been documented after successful recanalization in such patients *(31,32,34)*.

The time window for thrombolysis may be longer in the vertebrobasilar circulation. Many series have included patients up to 24 h *(29)*, 48 h *(31,35)*, and even 72 h *(29,32)* after symptom onset in patients with stuttering courses. An association between time to treatment and outcome has been suggested *(36)* but many series do not support this *(31,37,38)*. In fact, in some studies the time to treatment was actually longer in patients who survived or had good outcomes *(32,37)*. A longer time window may be because of a higher ischemic tolerance or improved collateralization in the posterior circulation. Cross and colleagues *(32)*, reporting on 20 patients with basilar artery thrombosis who received IA thrombolysis, found that better collateral blood flow was correlated with improved responses to thrombolysis and with longer tolerance of ischemia. Patients with proximal basilar artery thrombosis did not seem to have the same benefit.

Patients with vertebrobasilar ischemia often have chronic atherosclerotic disease which allows collaterals to develop over time. As hypothesized by Cross et al. *(32)*, there may be two distinct populations of patients with vertebrobasilar occlusion. Patients with a progressive stuttering course may have better collateral circulation and have better outcomes despite later treatment than patients with the sudden onset of severe deficits owing to poor collaterals even though they may be brought to treatment earlier.

Although some authors believe that patients with brainstem infarction on CT are not candidates for thrombolytic therapy *(29,31)* others have found no correlation with neurologic outcome *(32,37)*. In two separate series, none of the patients who had CT evidence for brainstem infarction developed a hemorrhage. However, because of the experience in the anterior circulation, caution should be used when considering thrombolysis in patients with early infarct signs on CT.

THE PROLYSE IN ACUTE CEREBRAL THROMBOEMBOLISM TRIALS (PROACT I AND PROACT II)

The only randomized, controlled multicenter trials of IA thrombolysis in acute ischemic stroke are PROACT I *(5)* and PROACT II *(6)*. In PROACT I the safety and recanalization efficacy of 6 mg r-proUK was examined in 40 patients with acute ischemic stroke of less than 6 h due to occlusion of the MCA. The control group received IA saline placebo. The recanalization rate was 57.7% in the r-proUK group and only 14.3% in the placebo group. Two doses of heparin were used in PROACT I. In the high heparin group (100 U/kg bolus followed by 1000 U per hour infusion) the recanalization rate was 80% but the symptomatic intracranial hemorrhage (ICH) rate was 27%. In the low heparin group the recanalization rate was 47% but the ICH rate was decreased to 6%. Although not a clinical efficacy trial, there appeared to be a 10–12% increase in excellent outcomes in the IA r-proUK group.

The follow-up clinical efficacy trial, PROACT II *(6)*, was launched in February, 1996 and completed in August, 1998. The results were first reported in February, 1999. PROACT II used an open design with blinded follow-up. Patients were screened with conventional angiography for occlusion of the MCA and had to have a National Institutes of Health Stroke Scale (NIHSS) score between 4 and 30. The patients in PROACT II had a very high baseline stroke severity with a median NIHSS of 17. Patients with early signs of an infarct in greater than one-third of the MCA territory (so-called ECASS criteria) on the baseline CT scan were excluded from the study. One hundred eighty patients were then randomized to receive either 9 mg of IA r-proUK plus low dose IV heparin or low dose IV heparin alone. The primary outcome measure was the percent of patients who achieved a modified Rankin score of ≤2 at 90 d, which signified slight or no neurologic disability. Secondary measures included the percentage of patients who had an NIHSS ≤1 at 90 d, angiographic recanalization, symptomatic intracerebral hemorrhage, and mortality. The median time from onset of symptoms to initiation of IA thrombolysis was 5.3 h.

In the r-proUK treated group there was a 15% absolute benefit in the number of patients who achieved a modified Rankin score of ≤2 at 90 d ($p = 0.043$). On average, seven patients with MCA occlusion would require IA r-proUK for one to benefit. The benefit was most noticeable in patients with a baseline NIHSS between 11 and 20. Recanalization rates were 66% at 2 h for the treatment group and 18% for the placebo group ($p < 0.001$). Symptomatic brain hemorrhage occurred in 10% of the r-proUK group and 2% of the control group. In PROACT II, as in the NINDS trial, despite the higher early symptomatic brain hemorrhage rate, patients overall benefited from the therapy and there was no excess mortality (r-proUK 24%, control 27%).

BRAIN HEMORRHAGE AND IA THROMBOLYSIS

Aggregate data indicate an 8.3% risk of symptomatic brain hemorrhage with IA thrombolysis in the carotid territory and a 6.5% risk in the vertebrobasilar territory *(28)*. There is no evidence that the rate of symptomatic brain hemorrhage is lower with IA thrombolysis than with IV thrombolysis but direct comparisons are difficult. In an uncontrolled series, Gönner et al. *(39)* reported a 4.7% rate of symptomatic brain hemorrhage in 42 patients treated with IA thrombolysis. This series differed from PROACT II in that only 26 out of the 42 patients received heparin; the remainder received aspirin. The higher rate of intracranial hemorrhage with neurological deterioration with IA rpro-UK in PROACT II (10.2%) compared to IV t-PA in NINDS (6.4%) *(1)*, ATLANTIS (7.2%) *(40)* and ECASS II (8.8%) *(41)* must be understood within the context of the greater baseline stroke severity, longer time to treatment and 66% MCA recanalization rate in PROACT II. The median baseline NIHSS score in ATLANTIS and ECASS II was 11, in NINDS 14 and in PROACT II 17. Greater baseline stroke severity was first associated with increased intracranial hemorrhage risk in NINDS and ECASS I. All symptomatic intracranial hemorrhages in PROACT II occurred in patients with a baseline NIHSS score ≥11 and in NINDS the rate of symptomatic brain hemorrhage in patients with a NIHSS >20 was 18%.

Although brain hemorrhage complicating thrombolysis for acute stroke likely reflects reperfusion of necrotic tissue, several series have found no direct relationship between recanalization and hemorrhage risk *(42,43)*. The amount of ischemic damage is a key factor in the development of brain hemorrhage after thrombolysis induced recanalization. Major early CT changes and severity of the initial neurological deficit, both indicators of the extent of ischemic damage, are some of the best predictors of the risk of hemorrhagic transformation *(43,44)*.

Several other factors have been associated with hemorrhage after thrombolysis for both stroke and MI, including thrombolytic dose *(45)*, blood pressure *(43,46,47)*, advanced age, prior head injury *(48)*, and blood glucose >200 mg/dl. Adjunctive antithrombotic therapy may also play a role during IA thrombolysis.

Age was the most important risk factor in one of the largest series of thrombolysis-related intracranial hemorrhage *(48)*. A relationship between advanced age and hemorrhage was demonstrated in the NINDS *(1)* and ECASS trials *(41,44)*. Although there is no strict age cut-off for administering thrombolytics for stroke, physicians need to take age into account especially in patients over age 75 when determining the risk of angiography and IA thrombolysis.

IV VS IA THROMBOLYSIS

There have been no randomized studies comparing recanalization rates and clinical outcomes between IV thrombolysis and IA thrombolysis. Limited data suggest, however, that IV t-PA may be relatively ineffective in patients with ICA or MCA occlusion. Tomsick et al. *(49)* reported that IV t-PA given <3 h from stroke onset was ineffective in patients with a baseline NIHSS score ≥10 and a hyperdense MCA sign (signifying MCA occlusion) on CT.

Endo et al. *(50)* retrospectively reviewed 33 consecutive patients with occlusion of the cervical internal carotid artery. The first 12 patients were treated with IV t-PA or IV urokinase with posttreatment angiograms or sonograms failing to show recanalization. Nine of these patients died and the remainder had a poor outcome (defined as being incapable of independent living). The remaining 21 patients were treated with IA thrombolysis, of these 8 successfully recanalized, 4 of whom recovered with no to minimal neurologic deficits. Of the 13 patients treated with IA thrombolysis who failed to recanalize all had poor outcomes similar to the IV thrombolysis group.

It may be feasible to combine IV and IA thrombolysis. The EMS Bridging Trial *(51)* employed a novel design to investigate the safety of combined IV and IA t-PA. Patients with a NIHSS ≥6 were randomized within 3 h from symptom onset to receive 0.6 mg/kg IV t-PA (*n* = 17) or placebo (*n* = 18) over 30 min followed by angiography. If a thrombus was present, patients in both groups then received local IA t-PA up to a total of 20 mg over 2 h. For patients with M1, M2, or PCA occlusion there was complete (*n* = 6) or partial (*n* = 3) recanalization in all IV + IA cases. For IA only cases, there were no cases of complete recanalization, four with partial and two with no recanalization. However, all three cases of major bleeding occurred in the combined IV + IA group.

A suggested treatment algorithm in patients with MCA occlusion is provided in Fig. 4. Patients presenting to hospital <3 h from stroke onset would undergo noninvasive screening to detect an MCA occlusion. IV t-PA would be given but if the MCA is still occluded between 3 and 6 h the patient would go to angiography for "rescue" IA thrombolysis. Alternatively, the patient could go directly to angiography if IA thrombolysis is available in <60 min, or a 0.6 mg/kg loading dose of IV t-PA could be initiated prior to angiography as in the Bridging Trial. This would allow outlying community hospitals to start IV t-PA and then transport the patient to a regional stroke center for definitive diagnosis and treatment.

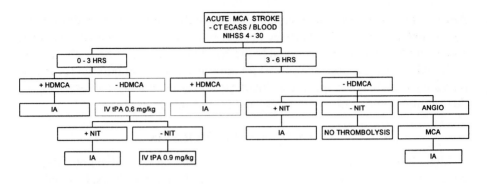

HDMCA = HYPERDENSE MIDDLE CEREBRAL ARTERY
NIT = NON-INVASIVE TESTS
NIHSS = NATIONAL INSTITUTES OF HEALTH STROKE SCALE
IA = INTRA-ARTERIAL THROMBOLYSIS
IV = INTRAVENOUS
tPA = TISSUE PLASMINOGEN ACTIVATOR
ECASS = EUROPEAN COOPERATIVE ACUTE STROKE STUDY

Fig. 4. Potential Thrombolysis Algorithm for Acute MCA Occlusion.

LIMITATIONS OF IA THROMBOLYSIS

A major issue regarding access to IA thrombolysis to treat acute ischemic strokes is that it requires the ready availability of a neurointerventionalist and a tertiary stroke team. Such expertise is not currently available in most community hospitals across the United States and is limited to large academic centers (52,53). Another limitation of IA thrombolysis is the additional time required to begin treatment compared to IV thrombolysis. In PROACT II the average time from arrival to the hospital to the initiation of IA r-proUK was 3 h. There are also concerns regarding the invasiveness of the technique and procedural risks not inherent to IV thrombolysis. However, serious procedural complications were uncommon in PROACT I and II, and cerebral angiography in experienced centers is associated with a morbidity of only 1.4% and a rate of permanent neurological complications and death of 0.1% and 0.02%, respectively.

SPECIAL SETTINGS FOR IA THROMBOLYSIS

IA thrombolysis may be useful in situations where IV thrombolysis carries an excessive bleeding risk. Patients with recent nonintracranial hemorrhage, recent surgery or arterial puncture, and patients on systemic anticoagulation were excluded from the NINDS trial because of their perceived increased risk of hemorrhagic complications. Intra-arterial thrombolysis, by delivering smaller doses of thrombolytics directly into the affected blood vessel, offers the potential to treat such patients with a lesser risk of hemorrhage. Katzan et al. (54) used IA thrombolysis to treat 6 patients who developed acute strokes in the postoperative period after open heart surgery. Although the series was small and only one patient improved dramatically, the authors were able to show the relative safety and feasibility of the procedure as only one minor bleeding complication occurred.

Cronqvist et al. in 1998 *(55)*, published their results on local intra-arterial fibrinolysis of thromboemboli occurring during endovascular treatment of intracerebral aneurysms. In 19 patients, iatrogenic occlusions occurred in either the middle cerebral artery, anterior cerebral artery, or basilar artery during the neurointerventional procedure. Utilizing a combination of urokinase and mechanical clot fragmentation, they were able to achieve complete recanalization in 10 patients (53%) and partial recanalization in the other 9 patients (47%). Fourteen patients (74%) had a good to excellent recovery and there was good correlation with complete recanalization and improved clinical outcome.

IV thrombolysis has not been studied in retinal ischemia. The series by Weber et al. *(56)* of 17 patients and the smaller series of 3 patients by Padolecchia et al. *(57)* have shown the safety and efficacy of super selective IA thrombolysis in cases of central retinal artery occlusion. In both groups there were no hemorrhagic complications and there were significant improvements in visual acuity. In the series by Weber et al., 17.6% of patients recovered completely and their patients fared better than historical controls.

SUMMARY AND FUTURE DIRECTIONS

IA thrombolysis is an established treatment option for patients with acute ischemic stroke resulting from large vessel cerebrovascular occlusions. In the carotid territory the efficacy of IA thrombolysis in patients with MCA occlusion of <6 h duration has been demonstrated in the PROACT trials. The thrombolytic agent used in the PROACT trials, r-proUK, is not FDA approved. Although there is no evidence that IA UK is superior to IA t-PA there is more aggregate experience with IA UK. More data are needed on the dosing and safety of IA t-PA and new thrombolytic agents such as TNK t-PA and reteplase in acute ischemic stroke.

Recanalization and clinical outcome are less predictable with occlusions at the internal carotid artery origin, the intracranial carotid T bifurcation or in the vertebrobasilar circulation. This may partly reflect the fact that most MCA occlusions are owing to soft clot from cardiac embolism or fresh thrombus from a proximal atherosclerotic plaque. The low TIMI 3 recanalization rate in PROACT II (20%) indicates residual thrombus is frequently present after IA thrombolysis. There is no consensus on how to deal with distal embolization, reocclusion, or underlying atherostenosis complicating IA stroke thrombolysis. These issues, and the role of clot composition in recanalization efficacy, require further study.

IA stroke thrombolysis is still evolving and there has been no standardization of patient selection, neurointerventional techniques or adjunctive therapy.

Mechanical clot removal, new catheter techniques, and new adjunctive antithrombotic agents should improve the degree, speed, and safety of IA recanalization. The number of patients subjected to unnecessary angiography can be reduced by the emergent performance of noninvasive screening, a capability many centers do not currently have. In addition, patient selection and the treatment window may be better defined by using new technologies such as perfusion-diffusion MRI *(58)*. Lastly, IA thrombolysis can be combined not only with IV thrombolysis, but also with cytoprotective strategies to improve patient outcomes after acute ischemic stroke.

REFERENCES

1. The National Institute of Neurological Disorders and Stroke rt-PA Stroke Study Group: Tissue Plasminogen Activator for Acute Ischaemic Stroke. *N Engl J Med* 1995;333:1581–1587.
2. Wolpert SM, Bruckmann H, Greenlee R, et al. Neuroradiology evaluation of patients with acute stroke treated with recombinant tissue plasminogen activator. AJNR 1993;14:3–13.
3. Tomsick T, Brott T, Barsan W, et al. Thrombus localization with emergency CT. *Am J Neuroradiol* 1992;12:257–263.
4. Higashida RT, Halbach VV, Tsai FY, Dowd CF Hieshima GB. Interventional neurovascular techniques in acute thrombolytic therapy for stroke. In: *Thrombolytic Therapy in Acute Ischemic Stroke III*, Yamagushi T, Mori E, Minematsu K, del Zoppo GJ, eds. Springer-Verlag: Tokyo. 1995; pp. 294–300.
5. del Zoppo GJ, Higashida RT, Furlan AJ, et al. PROACT: A Phase II Randomized Trial of recombinant pro-urokinase by direct arterial delivery in acute middle cerebral artery stroke. *Stroke* 1998;29:4–11.
6. Furlan A, Higashida RT, Wechsler L, Gent M, and the PROACT Investigators, et al. Intra-arterial prourokinase for acute ischemic stroke: The PROACT II study: A Randomized Controlled Trial. *JAMA* 1999;282:2003–2011.
7. Wallace RC, Furlan AJ, Moliterno DJ, et al. Basilar artery rethrombosis: Successful treatment with platelet glycoprotein IIb/IIIa receptor inhibitor. *AJNR* 1997;18:1257–1260.
8. Abciximab in Ischemic Stroke Investigators. Abciximab in Acute Ischemic Stroke. Randomized, Double-Blind, Placebo-controlled, Dose-Escalation Study. *Stroke* 2000;31:601–609.
9. Pessin M, del Zoppo GJ, Furlan AJ. Thrombolytic treatment in acute stroke: review and update of selective topics. In: *Cerebrovascular Diseases*, Moskowitz MA, Caplan LR, eds. Nineteenth Princeton Stroke Conference. Butterworth-Heinemann: Boston. 1995; pp. 409–418.
10. del Zopo GJ, Sasahara AA. Interventional use of plasminogen activators in central nervous system diseases. *Med Clin N Am* 1998;82(3):545–568.
11. Hoffman AI, Lambiase RE, Haas RA, Rogg JM, Murphy TP. Acute vertebrobasilar occlusion: Treatment with high-dose intra-arterial urokinase. *AJR* 1999;172:709–712.
12. Cross DT, Moran CJ, Akins PT, et al. Intra-arterial thrombolysis in vertebrobasilar occlusion. *AJNR* 1996;17:255–262.
13. Sussman BJ, Fitch TSP. Thrombolysis with fibrinolysin in cerebral arterial occlusion. *JAMA* 1958;167:1705.
14. Atkin N, Nitzberg S, Dorsey J. Lysis of intracerebral thromboembolism with fibrinolysin. Report of a case. *Angiology* 1964;15:436.
15. Labauge R, Blard JM, Salvaing P et al. Traitment fibrinolytique et anticoagulant dans 37 cas d'occlusions arterielles, cervicocerebrales d'origin thrombo-embolique. In: Proceedings of the fifth international congress on thromboembolism. Bologna, 1978. Pisa, Quaderni della Coagulazione, 1980, pp. 362–364.

16. Zeumer H, Hundgen R, Ferbert A, Ringelstein EB. Local intra-arterial fibrinolytic therapy in inaccessible internal carotid occlusion. *Neuroradiology* 1984;26:315–317.
17. del Zoppo GJ, Ferbert A, Otis S, Bruckman H, Hacke W, Zyroff J, Harker LA, Zeumer H. Local intra-arterial fibrinolytic therapy in acute carotid territory stroke. A pilot study. *Stroke* 1988;19:307–313.
18. Mori E, Tabuchi M, Yoshida T, Yamadori A. Intracarotid urokinase with thromboembolic occlusion of the middle cerebral artery. *Stroke* 1988;19:802–812.
19. Theron J, Courtheoux P, Casasco A, Alachkar F, Notari F, Ganem F, Maiza D. Local intra-arterial fibrinolysis in the carotid territory. *AJNR* 1989;753–765.
20. Zeumer H, Freitag HJ, Zanella F, Thie A, Arning C. Local intra-arterial fibrinolytic therapy in patients with stroke: urokinase versus recombinant tissue plasminogen activator (rt-PA). *Neuroradiology* 1993;35:159–162.
21. Higashida RT, Halbach VV, Barnwell SL, Dowd CF, Hieshima GB. Thrombolytic therapy in acute stroke. *J Endovascular Surg* 1994;1:4–15.
22. Freitag HJ, Becker V, Thie A, Tilsner V, Philapitsch A, Schwarz HP. Plasminogen plus rt-PA improves intra-arterial thrombolytic therapy in acute ischemic stroke. In: *Thrombolytic Therapy in Acute ischemic Stroke ILL*, Yamugushi T, Mori E, Minematsu K, del Zoppo GJ, eds. Springer-Verlag: Tokyo. 1995; pp. 271–278.
23. Matsumoto K, Satoh K. Intra-arterial therapy in acute ischemic stroke. In: *Thrombolytic Therapy in Acute Ischemic Stroke III*, Yamagushi T, Mori E, Minematsu K, del Zoppo GJ, eds. Springer-Verlag: Tokyo. 1995; pp. 279–287.
24. Goto K, Ogata N. "Central" intra-arterial thrombolysis using a newly developed low friction guidewire/catheter system. In: *Thrombolytic Therapy in Acute Ischemic Stroke III*, Yamagushi T, Mori E, Minematsu K, del Zoppo, GJ, eds. Springer-Verlag: Tokyo. 1995; pp. 301–306.
25. Gönner F, Remonda L, Mattle H, Sturzenegger M, et al. Local intra-arterial thrombolysis in acute ischemic stroke. *Stroke* 1998;29:1894–1900.
26. Lansberg MG, Tong DC, Norbash AM, Yenari MA, Moseley ME. Intra-arterial rtPA treatment of stroke assessed by diffusion- and perfusion-weighted MRI. *Stroke* 1999;30:678–680.
27. Furlan AJ. Natural history of atherothromboembolic occlusion of cerebral arteries: carotid versus vertebrobasilar territories. In: *Thrombolytic Therapy in Acute Ischemic Stroke*, Hacke W, del Zoppo GJ, Hirschberg M, eds. New York: NY. Springer-Verlag: 1991; pp. 71–76.
28. Katzan IL, Furlan AJ. Thrombolytic therapy. In: *Current Review of Cerebrovascular Disease* 3rd Edition, Fisher M, Bogousslavsky J, eds. Butterworth Heinemann: Boston: 1999; pp. 185–193.
28a. Rasmussen PA, Perl J, Barr J, Markarian GZ, et al. Stent-assisted angioplasty of intracranial vertebrobasilar atherosclerosis: An initial experience. *J Neurosurg* 2000;92:771–778.
29. Hacke W, Zeumer H, Ferbert A, et al. Intra-arterial thrombolytic therapy improves outcome in patients with acute vertebrobasilar occlusive disease. *Stroke* 1988;19:1216–1222.
30. Schumacher M, Siekmann R, Radu W, Wakhloo AK. Local intra-arterial fibrinolytic therapy in vetebrobasilar occlusion. In: BL Bauer, M. Brock, M Klinger. *Advances in Neurosurgery* 1994;22:30–34.
31. Brandt T, von Kummer R, Muller-Kuppers M, et al. Thrombolytic therapy of acute basilar artery occlusion, variables affecting recanalization and outcome. *Stroke* 1996;27:875–881.
32. Cross DT, Moran CIJ, Akins P, et al. Relationship between clot location and outcome after basilar artery thrombolysis. *AJNR* 1997;18:1221–1228.
33. Huemer M, Niederwieser V, Ladurner G. Thrombolytic treatment for acute occlusion of the basilar artery. *J Neurol Neurosurg Psychiatry* 1995;58:227–228.
34. Wijdicks EF, Nichols DA, Thielen KR, et al. Intra-arterial thrombolysis in acute basilar artery thromboembolisms: The initial Mayo Clinic experience. *Mayo Clin Proc* 1997;72:1005–1013.

35. Clark W, Barnwell S, Nesbit G, et al. Efficacy of intra-arterial thrombolysis of basilar artery stroke (abstr). *J Stroke Cerebrovasc Dis* 1997;6:457.
36. Zeumer H, Freitag HJ, Grzyska U, et al. Local intra-arterial fibrinolysis in acute vertebrobasilar occlusion. *Neuroradiology* 1989;31:336–340.
37. Becker KJ, Monsein LH, Ulatowski J, et al. Intra-arterial thrombolysis in vertebrobasilar occlusion. *AJNR* 1996;17:255–262.
38. Mitchell PJ, Gerraty RP, Donnan GA, et al. Thrombolysis in the vertebrobasilar circulation: the Australian urokinase stroke trial. *Cerebrovasc Dis* 1997;7:94–99.
39. Gönner F, Remonda L, Mattle H, Sturzenegger M, et al. Local intra-arterial thrombolysis in acute ischemic stroke. *Stroke* 1998;29:1894–1900.
40. Clark W, Wissman S, Albers G, Jhamandas J, Madden K, Hamilton S, for the ATLANTIS Investigators. Recombinant Tissue-Type Plasminogen Activator (Alteplase) for Ischemic Stroke 3 to 5 Hours After Symptom Onset. *JAMA* 1999;282:2019–2024.
41. Hacke W, Kaste M, Fieschi C, et al. Randomized double-blind placebo-controlled trial of thrombolytic therapy with intravenous alteplase in acute ischemic stroke (ECASS II). *Lancet* 1998;352:1245–51.
42. von Kummer R, Hacke W. Safety and efficacy of intravenous tissue plasminogen activator and heparin in acute middle cerebral artery stroke. *Stroke* 1992;23:646–652.
43. The NINDS t-PA Stroke Study Group. Intracerebral hemorrhage after intravenous t-PA therapy for ischemic stroke. *Stroke* 1997;28:2109–2118.
44. Hacke W, Kaste M, Fieschi C, Toni D, et al. Intravenous thrombolysis with recombinent tissue plasminogen activator for acute hemispheric stroke. The European Cooperative Acute Stroke Study (ECASS). *JAMA* 1995;274:1017–1025.
45. Gore JM, Sloan M, Price TR, et al. Intracerebral hemorrhage, cerebral infarction, and subdural hematoma after acute myocardial infarction and thrombolytic therapy in the thombolysis in myocardial infarction study. Thrombolysis in myocardial infarction, phase II, pilot and clinical trial. *Circulation* 1991;83:448–459.
46. Simoons MI, Maggioni AP, Knatterud G et al. Individual risk assessment for intracranial hemorrhage during thrombolytic therapy. *Lancet* 1993;342:1523–1528.
47. Anderson JL, Karagounis L, Allen A, et al. Older age and elevated blood pressure are risk factors for intracerebral hemorrhage after thrombolysis. *Am J Cardiol* 1991;68:166–170.
48. Gebel M, Sila CA, Sloan MA et al. Thrombolysis-related intracranial hemorrhage: A radiographic analysis of 244 cases from the GUSTO-1 trial with clinical correlation. *Stroke* 1998;29:563–569.
49. Tomsick T, Brott T, Barsan W, et al. Prognostic value of the hyperdense middle cerebral artery sign and stroke scale score before ultra early thrombolytic therapy. *AJNR* 1996;17:79–85.
50. Endo S, Kuwayama N, Hirashima Y, Akai T, Nishijima M, Takaku A. Results of urgent thrombolysis in patients with major stroke and atherothrombotic occlusion of the cervical internal carotid artery. *AJNR* 1998;19:1169–1175.
51. Emergency Management of Stroke (EMS) Investigators: Combined intra-arterial and intravenous tPA for stroke (abstract). *Stroke* 1997; 28:273.
52. Grotta J. t-PA-The best current option for most patients. *N Engl J Med* 1997;337:1310–1312.
53. Caplan LR, Mohr JP, Kitler JP, et al. Should thrombolytic therapy be the first-time treatment for acute ischemic stroke? Thrombolysis—not a panacea for ischemic stroke. *N Engl J Med* 1997;337:1309–1310.
54. Katzan IL, Masaryk TJ, Furlan AJ, Sila CA, Perl II J, et al. Intra-arterial thrombolysis for perioperative stroke after open heart surgery. *Neurology* 1999;52:1081–1084.
55. Cronqvist M, Pierot L, Boulin A, et al: Local intraarterial fibrinolysis of thromboemboli occurring during endovascular treatment of intracerebral aneurysm: A comparison of anatomic results and clinical outcome. *AJNR* 19:157–165, 1998.

56. Weber J, Remonda L, Mattle HP, Koerner U, et al. Selective intra-arterial fibrinolysis of acute central retinal artery occlusion. *Stroke* 1998;29:2076–2079.
57. Padolecchia R, Puglioli M, Ragone MC, Romani A, Collavoli PL. Superselective intra-arterial fibrinolysis in central retinal artery occlusion. *AJNR* 1999;20:565–567.
58. Albers GW. Expanding the time window for thrombolytic therapy in acute stroke. The potential role of acute MRI for patient selection. *Stroke* 1999;30:2230–2237.

11

Combinations of Intravenous and Intra-Arterial Thrombolysis

Joseph Broderick, MD
and Rashmi Kothari, MD

CONTENTS

INTRODUCTION
INTRAVENOUS TISSUE PLASMINOGEN ACTIVATOR (T-PA)
    FOR ACUTE ISCHEMIC STROKE—
    EFFICACY AND KNOWN LIMITATIONS
INTRA-ARTERIAL THROMBOLYTIC THERAPY—
    POTENTIAL ADVANTAGES AND KNOWN LIMITATIONS
COMBINED INTRAVENOUS AND INTRA-ARTERIAL T-PA—
    RATIONALE AND PRIOR EXPERIENCE
COMBINED IV/IA APPROACH—CARDIOLOGY EXPERIENCE
WHICH IS BETTER—A COMBINED IV/IA
    OR THE CURRENTLY APPROVED DOSE OF IV T-PA?
REFERENCES

INTRODUCTION

The purpose of this chapter is to introduce physicians to the concept of a combined intravenous/intra-arterial approach to recanalization. Current experience is limited but the concept is attractive and worthy of further study. To understand the potential advantages of a combined approach, it is helpful to first examine the known advantages and limitations of intravenous (iv) and intra-arterial (IA) delivery of thrombolytic agents. The basic rationale for IA thrombolysis is presented in Chapter 10. Here we will discuss some of the limitations of IA therapy.

From: *Thrombolytic Therapy for Stroke*
Edited by: P. D. Lyden © Humana Press Inc., Totowa, NJ

INTRAVENOUS TISSUE PLASMINOGEN ACTIVATOR (t-PA)
FOR ACUTE ISCHEMIC STROKE—
EFFICACY AND KNOWN LIMITATIONS

Intravenous recombinant tissue plasminogen activator (rt-PA) administered within 3 h of symptom onset is the only FDA-approved treatment for acute ischemic stroke *(1)*. The time from stroke onset to initiation of thrombolytic therapy has been demonstrated to be the most critical predictor of effectiveness *(2)*. Six other moderate-sized randomized studies of iv thrombolytic therapy, three studies of streptokinase, and three of rt-PA, have been reported in which most patients were treated more than 3 h after stroke onset *(3–8)*. These studies did not demonstrate any significant benefit for thrombolytic therapy when administered beyond 3 h from onset as measured by the primary study end points *(3–8)*.

Does the time to treatment within the first 3 h after onset affect the effectiveness of t-PA? In the initial analysis of the NINDS t-PA Stroke Trial, the only difference between the two time stratum (0–90 min and 91–180 min) was a significantly increased likelihood of a 4 or more point improvement in the National Institute of Health Stroke Scale Score (NIHSSS) from baseline to 24 h in patients treated with t-PA within 90 min of onset, as compared to placebo patients *(1)*. An increased likelihood of a 4 or more point improvement in the NIHSSS was not seen in patients treated with t-PA at 90–180 min after onset. However, t-PA was clearly effective at improving the likelihood of an excellent outcome at 3 mo for patients treated in the two time tiers.

Further analysis subsequently was performed to test whether there was an effect of "time to treatment" on 24-h improvement, 3-mo favorable outcome, or the rate of intracranial hemorrhage (ICH), after adjusting for potential confounders that may have masked a relationship between time-to-treatment and effectiveness of t-PA *(2)*. When the difference in patient baseline characteristics were considered, patients treated with t-PA within 0–90 min from stroke onset were more likely to show improvement at 24 h and at 3 mo, compared to placebo-treated patients, than patients who were treated with t-PA at 90–180 min. No relationship between time-to-treatment and occurrence of ICH was seen, possibly owing to low power *(2)*. Thus, time to initiation of thrombolytic therapy and restoration of blood flow is critical for clinical benefit, even within the first 3 h after onset.

Intravenous t-PA has known limitations. For example, iv t-PA administered within 8 h from symptom onset, reopens only 30–40% of occluded major intracranial trunk arteries within the first 1–2 h after initiation of treatment as determined by cerebral angiography *(9–11)*. In the NINDS t-PA Stroke Trial, patients with a high NIHSS Score (severe stroke) did better overall with iv t-PA than with those patients who were treated with placebo *(1)*. Although these patients with high NIHSS scores did better with t-PA, the overall prognosis of these patients after t-PA therapy in the NINDS t-PA Trial was poor *(12)*. For example, only 21% of patients with an NIHSSS ≥10 at the start of iv t-PA treatment had an NIHSSS of 0 or 1 at 3 mo. In addition, patients with a high NIHSSS (i.e., a large ischemic stroke) are highly likely to have an occlusion of a major intracranial and/or major extracranial artery *(13)*.

Given that the large majority of patients with a high NIHSS score have an occlusion of a major extracranial or intracranial trunk artery *(13)* and that iv t-PA alone often does not open up major arterial occlusions during the first several hours, the overall poor response in patients with high NIHSSS in the NINDS t-PA Trial is not surprising. Patients with a high NIHSSS in the NINDS t-PA Stroke Trial who received iv t-PA (dose 0.9 mg/kg) were also at increased risk for intracranial hemorrhage *(14)*. Thus, the likely explanation for poor outcome in patients with a moderate to high NIHSSS, despite rapid administration of iv t-PA, is that most large arteries are not recanalized by iv t-PA in the time window necessary to prevent brain infarction.

INTRA-ARTERIAL THROMBOLYTIC THERAPY— POTENTIAL ADVANTAGES AND KNOWN LIMITATIONS

Intra-arterial therapy by a selective microcatheter has the advantage of delivery of a thrombolytic agent directly at the site of an occluded intracranial artery (see Chapter 10). This is true even if a more proximal artery, such as the internal carotid artery, is occluded.

Administration of t-PA or urokinase via microcatheter at the site of the thrombus has been reported to fully or partially recanalize occluded arteries in approx 50–82% of patients *(15–20)*. The rate of symptomatic intracerebral hemorrhage in these uncontrolled series of IA thrombolytic therapy has been relatively low (an average rate of approx 10%). Heparin administration has generally been part of the protocol of these IA thrombolytic studies.

The only two published randomized studies of IA thrombolytic therapy are the PROACT I and II studies *(15,17)*, which compared pro-urokinase plus iv heparin to IA placebo plus iv heparin. PROACT I demonstrated a recanalization rate of 58% after 2 h of infusion of pro-urokinase plus heparin in 26 patients compared to 14% after an infusion of a placebo plus heparin in 14 patients *(17)*. The rate of symptomatic hemorrhage in the group that was treated with 6 mg of pro-urokinase plus, a 100 u/kg bolus of heparin followed by 1000 U of heparin/hour for 4 h, was 27%. For this reason, the heparin dose was decreased to a 2000 unit bolus followed by a 500 u/hour infusion of heparin for 4 h. The hemorrhage rate in the patients treated with 6 mg of pro-urokinase and "low dose" heparin was 7%. Although the recanalization rate in the pro-urokinase treated group was significantly greater than in placebo-treated patients, neurologic outcome was not significantly different between pro-urokinase and placebo-treated patients.

The PROACT II Study was published in December 1999 (15). One-hundred-twenty-one patients with M-1 or M-2 occlusions by angiography were randomized within 6 h of symptom onset to receive 9 mg of pro-urokinase plus heparin (low-dose) vs fifty-nine patients who received placebo plus low-dose heparin. Of patients in the pro-urokinase group, 40% had a Rankin of 0–2 at 3 mo compared to 25% of control patients ($p = 0.04$, stratified by NIHSSS at baseline). Only 19% of patients who received pro-urokinase had TIMI grade III flow (complete opening of the arterial occlusions) after 2 h of therapy as compared to 2% of placebo patients. But 66% of patients who received pro-urokinase did have TIMI 2 or 3 flow (complete or partial reopening). The symptomatic rate of ICH in the pro-urokinase group was 10%. Even though the absolute difference between groups was moderate in effect, the FDA requested an additional study because of the borderline statistical significance of the overall result. In addition, the small number of control patients in the study ($n = 59$, 2 to 1 randomization design) makes it difficult to adjust for differences in baseline variables between the two groups that may affect the interpretation of the study results.

IA administration of thrombolytic agents appears to have higher rates of recanalization than iv t-PA, and the rate of intracerebral hemorrhage is similar to that seen in the NINDS t-PA Stroke Trial, but the IA approach also has limitations. The most important limitation of IA therapy has been the time from onset of symptoms to initiation of therapy and the time to recanalization once therapy has begun. For example, in the PROACT II study, the time from onset of symptoms to initiation of IA treatment was >5 h and only 4 patients had pro-urokinse started within 3 h (personal communication Anthony Furlan, P.I., PROACT II Study) (15). In addition, the median time for recanalization in IA studies in which times are reported is about 2 h. Two published reports of IA thrombolytic therapy from Japan and Switzerland (18,20) indicate that treatment begun within 3–4 h of symptom onset is associated with higher rates of recanalization and better outcome.

In summary, iv t-PA administered within 3 h of onset is the only FDA-approved treatment for acute ischemic stroke. The major limitation of this approach is that iv t-PA opens a minority of large intracranial arterial occlusions in a time frame that is likely to improve patient outcome. Intravenous t-PA also carries a risk of symptomatic intracerebral hemorrhage, particularly in patients with large strokes as measured by the NIHSSS. Intra-arterial therapy has higher reported rates of arterial recanalization, but it is associated with a long time window from symptom onset to recanalization. The PROACT II Study suggests that IA thrombolytic therapy alone at longer time windows may be effective in highly selected groups of patients with acute ischemic stroke. Whatever method of recanalization is used, the time from symptom onset to recanalization of the artery appears to be the key determinant of effectiveness.

COMBINED INTRAVENOUS AND INTRA-ARTERIAL t-PA— RATIONALE AND PRIOR EXPERIENCE

Combined iv and IA delivery of thrombolytic drug has several potential advantages. First, a combined approach looks to start iv thrombolytic therapy as quickly as possible in order to minimize the time from stroke onset to recanalization. The addition of IA therapy following iv t-PA has the advantage of demonstrating whether or not a clot is still present and whether more thrombolytic drug or other methods to recanalize the occluded artery are needed. The potential risks of a combined approach would be that one needs to perform a femoral artery puncture after recent administration of intravenous t-PA or other thrombolytic agent.

From 12/94–12/95, and prior to approval of iv t-PA for acute ischemic stroke, several of the investigators from the NINDS t-PA Stroke Trial initiated a study which attempted to combine the advantages of iv and IA t-PA *(13)*. The Emergency Management of Stroke (EMS) Trial, a randomized controlled study, was designed to test the feasibility and provide preliminary data regarding the relative benefits and risks of combined iv t-PA (0.6 mg/kg over 30 min) and IA t-PA therapy (administered only if a clot was demonstrated by angiography at a dose of up to 20 mg at the site of the clot over 2 h), as compared to iv placebo and IA t-PA therapy. Intravenous treatment in the EMS Study had to be started within 3 h of onset. The inclusion/exclusion criteria for the EMS Pilot Trial were identical to that of the NINDS t-PA randomized Trial except that patients had to have an NIHSSS of 5 or more (patients had a slightly higher median NIHSSS), a higher systolic blood pressure at baseline was allowed (190 systolic as compared to 185 systolic in the NINDS trial), and patients greater than 85-yr-of-age were not treated (the NINDS trial had no upper age limit). The only computed tomography (CT) exclusion for either trial was the presence of hemorrhage on the baseline CT.

The total number of patients in the EMS study was small (total $n = 35$, combined iv/IA t-PA group = 17 and iv placebo and IA t-PA =18). The pilot study was not powered to examine differences in efficacy between the two treatment groups. The combined IV/IA t-PA group had a higher median NIHSSS (16, interquartile range 9–21) than the IA t-PA alone group (11, interquartile range 9–16). This imbalance in NIHSS scores is important for the interpretation of angiographic results in the EMS Study since the baseline NIHSSS correlated extremely well with the presence or absence of a clot at angiography. For example, 78% of patients with an NIHSSS ≥10 had a demonstrable IA clot at angiography.

Despite the imbalance in the baseline NIHSS scores between the two treatment groups, recanalization in the combined IV/IA t-PA treatment group was more complete than recanalization in the IA alone group, although the difference was not significant. For those patients who had a clot at angiogram, recanaliza-

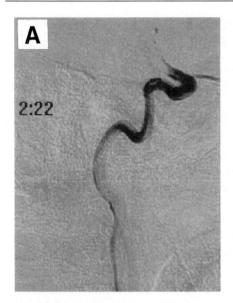
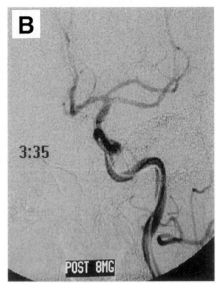

Fig. 1. (A) Intraluminal clot in ICA terminus 60 min after iv t-PA began and 2 h and 20 min after onset of stroke symptoms. **(B)** Complete recanalization after additional IA t-PA 3 h and 30 min after onset of stroke symptoms.

tion was significantly greater in the combined IV/IA group than in the IA alone group (Fig. 1, Table 1). The proportion of improved outcomes (prospectively defined as a seven point improvement of the NIHSSS at 7–10 d) was not significantly greater in the combined IV/IA treatment group as compared to the IA alone group (both groups = 24%).

The prospectively determined primary safety measure for the EMS Study was life-threatening bleeding events during the first 24 h after start of therapy. There were no symptomatic or asymptomatic intracerebral hematomas in the 35 EMS patients. One symptomatic hemorrhagic infarction occurred among the 18 patients treated with placebo/IA t-PA therapy during the first 24 h. One confused patient in the combined iv/IA treatment group removed her femoral sheath post-procedure and had a retroperitoneal hemorrhage during the first 24 h with resulting hypotension requiring transfusion of blood. She subsequently developed myocardial ischemia and eventually died. Finally, one patient in the combined group had an unrecognized aortic dissection and developed a hemopericardium following iv-t-PA and prior to IA therapy.

Two symptomatic hemorrhagic infarctions occurred in the combined iv/IA group during 24–72 h after treatment. Asymptomatic intracerebral hemorrhagic infarction during the first 72 h was also noted more frequently in the iv/IA group ($n = 5$) as compared to the IA group alone ($n = 1$). The mean dose of t-PA that

Table 1
Post-Treatment Arterial Patency in EMS Study
(results in those with clot on initial angiogram)

	iv/IA* N = 11 (with clot)		Placebo N = 10 (with clot)	
TIMI Score	N (%)	(artery)	N (%)	(artery)
0	0 (0%)		2 (20%)	M_2, M_1
1	2 (18%)	2-ICA	3 (30%)	M_1, ICA, M_1+ICA
2	3 (27%)	2-M_1, M_2	4 (40%)	2-M_2,2-M_1, Basilar
3	6 (54%)	3-M_1, 2-M_2, 1-M_1	1 (10%)	ICA

*IV/IA Group has better arterial patency by regression analysis at $p = 0.03$ using a central interpretation of the angiograms.
M_1 – first part of middle cerebral artery.
M_2 – second part of middle cerebral artery.
ICA - internal carotid artery.

Table 2
Time Intervals–EMS Study

	Median number of hours	
	iv/IA	Placebo/IA
Time from stroke onset to iv treatment ($n = 35$)	2.6	2.7
Time from stroke onset to start of angiogram ($n = 35$)	3.3	3.0
Time from stroke onset to recanalization for those who had clot at angiogram	6.3	5.7

was administered in the iv/IA group was 56 mg ± 11 mg as compared to a mean dose of 11 mg ± 10 in the IA only treatment group.

The median time from symptom onset to initiation of iv therapy was 2.6 h. Delays in initiating angiography, getting the catheter to the site of the occluded artery to begin IA therapy and to recanalization are presented in Table 2.

We compared the results of combined iv-IA t-PA in the EMS Study for patients with an M-1 or M-2 occlusion with the results of the PROACT II Study. The number of patients is very small but there is a trend toward better outcomes (Rankin of 0 or 2–57% EMS, 40% PROACT, same median NIHSSS at baseline for EMS and PROACT II patients) and better rates of TIMI Grade III flow (complete recanalization) in the patients treated with combined iv/IA t-PA as shown in Table 3.

More recent experiences of 20 patients treated with the iv/IA approach at the University of Cincinnati demonstrate that the median time to start iv therapy can be decreased to a median time of 2.1 h and that IA therapy can be started at a median of 3.5 h from onset of symptoms (unpublished data). Figure 1 illustrates

Table 3
EMS vs PROACT: Patients with M_1 M_2 Clots–TIMI Flow After Therapy

	% TIMI Grade 3	% TIMI Grade 2 or 3
PROACT II		
Placebo (n = 59)	2%	18%
PROACT II		
ProUK (n = 121)	19%	66%
EMS		
iv/IA t-PA (n = 9)	67%	100%
IA t-PA alone (n = 6)	0%	50%
Total (n = 15)	40%	80%

a patient at the University of Cincinnati who was recently treated with combined iv/IA and had intravenous t-PA begun within 95 min of onset at a local community hospital by a stroke-team physician and then was transferred to University Hospital where a cerebral angiogram was performed immediately. At angiography (and after 30 mg of intravenous t-PA) she had an occlusion of the left internal carotid artery terminus and middle cerebral artery (MCA) (Fig. 1A). Only 12 mg of additional t-PA at the site of the clot plus mechanical manipulation via the guidewire and catheter were needed to completely restore blood flow in these arteries at 3 h and 20 min from the onset of her symptoms (Fig. 1B). The patient's baseline NIHSS score was 24. After restoration of blood flow, she immediately improved on the table when her arteries reopened at 15:20 PM (turned to physician and asked "What happened?") and at 24 h after stroke onset had an NIHSSS score of 1 with a normal CT (Fig. 2).

1200 PM–Patient witnessed to have a sudden onset of aphasia, and right sided weakness.
1208 PM–911 called
1215 PM–Ambulance at patient's home
1228 PM–Patient arrives at Emergency Room of community hospital
1240 PM–Stroke Pager Called, CT Scan ordered
1248 PM–CT Scan completed: Hyperdense L MCA, no hemorrhage.
1300 PM–Stroke team physician arrives. NIHSSS 24
1318 PM–IV t-PA Bolus given. Infusion begun.
1333 PM–Leaves outside ED in Ambulance for University of Cincinnati
1349 PM–Arrives at University of Cincinnati
1403 PM–Angiography begun
1420 PM–At clot. ICA Terminus clot with extension into MCA. 4 mg bolus given intraclot.
           Infusion at 10 mg/h of t-PA begun IA.
1515 PM–Trickle of flow seen in MCA. NIHSSS 23

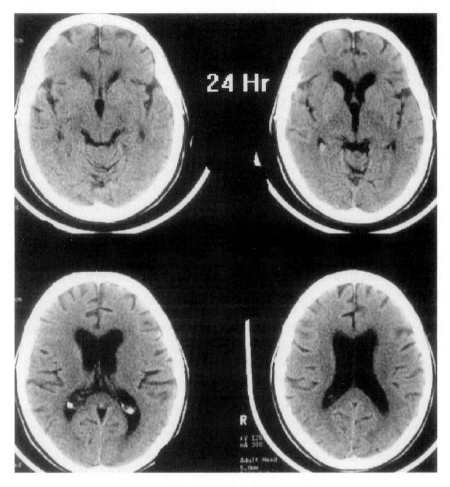

Fig. 2. 24-h CT of patient treated with combined iv/IA t-PA.

1520 PM–Complete opening of ICA and MCA. NIHSSS 7
1550 PM–Arrives in ICU. NIHSSS 3
1200 PM–24 h NIHSSS 1
Discharged home 6 d later with NIHSSS–0.

These data illustrate that a combined approach can help to minimize the time to treatment and recanalization, can be used to help titrate the amount of thrombolytic drug, and can be associated with excellent outcome.

COMBINED IV/IA APPROACH—CARDIOLOGY EXPERIENCE

Many investigators in cardiology have already embraced the concept of a combined iv/IA approach in patients with acute myocardial infarction. This combined iv/IA approach is illustrated by the plasminogen activator-angioplasty compatibility trial (PACT) *(21)*. This double-blind, randomized trial addressed: 1) angiographic patency following lower-dose t-PA (50 mg) or placebo, and 2) the need for rescue angioplasty. Time-to-treatment in the 606 randomized patients was 2.7 h. TIMI-3 flow (full perfusion) at the first angiogram (median 50 min after treatment) was achieved in 33% of the lower dose t-PA patients compared to 15% of the placebo patients. There was no clinically significant differences in safety end points including groin hematoma (a peripheral bleeding complication rate of 8% in both groups). These patency results for lower dose t-PA in the PACT study are almost identical to the 60-min patency results reported recently in the RAPID trial for full dose t-PA *(22)*. In the RAPID trial, 100 mg of alteplase was administered over 3 h to patients with acute myocardial infarction (AMI) as part of a randomized comparison study of t-PA (alteplase) with reteplase. TIMI-3 patency was achieved in 33% of the 101 patients randomized to t-PA. In summary, twice as many patients treated with iv t-PA compared to placebo-treated patients had restored blood flow by the time of angiography which obviated the need for angioplasty.

The results support the concept of a combined iv/IA approach as opposed to an IA-alone approach and provide evidence for comparable clot-lysis capability of lower-dose iv t-PA as compared to full dose iv t-PA. These studies also support data in ischemic stroke patients that iv t-PA alone recanalizes only a third of occluded intracranial arteries.

WHICH IS BETTER—A COMBINED IV/IA OR THE CURRENTLY APPROVED DOSE OF IV t-PA?

There is no randomized trial that has compared combined IV/IA t-PA to the currently approved dose of iv t-PA nor even to placebo. Thus, the efficacy of a lower dose of iv t-PA followed by IA delivery of t-PA has yet to be demonstrated. Whether the higher rates of recanalization demonstrated in the EMS study are associated with improved efficacy as compared to full dose iv t-PA will need to be tested in a randomized study. The patient selection for such a randomized study would be critical. It is likely that patients with a small NIHSSS and a smaller area of affected brain would be best treated with iv t-PA since they are much less likely to have occlusions of major intracranial arteries as a cause of their stroke. A recently NINDS funded multicenter pilot study "Interventional Management of Stroke" or "IMS Study" will limit iv/IA treatment of patients to those with a NIHSSS ≥10 because they have a high likelihood of a major IA occlusion. The IMS Study will also address the logistical issues that need to be addressed such as decreasing the time to initiation of iv and IA t-PA as well as better ways of recanalization of the occluded artery. Solving these logistical issues will be important prior to embarking on a large randomized study.

At best, the combined iv/IA t-PA approach may offer a modest improvement to the currently approved dose of iv t-PA. Other innovative means of recanalization of the artery will assume greater importance in the coming years. These include mechanical devices to remove or break-up clots via the catheter *(23)*, the addition of other agents such as the G II b/III a platelet receptor antagonist *(24,25)* or substrates for t-PA such as plasminogen *(26)*. Whatever combination of agents or methods is tested, the primary goal will be to shorten the time from onset of symptoms to recanalization of the artery. We will likely follow the steps of the cardiologists who have used a multi-pronged approach to reopen occluded coronary arteries that involves drugs and mechanical devices, and that depends upon the availability of technology and expertise at a given hospital.

REFERENCES

1. The National Institutes of Neurological Disorders and Stroke rt-PA Stroke Study Group. Tissue plasminogen activator for acute ischemic stroke. *N Engl J Med* 1995;333:1581–1587.
2. Marler J, Tilley B, Lu M, Broderick J, Brott T, Lyden P, for the NINDS rt-PA Stroke Study Group. Earlier treatment associated with better outcome: the NINDS t-PA Stroke Study. *Neurology*, 2000; 55:1649–1655.
3. Multicentre Acute Stroke Trial-Italy (MAST-1) Group. Randomized controlled trial of streptokinase, aspirin, and combination of both in treatment of acute ischemic stroke. Lancet 1995;346:1509–1514.
4. Multicentre Acute Stroke Trial-European Study Group. Thrombolytic therapy with streptokinase in acute ischemic stroke. *N Engl J Med* 1996;335:145–150.
5. Donnan GA, Davis SM, Chambers BR, Gates PC, Hankey GJ, McNeil JJ, et al. Letter to the Editor. *Lancet* 1995;345:578–579.
6. Hacke W, Kaste M, Fieschi, C, et al. Intravenous thrombolysis with recombinant tissue plasminogen activator for acute hemispheric stroke. *JAMA* 1995; 274:1017–1025.
7. Hacke W, Kaste M, Fieschi C, et al. Randomised, double-blind, placebo-controlled trial of thrombolytic therapy with intravenous alteplase in acute ischemic stroke (ECASS II). *Lancet* 1998;352:1245–1251.
8. Clark WM, Wissman S, Albers GW, Jhamandas JH, Madden KP, Hamilton S, for the ATLANTIS Study Investigators. Recombinant tissue-type plasminogen activator (Alteplase) for ischemic stroke 3 to 5 hours after symptom onset: The ATLANTIS Study: A Randomized Controlled Trial. *JAMA* 1999;282:2019–2026.
9. Wolpert SM, Bruckmann H, Greenlee R, Wechsler L, Pessin MS, del Zoppo GJ, and the rt-PA Acute Stroke Study Group. Neuroradiologic evaluation of patients with acute stroke treated with recombinant tissue plasminogen activator. *AJNR* 1993;14:3–13.
10. Yamaguchi T, Hayakawa T, Kiuchi H, for the Japanese Thrombolysis Study Group. Intravenous tissue plasminogen activator ameliorates the outcome of hyperacute embolic stroke. *Cardiovascular Dis* 1993;3:269–272.
11. Mori E, Yoneda Y, Tobuchi M, et al. Intravenous recombinant tissue plasminogen activator in acute carotid artery territory stroke. *Neurology* 1992;42:976–982.
12. NINDS t-PA Acute Stroke Investigators. Generalized efficacy of t-PA for acute stroke: Subgroup analysis of the NINDS t-PA stroke study. *Stroke* 28:2119–2125, 1997.
13. Lewandowski CA, Frankel M, Tomsick T, Broderick J, Frey J, Clark W, and the EMS Bridging Trial Investigators. Combined intravenous and intra-arterial rt-PA versus intra-arterial therapy of acute ischemic stroke. Emergency Management of Stroke (EMS) Bridging Trial. *Stroke* 1999;30:2598–2605.

14. NINDS t-PA Stroke Study Group. t-PA and the risk of intracerebral hemorrhage inpatients with ischemic stroke: The NINDS t-PA Stroke Study. *Stroke* 1997;28:2109–2118.
15. Furlan A, Higashida R, Wechsler L, et al. for the PROACT Investigators. Intra-arterial prourokinase for acute ischemic stroke. The PROACT II Study: A randomized controlled trial. *JAMA* 1999;282:2003–2011.
16. Brott T, Hacke W. Thrombolytic and Defibrinogenating Agents for Ischemic and Hemorrhagic Stroke. In: *Stroke: Pathophysiology, Diagnosis, and Management*, Barnett HJ, Stein BM, Mohr JP, Yatsu FM, eds. Churchill and Livingston: 1992; pp. 953–965.
17. del Zoppo GJ, Higashida RT, Furlan AJ, Pessin MS, Rowley HA, Gent M, and the PROACT Investigators. PROACT: a phase II randomized trial of recombinant pro-urokinase by direct arterial delivery in acute middle cerebral artery stroke. *Stroke* 1998;29:4–11.
18. Gonner F, Remonda L, Mattle H, Sturzenegger M, Ozboda C, Lovblad K-O, et al. Local intra-arterial thrombolysis in acute ischemic stroke. *Stroke* 1998;29:1894–1900.
19. Zeumer H, Freitag H-J, Zanella F, Thie A, Arning C. Local intra-arterial fibrinolytic therapy in patients with stroke: Urokinase versus recombinant tissue plasminogen activator (r-TPA). *Neuroradiology* 1993;35:159–162.
20. Endo S, Kuwayama N, Hirashima Y, Akai T, Nishijima M, Takaku A. Results of urgent thrombolysis in patients with major stroke and atherothrombotic occlusion of the cervical internal carotid artery. *AJNR* 1998;19:1169–1175.
21. Ross AM, Coyne KS, Reiner JS, Greenhouse SW, Fink C, Frey A, et al. A randomized trial comparing primary angioplasty with a strategy of short-acting thrombolysis and immediate planned rescue angioplasty in acute myocardial infarction: The PACT trial. PACT investigators. *J Am Coll Cardiol* 1999 Dec;34(7):1954–62.
22. Smalling R, Bode C, Kalbfleisch J, Sen S, Limbourg P, Forycki F, et al. More rapid, complete, and stable coronary thrombolysis with bolus administration of reteplase compared with alteplase infusion in acute myocardial infarction. *Circulation* 1995;91:2725–2732.
23. Clark WM, Buckley LA, Nesbit GM, Lutsep HL, Barnwell SL, Doherty AJ, et al. Intra-arterial laser thrombolysis therapy for clinical stroke: A feasibility study. *Stroke* 2000;31:307 (abstract).
24. Wallace R, Furlan A, Molterno D, Stevens G, Masaryk T, Perl Jn. Basilar artery rethrombosis: Successful treatment with platelet glycoprotein IIb/IIIa receptor inhibitor. *Am J Neuroradiol* 1998;18:125–160.
25. The EPILOG Investigators: Effect of the platelet glycoprotein IIb/IIIa receptor inhibitor abciximab with lower heparin doses in ischemic complications of percutaneous coronary revascularization. *New Engl J Med* 1997;336:1689–1696.
26. Freitag H, Becker V, Thie A, et al. Lys-plasminogen as an adjunct to local intra-arterial fibrinolysis for carotid territory stroke. *Neuroradiology* 1996;38:181–185.

III USING THROMBOLYSIS FOR ACUTE STROKE

12 The Case for Thrombolytic Therapy in Stroke Patients

Patrick D. Lyden, MD

CONTENTS

INTRODUCTION
T-PA IS COST EFFECTIVE
THROMBOLYTIC THERAPY CAN BE GIVEN OUTSIDE
    OF ACADEMIC MEDICAL CENTERS
THE ORIGINAL RESULTS ARE CONFIRMED
    ON LONG-TERM FOLLOW-UP
VASCULAR IMAGING IS UNNECESSARY PRIOR
    TO THROMBOLYTIC THERAPY
SUBGROUP SELECTION IS NOT JUSTIFIED
THE POSITIVE RESULTS HAVE BEEN CONFIRMED
    USING OTHER PROTOCOLS, OTHER DRUGS
CONCLUSIONS
ACKNOWLEDGMENTS
REFERENCES

INTRODUCTION

The use of thrombolysis for acute stroke was proven safe and effective in the National Institutes of Neurologic Disorders and Stroke (NINDS) study of tissue-plasminogen activator (t-PA) for acute stroke, published in 1995 *(1)*. The therapy was approved by FDA in 1996, and endorsed by the American Heart Association, American Academy of Neurology, and National Stroke Association in 1997 *(2–4)*. Nevertheless, some authorities argued that thrombolytic therapy with t-PA for stroke was not ready for general use, leaving the practitioner in an awkward position *(5)*. Since a previous review of this topic *(4)*, there have been several reports that bear on some of the questions raised by skeptics. What have we

From: *Thrombolytic Therapy for Stroke*
Edited by: P. D. Lyden © Humana Press Inc., Totowa, NJ

211

learned since the original study to answer remaining concerns about thrombolytic stroke therapy? Are data available now, that were not available previously, to reassure neurologists that now is the time to begin expanding their use of thrombolytic therapy for stroke patients? The case for limiting the use of thrombolytic therapy is eloquently made by Dr. Lou Caplan in the Chapter 13. Here, we will present the case in favor of thrombolytic therapy.

Recent publications support six basic contentions: 1) t-PA for stroke therapy is cost effective, despite the high cost of the drug itself and the stroke teams to give it; 2) Community-based practicing neurologists can use t-PA for acute stroke and obtain the same good results seen in the original research study; 3) Additional support for the first study conclusions comes from long-term follow-up of the original patients and from analysis of the computed tomography (CT) scan data; 4) Angiograms are probably not necessary prior to administering t-PA; 5) There are no particular subgroups from whom t-PA should be withheld, such as those with very large strokes; 6) Other groups, using other drugs such as pro-urokinase, have found beneficial effects of thrombolytic therapy for stroke. On the other hand, there still remains considerable room for improvement, and we are far from having the ideal thrombolytic agent. Let us consider these contentions in turn.

t-PA IS COST EFFECTIVE

Since the initial publication of the NINDS t-PA Stroke Trial results, the NINDS investigators have published additional data and analyses, which is presented in Chapter 9. It is critical to understand that in that analysis, rigorous methodology was used to estimate the likelihood that the cost estimates were correct. Certain assumptions about stroke costs and outcomes were based on data from the literature and from the original study. Then, to account for possible errors in those assumptions, a simulation method was used to vary the values of those assumptions. For example, the authors estimated that the cost of in-patient rehabilitation might be $21,233, but in the simulation, this assumption was varied from $10,000 to $40,000. For a cohort of 1000 t-PA-treated patients, the net cost savings in the first year were estimated to be $4 million; the sensitivity analysis from the simulations indicated a probability of 93% that the estimate is correct. Thus, thrombolytic stroke therapy joins a very small number of therapies that not only saves disability, but also saves dollars. To put these results in perspective, it is important to remember how few other therapies result in net cost savings to the health care system; two traditional examples are prenatal care and early childhood vaccinations (6–10). These therapies cost money to administer, but overall there is a net cost reduction owing to lower disease incidence.

THROMBOLYTIC THERAPY CAN BE GIVEN OUTSIDE OF ACADEMIC MEDICAL CENTERS

It has been stated that the NINDS investigators were a select group of neurologists with special expertise, and that the study hospitals were unusual places where t-PA could be used safely *(11,12)*. It was hypothesized that in wider clinical practice the risk of the drug, a hemorrhage rate of 6.4%, would be higher, fewer patients would benefit, and practicing neurologists would not meet the strict requirement for prompt evaluation and treatment *(5)*. In support of this, the Cleveland area Stroke Team surveyed local hospitals about their experience with thrombolytic therapy *(13)*. A total of 3948 patients were admitted with a primary diagnosis of stroke (using the International Classification of Diseases, Ninth Revision, code 434 or 436). Of these patients, the authors could find records and study the use of t-PA in 70 patients (1.8%). Of these, in 50% there were protocol variations, and in 11 (15.7%) there were symptomatic hemorrhages. These data suggest that perhaps the benefit of the thrombolytic stroke therapy may not accrue in a community application. In many respects, however, the study was flawed. Most importantly, the charts were located and reviewed retrospectively, so there is a high likelihood of selection bias: bad cases are more likely to be found than good cases. The study does illustrate nicely, however, that few patients are receiving t-PA for their stroke. Similarly, in Rio de Janiero, only 5 of 56 evaluated patients could be treated, primarily owing to lack of symptom recognition, transfer delay, or late CT scan *(14)*. In a distressing eight patients, the CT scan could not be performed in a timely manner.

Although it is true that all investigators in the original study were trained to follow the study protocol properly, including video certification using the NIH Stroke Scale *(15,16)*, it is also true that a majority of patients were enrolled at community hospitals, not academic medical centers. In the original trial, over two-thirds of the patients were enrolled at non-academic medical centers. The investigators involved, however, were trained by the investigative team, and could have enjoyed some special advantage that would not be available in wider clinical use. To determine whether the study results could be replicated in practice, several groups have studied thrombolytic therapy in large numbers of stroke patients, known as postmarketing or Phase IV studies. It is now clear that community-based neurologists can deliver the drug with statistics that mirror the original study.

In Alberta, Canada, the stroke center examined 68 consecutive patients treated by general neurologists (nonstroke specialists) in an academic medical center *(17)*. A favorable outcome, as defined by the NIH stroke scale, was noted in 38% by 3 mo after treatment. Using the Rankin scale, a favorable outcome occurred in 57% by 3 mo. Symptomatic hemorrhages occurred more often in patients in whom the protocol was violated (27%) than in those in whom the protocol was followed (5%). In Oregon, the stroke center collected results on 33 patients seen in 6 medical centers *(18)*. Of these, one is an academic, tertiary referral center, one is a Veteran's Administration hospital, and four are private community hospitals. The overall rate of symptomatic hemorrhage was 9%, and the rate of successful outcome was 36%, both numbers similar to the original study. In

Houston, Chiu and colleagues *(19)* found a hemorrhage rate of 7% in two community hospitals and one university hospital. Full recovery was seen in 37%, mirroring the data seen in the original study. Time to treatment (door-to-needle) was about 100 min, and there was no significant difference between the community and university settings. Tanne and colleagues *(20)* pooled 189 consecutive patients from several community and academic hospitals. In this series, the rate of full recovery by discharge was 34%, rate of return home was 48%, and the symptomatic hemorrhage rate was 3%, all of which is consistent with the original study. On the other hand, hemorrhages occurred in 11% of the patients who were not treated according to protocol *(21)*. In Cologne, Germany, similar results have been reported from a study of community hospitals where the symptomatic hemorrhage rate was 5% and the favorable response rate was 40 to 53% *(22)*. In Lyon, France, 43 consecutive patients were studied prospectively with similar results *(23)*.

The largest Phase IV study of thrombolytic therapy was organized by the maker of t-PA, Genentech *(24)*. This prospective, multicenter study was conducted at 57 medical centers in the United States, of which 24 were academic and 33 were community. In this series, the hemorrhage rate was 3.3%, and as expected, one-half of these patients died. After 30 d, 35% of the patients had very favorable outcomes; 43% were functionally independent. Protocol violations were noted in 32.6%.

These reports of community experiences are limited by the unavoidable fact that they cannot be blinded or placebo-controlled. At this time, however, it is fair to conclude that if the NINDS protocol is followed scrupulously, then outcome results similar to the original study can be obtained in community hospitals. It remains speculative, but a reasonable presumption, that violating the protocol necessarily results in higher rates of complications. The notion that somehow the investigators in the original trial treated patients differently than practicing clinicians has been put to rest. No matter what the background, training or experience of the physician, if the protocol is followed, the same benefits will accrue.

THE ORIGINAL RESULTS ARE CONFIRMED ON LONG-TERM FOLLOW-UP

There is always a question as to whether good results seen early after therapy can still be detected some time after the therapy. In the initial report, the effect of thrombolysis was confirmed 3 mo after stroke. Now, the beneficial effects of thrombolytic stroke therapy have been confirmed by following the patients in the original study for up to 1 yr *(25)*. These data are presented in more detail in Chapter 9. Only 22 patients (out of 624) were lost to follow-up, 14 in the t-PA group and 8 in the placebo group. In order to avoid biasing the results toward benefit in the t-PA group, each of these missing patients was assigned the most unfavorable outcome; that is, the analysis was slightly biased in favor of the placebo group. When the patients were assessed 6 and 12 mo after thrombolytic stroke therapy, the results were nearly exactly the same as in the original publication, which reported on follow-up data 3 mo after stroke. Using a global test to simultaneously describe the results of three outcome measures, the odds ratio of a near complete recovery after t-PA was 1.7 (95% CI 1.3 to 2.3), compared to placebo ($p = 0.0013$). Looking at the individual measures of outcome, patients are 30% to 50% more likely than placebo-treated patients to have minimal or no disability 1 yr after thrombolytic stroke therapy. In addition to the long-term functional data, the volume of infarction seen on CT scans 3 mo after thrombolytic therapy was analyzed. A preliminary report of the data communicated a significant effect: median stroke volume was 25.5 cm^3 in placebo treated, vs 15.5 cm^3 in t-PA treated, patients ($p = 0.039$). A final report of this data analysis is in preparation.

These data show that the beneficial effects of thrombolytic therapy are maintained up to one year after treatment.

VASCULAR IMAGING IS UNNECESSARY PRIOR TO THROMBOLYTIC THERAPY

The need for vascular imaging prior to stroke thrombolysis remains controversial, at least for some (*see* Chapter 13) *(5)*. The argument may be summarized by the contention that thrombolytic therapy could be given needlessly to some patients unless an image of the occluded artery is first obtained. That is, if the patient has no documented vascular occlusion, then thrombolytic therapy should not be used. In rebuttal, consider two important points: First, using the NINDS thrombolysis protocol, very few patients were treated "needlessly." In the placebo group, only 2% of patients exhibited no neurologic deficit (NIHSS = 0) when examined 24 h after stroke *(1)*. These 2% of patients included patients with transient ischemic attack (TIA) and perhaps other nonstroke etiologies. No hemorrhages or other side effects occurred in these patients. At 3 mo after their strokes, all of these patients were independent in activities of daily living; none suffered hemorrhage. Thus, it seems unlikely that vascular imaging prior to thrombolytic stroke therapy would add any benefit, since the protocol allows the proper selection of suitable patients. That is, if the protocol is followed correctly, there is only a 2% chance of treating a nonstroke etiology with thrombolysis. No harm occurred to any of the "TIA" patients who received t-PA.

The second rebuttal point is that the press of time requires prompt intervention, and vascular imaging requires precious time. An angiography team requires at least 60 min to mobilize and obtain the first images, even in the most dedicated centers (see Chapter 11) *(26)*. During those 60 min, brain cell death continues and the chances for a good outcome probably decline. Alternatives to invasive angiography await further development. Transcranial ultrasound techniques are improving, but do not visualize the intracerebral circulation in a majority of acute stroke patients. Novel techniques, such as spiral CT angiography and xenon enhanced CT may hold promise, but will require carefully designed, properly controlled trials to assure reliability. In the meantime, vascular imaging seems to be neither required, nor desirable, prior to thrombolytic stroke therapy.

The advantage of intravenous thrombolytic therapy is that active treatment is delivered to patients within a reasonable time frame. Is it harmful to administer t-PA to patients in whom no blockage can be documented on angiogram to respond to therapy? The evidence is to the contrary: in the subgroup analysis of the NINDS t-PA study the group of patients who were thought to have lacunes responded to therapy as well as or better than other subgroups *(27)*. It is well-appreciated that for patients with lacunar-syndrome presentations, angiography is inadequate to document the level of arterial occlusion. Since these patients responded to thrombolytic therapy, it can be inferred that thrombosis occurs in lacunar syndromes and that angiography will not document this thrombus. Further, the safety of thrombolytic therapy in this subgroup of "angio-negative" strokes is proven.

On the other hand, one important advantage of angiography is that intra-arterial therapy could be delivered directly into the clot *(28)*. Recently a large trial of intra-arterial pro-urokinase (PROACT) was reported: The authors found that the combination of pro-urokinase plus standard dose heparin was hazardous, resulting in hemorrhages in 27.3% of treated patients, compared to 20% in patients who received only standard heparin *(26)*. Patients who received low doses of Heparin did not suffer such a high degree of hemorrhages (6.7%), but also did not enjoy rapid thrombolysis of their clots. Using this preliminary safety and efficacy data, the study was revised and reconducted (PROACT II): 180 patients were treated within 6 h of stroke onset with intravenous low-dose heparin and intra-arterial pro-urokinase *(29)*. Intra-arterial pro-urokinase significantly improved the proportion of good outcomes from 25% to 40% ($p < 0.05$). Hemorrhages were seen in 10%, consistent with other thrombolytic trials. This study demonstrated that thrombolysis with intra-arterial pro-urokinase is safe and effective up to 6 h after stroke. (These studies are presented in detail in Chapters 10 and 11.)

SUBGROUP SELECTION IS NOT JUSTIFIED

It may be argued that because the full range of potentially salvageable stroke patients is not known, we should treat no one until we know precisely which patient subgroups do respond to thrombolytic therapy. This argument can be supported by examining the response rate in the original report and in subsequent analyses: a minority (30 to 50%) of t-PA treated patients enjoys a full recovery.

Further, every clinician desires to find the best possible candidate for therapy, and to attempt to "target" treatment at the subgroup of patients that is most likely to respond. Recent analysis, however, has been published to show that a majority of patients enjoy some benefit from t-PA, albeit not a complete cure *(27)*. This discrepancy derives from the statistical method that was used in the original report; the outcomes were reported in terms of the numbers of complete or nearly complete recoveries. The original report did not mention the benefits accrued in those patients who had less than a complete recovery. For example, patients who have a severe deficit on admission (pretreatment) and are over the age of 75, appear to improve significantly compared to placebo-treated patients in the same subgroup (see Fig. 4 in Chapter 9). These patients do not achieve the criteria for a complete recovery with either placebo or t-PA treatment, but there are more patients with a mild deficit, and fewer patients with a moderate or severe deficit, in the t-PA treated group *(27)*. That is, patients in this subgroup are too ill to recover completely, but t-PA treatment may improve their outcome from severe to mild. Similar analyses can be presented for other types of patients as well. The NINDS investigators have examined the original data for ANY subgroup of patients in whom t-PA was unlikely to benefit, and therefore could be withheld *(27)*. A similar analysis was conducted to try to identify subgroups of patients who were more likely than others to suffer hemorrhagic complications *(30)*. The analysis included multiple sequential statistical analyses, and various combinations of baseline data were analyzed. From the analyses of baseline variables, such as age, stroke deficit, presence of diabetes, presence of prior stroke, and other important factors, no subgroup could be identified for whom thrombolytic stroke therapy can be particularly recommended or prohibited. At present, therefore, the wisest course for the active clinician is to prescribe t-PA to patients who fulfill the criteria as outlined in the original protocol. Withholding therapy in some subgroup of patients hoping to target treatment to a more-likely-to-respond group is unwise.

THE POSITIVE RESULTS HAVE BEEN CONFIRMED USING OTHER PROTOCOLS, OTHER DRUGS

Since the original report of the NINDS t-PA Stroke Trial, there have now been published additional confirmations of the value of thrombolytic therapy for stroke including the pro-urokinase trial that was discussed above. In the first report of the European Cooperative Acute Stroke Study (ECASS), there was no statistically significant benefit for t-PA. Upon reanalysis, however, using the data methods developed for the NINDS study, a clear benefit was seen: the global odds ratio for favorable outcome was 1.5 (95% CI 1.1 to 2.0, $p = 0.008$) *(31)*. Further, in ECASS, most patients were enrolled within 6 h of stroke onset, but 87 patients were enrolled within the 3-h time limit used in the NINDS study *(32)*.

In these patients, the global odds ratio for favorable outcome was 2.3 (95% CI 0.9–5.3, $p = 0.07$), which is not statistically significant owing to the small sample size. To examine these potentially positive findings further, a confirmatory study was conducted (ECASS II) *(33)*. The primary end point of this study, the global odds ratio for a favorable outcome (score of 0 or 1) on the modified Rankin Scale, was negative. However, there were significantly more patients who scored well on the Rankin (score of 0, 1, or 2) in the t-PA treated (54.3%) vs placebo-treated (46.0%) patients, ($p = 0.024$). In this trial there were quite conservative inclusion criteria, resulting in an excess of mild patients in the study. For this reason, the beneficial effect of t-PA could have been diluted, resulting in lower statistical power.

Using a completely different type of drug, the defibrinogenating agent ancrod, a group of investigators also found benefit for patients treated within 3 h. Ancrod causes a reduction in fibrinogen, prolongation of the prothrombin time, reduced serum viscosity, and perhaps a thrombolytic effect *(34)*. In this trial, patients were treated within 3 h of stroke onset with a 72-h infusion of ancrod; the dose was adjusted to lower the fibrinogen to a target level. Preliminary data indicated a treatment benefit: there was a favorable outcome (modified Rankin of 0 or 1) in 41.1% of patients, compared to 35.3% in placebo-treated patients ($p > 0.05$) *(35)*. Unfortunately, if the fibrinogen were lowered excessively, there were more symptomatic intracranial hemorrhages.

CONCLUSIONS

The data collected and analyzed during the first years of the stroke thrombolytic era suggest that this new therapy withstands the test of time. The benefits persist over the long term, and are realized by clinically active neurologists practicing in typical community settings. Several groups have confirmed the value of thrombolytic stroke therapy when given within 3 h of stroke onset; treatment between 3 and 6 h after stroke appears to lack benefit, but may also lack significant risk. No specific subgroup can be found at particularly increased risk or benefit, suggesting that the original guidelines for selecting patients must be followed. Yet, the success of thrombolytic therapy, even at a distance of a few years, still raises a number of questions. Did we test the right dose and timing of drug administration? Might other thrombolytic drugs, or other dosing schedules, prove more beneficial? How can we increase the success rate to something greater than 50%? Will neuroprotectants add benefit or reduce risk, when combined with thrombolytic therapy? Is the 3-h time limit absolute, or is there some way to find patients in whom therapy could be given later? Most importantly, what can be done to educate more patients and potential stroke-witnesses about the signs of stroke and the need for immediate medical attention?

Thrombolytic stroke therapy represents something of a novel situation for clinically active neurologists. Heretofore, the general strategy in neurology has been to minimize disability although doing no harm. It is a rare situation when the active neurologist must choose between a therapy that has side effects but also has a net benefit: The first therapy for stroke is also the first therapy for which neurologists must urgently present difficult choices to patients and families for an immediate decision. Without question, this is an uncomfortable situation for all. However, now that the results of the NINDS t-PA study have been well digested, criticized, confirmed, supplemented with additional data, and diffused widely, it is time to take this bull by the horns. It is no longer appropriate to wait for further developments in this field: more than 11 patients per hour have a disabling stroke in America. Although more and more stroke patients receive thrombolytic therapy, it is still true that a majority of eligible patients do not receive it. The dictum *primum no nocere* still applies: we must do no harm, either by actively committing an act or by withholding a proven therapy through inaction.

ACKNOWLEDGMENTS

This work was supported by N01-NS02377 and the Veteran's Affairs Medical Research Service. These opinions are the author's, and do not necessarily reflect a consensus of the NINDS t-PA Stroke Study Group.

REFERENCES

1. NINDS rt-PA Stroke Study Group. Tissue plasminogen activator for acute ischemic stroke. *N Engl J Med* 1995;333:1581–1587.
2. Report of the Quality Standards Subcommittee of the American Academy of Neurology. Thrombolytic therapy for acute ischemic stroke—Summary Statement. *Neurology* 1996; 47:835–839.
3. Adams HP Jr, Brott TG, Furlan AJ, Gomez CR, Grotta J, Helgason CM, et al. Guidelines for thrombolytic therapy for acute stroke: A supplement to the guidelines for the management of patients with acute ischemic stroke. *Circulation* 1996;94:1167–1174.
4. Lyden PD, Grotta JC, Levine SR, Marler JR, Frankel MR, Brott TG. Intravenous thrombolysis for acute stroke. *Neurology* 1997;49:14–29.
5. Caplan L, Mohr JP, Kistler JP, Korosue K. Should thrombolytic therapy be the first-line treatment for acute ischemic stroke? thrombolysis—not a panacea for ischemic stroke. *New Engl J Med* 1997;337:1309–1310.
6. Avruch S, Cackley AP. Savings achieved by giving WIC benefits to women prenatally. *Public Health Rep* 1995;110:27–34.
7. Schoenbaum SC, Hyde JN, Baroshesky L, Crampton K. Benefit-cost analysis of rubella vaccination policy. *N Engl J Med* 1976;294:306–310.
8. Koplan JP, Schoenbaum SC, Weinstein MC, Fraser DW. Pertussis vaccine—an analysis of benefits, risks and costs. *N Engl J Med* 1979;301:906–911.
9. Koplan JP, Preblud SR. A benefit-cost analysis of mumps vaccine. *Am J Dis Child* 1982;136:362–364.
10. Cutting WA. Cost-benefit evaluations of vaccination programmes. *Lancet* 1980; 8195 pt 1:634–635.
11. Furlan A, Kanoti G. When is thrombolysis justified in patients with acute ischemic stroke? A Bioethical Perspective. *Stroke* 1997;214–218.

12. del Zoppo, G. Acute stroke: on the threshold of a therapy? New Engl J Med 1995;333:1632–1633.

13. Katzan I, Furlan A, Lloyd L, Frank J, Harper D, Hinchey J, et al. Use of tissue-type plasminogen activator for acute ischemic stroke: The Cleveland Area Experience. *JAMA* 2000;283:1151–1158.

14. Andre C, Moraes-Neto J, Novis S. Experience with t-PA treatment in a large South American city. *J Stroke Cerebrovasc Dis* 1998;7:255–258.

15. Albanese MA, Clarke WR, Adams HP Jr, Woolson RF. Ensuring reliability of outcome measures on multicenter clinical trials of treatments for acute ischemic stroke: the program developed for the trial of ORG 10172 in acute stroke treatment (TOAST). *Stroke* 1994; 25:1746–1751.

16. Lyden P, Brott T, Tilley B, Welch KMA, Mascha EJ, Levine S, et al., NINDS TPA Stroke Study Group. Improved reliability of the NIH stroke scale using video training. *Stroke* 1994;25:2220–2226.

17. Buchan A, Barber P, Newcommon N, Karbalai H, Demchuk A, Hoyte K, et al. Effectiveness of t-PA in acute ischemic stroke. *Neurology* 2000;54:679–684.

18. Egan R, Lutsep HL, Clark WM, Quinn J, Kearns K, Lockfeld A, et al. Open label tissue plasminogen activator for stroke: The Oregon experience. *J Stroke Cerebrovasc Dis* 1999;8:287–290.

19. Chiu D, Krieger D, Villar-Cordova C, Kasner SE, Morgenstern LB, Bratina P, et al. Intravenous tissue plasminogen activator for acute ischemic stroke feasibility, safety, and efficacy in the first year of clinical practice. *Stroke* 1998;29:18–22.

20. Tanne D, Bates V, Verro P, Kasner SE, Binder J, Patel S, et al. Initial clinical experience with IV tissue plasminogen activator for acute ischemic stroke: a multicenter survey. *Neurology* 1999;53:424–427.

21. Tanne D, Verro P, Mansbach H, Levine S. Overview and Summary of phase IV data on use of t-PA for acute ischemic stroke. *Stroke Interventionalist* 1998;1:3–5.

22. Grond M, Rudolf J, Schmulling S, Stenzel C, Neveling M, Heiss WD. Early intravenous thrombolysis with recombinant tissue-type plasminogen activator in vertebrobasilar ischemic stroke. *Arch Neurol* 1998;55:466–469.

23. Trouillas P, Nighoghossian N, Getenet J-C, Riche G, Neuschwander P, Froment J-C, et al. Open trial of intravenous tissue plasminogen activator in acute carotid territory stroke: Correlations of outcome with clinical and radiological data. *Stroke* 1996;27:882–890.

24. Albers GW, Bates V, Clark W, Bell R, Verro P, Hamilton S. Intravenous tissue-type plasminogen activator for treatment of acute stroke: The standard treatment with alteplase to reverse stroke (STARS) study (STARS). *JAMA* 2000;283:1145–1150.

25. Kwiatkowski TG, Libman R, Frankel M, Tilley B, Morgenstern LB, Lu M, et al., NINDS rt-PA Stroke Study Group. Effects of tPA for acute ischemic stroke at one year. *NEJM* 1999; 340:1781–1787.

26. del Zoppo G, Higashida RT, Furlan AJ, Pessin MS, Rowley HA, Gent M, and the PROACT Investigators. PROACT: A Phase II randomized trial of recombinant pro-urokinase by direct arterial delivery in acute middle cerebral artery stroke. *Stroke* 1998;29:4–11.

27. NINDS TPA Stroke Study Group. Generalized efficacy of t-PA for acute stroke. *Stroke* 1997;28:2119–2125.

28. Hacke W, Zeumer H, Ferbert A, Bruckmann H, del Zoppo G. Intra-arterial thrombolytic therapy improves outcome in patients with acute vertebrobasilar occlusive disease. *Stroke* 1988;19:1216–1222.

29. Furlan AJ, Higashida RT, Wechsler L, Gent M, Rowly H, Kase C, et al. Intra-arterial pro-urokinase for acute ischemic stroke. The PROACT II study: a randomized controlled trial. *JAMA* 1999;282:2003-2011.

30. NINDS TPA Stroke Study Group. Intracerebral hemorrhage after intravenous t-Pa therapy for ischemic stroke. *Stroke* 1997;28:2109–2118.

31. Hacke W, Bluhmki E, Steiner T, Tatlisumak T, Mahagne M-H, Sacchetti ML, Meier D. Dichotomized efficacy end points and global end-point analysis applied to the ECASS intention-to-treat data set. *Stroke* 1998;29:2073–2075.

32. Steiner T, Bluhmki E, Kaste M, Toni D, Trouillas P, von Kummer R, Hacke W, ECASS Study Group. The ECASS 3-Hour Cohort. *Cerebrovasc Dis* 1998;8:198–203.

33. Hacke W, Kaste M, Fieschi C, von Kummer R, Davalos A, Meier D, et al. Randomised double-blind placebo-controlled trial of thrombolytic therapy with intravenous alteplase in acute ischaemic stroke (ECASS II). *Lancet* 1998;352:1245–1251.

34. The Ancrod Stroke Study Investigators. Ancrod for the treatment of acute ischemic brain infarction. *Stroke* 1994;25:1755–1759.

35. Sherman D, Atkinson R, Chippendale T, Levin K, Ng K, Futrell N, Hsu C, Levy D, and the STAT Writers Group. Intravenous ANCROD for Treatment of Acute Stroke. *JAMA* 2000;283:2395–2403.

13 The Case Against the Present Guidelines for Stroke Thrombolysis

The Present Recommendations for Clinical Use Should Be Modified

Louis R. Caplan, MD

CONTENTS

INTRODUCTION
THERE IS MUCH THAT WE DO NOT KNOW
   ABOUT STROKE THROMBOLYSIS
NONRANDOMIZED TRIALS SUGGEST
   THAT DIFFERENT VASCULAR LESIONS
   AND DIFFERENT MECHANISMS RESPOND DIFFERENTLY
   TO THROMBOLYTIC DRUGS
SOME PATIENTS THAT MEET PRESENT CRITERIA
   FOR USE OF THROMBOLYTIC DRUGS
   DO NOT HAVE OCCLUSIVE VASCULAR LESIONS
ETHICAL CONSIDERATIONS
SUGGESTIONS FOR NEW RECOMMENDATIONS FOR THROMBOLYSIS
REFERENCES

INTRODUCTION

Thrombolytic agents offer great promise as therapeutic agents for selected patients with acute cerebrovascular symptoms. Preliminary data show that thrombolytic drugs, as a whole, are probably effective when given early enough to the appropriate patients with occlusive vascular lesions who have brain at-risk for further infarction. Unfortunately, thrombolysis can also cause brain and systemic

From: *Thrombolytic Therapy for Stroke*
Edited by: P. D. Lyden © Humana Press Inc., Totowa, NJ

hemorrhage, at times fatal. As physicians our most important rule is *Primum non nocere*—do no harm. We must protect patients who do not have vascular lesions that might respond to thrombolytic drugs from receiving a potentially lethal treatment that has no prospect of helping them.

I believe that thrombolytic drugs should be used for stroke patients but only by experienced individuals and after testing that clarifies both the state of the brain ischemia and the causative cerebrovascular lesion. I do not agree with the present recommendations for thrombolytic use issued by committees of the American Heart Association (AHA) *(1)* and the American Academy of Neurology *(2)*. These recommendations are all based on the NINDS protocol and trial *(3)* results and are substantially the same. I believe that more trials and more experience are needed in thoroughly studied patients with well-defined vascular lesions, treated with various agents at various doses by thrombolytic drugs given both intravenously and intra-arterially and that this thrombolytic treatment should be compared with other therapeutic alternatives *(4)*.

THERE IS MUCH THAT WE DO NOT KNOW ABOUT STROKE THROMBOLYSIS

The trials published to date and experience have not clarified many important issues concerning stroke thrombolysis.

What Is the Role of Hematological-Coagulation Factors?

The most commonly used thrombolytic drug, rt-PA, is an activator of plasminogen, a naturally occurring substance present within the blood stream of patients given the treatment. Levels of this substrate—plasminogen—vary. Patients also have a naturally occurring inhibitor-plasminogen activator inhibitor (PAI), that is also present at variable levels. Does the level of plasminogen substrate and the level of PAI influence treatment? Must some patients be given plasminogen as well as t-PA for effectiveness, and, if so, will this use cause complications?

Also unknown is the effect of levels of other substances that are active in the coagulation and fibrinolytic processes: platelet count, platelet functions (especially in patients who were taking antiplatelet aggregants), fibrinogen levels, levels of antithrombin III, protein C, protein S, activated protein C, Factors VII, VIII, and Xa, prothrombin time, partial thromboplastin time (PTT), and markers of active thrombolysis, e.g., fibrinopeptide A (FpA) and D-dimer. More data are needed concerning the hematological and coagulation aspects of treatment.

What Is the Best Drug to Use, and at What Dose?

A number of agents are available. The most commonly used agents are activase and urokinase but other agents are being synthesized and on the drawing board. Clot specificity is crucial and systemic fibrinolysis should be minimized. One dose of rt-PA (0.9 mg/kg) is being used and recommended but this dose has not been tested adequately for efficacy/safety vs other doses that might be equally effective but safer.

How Should Thrombolytic Drugs Be Given? Intravenously Always? Intra-Arterially to Patients With Selected Vascular Lesions?

Preliminary experience but not from properly conducted randomized trials indicates that intra-arterial treatment might be more effective than intravenous therapy for some vascular lesions, e.g., occlusions of the basilar artery. Preliminary data also show that intravenous therapy is mostly ineffective for some vascular occlusive lesions, e.g., occlusion of the internal carotid artery. Intravenous application has not been tested directly against intra-arterial treatment in patients with vascular lesions that were defined prior to treatment. We do not know the relative clinical effectiveness or the rate of recanalization with these two routes of administration.

Is Thrombolysis Better Than Other Strategies for Various Patients With Various Vascular Lesions and Stroke Pathophysiology?

Preliminary trials have studied thrombolytic drugs vs placebo. Thrombolytic agents have not been compared to other therapies now in use or also under investigation. These include anticoagulants (heparin, low-molecular-weight heparin, heparinoids); antiplatelet aggregants (aspirin, clopidogrel, aspirin-dipyridamole, GP llb/llla inhibitors); and ancrod.

What Other Treatments Should Be Used in Selected Patients at the Time of Thrombolysis or Following Thrombolysis?

Preliminary data show rather conclusively that intracranial arteries that are occluded by emboli are more consistently recanalized after application of thrombolytic drugs than arteries that harbor *in situ* thrombi engrafted upon local atherostenotic lesions. Should angioplasty, with or without a stent, be used at the time of thrombolysis? Should heparin be used after thrombolysis? Should it be used in all patients or only in selected patients and, if so, when and how much is effective and safe? Would antiplatelet agents e.g., GP llb/llla inhibitors or aspirin be used instead?

NONRANDOMIZED TRIALS SUGGEST THAT DIFFERENT VASCULAR LESIONS AND DIFFERENT MECHANISMS RESPOND DIFFERENTLY TO THROMBOLYTIC DRUGS

From our knowledge about thrombolytic drugs, there is no reason to posit that patients without occlusive vascular lesions will respond to thrombolytics. Trials and observational studies that have defined the occlusive vascular lesions before and after thrombolysis have distinct advantages over trials and observations that do not include vascular data. The treated patients have, by definition, occlusive lesions, otherwise they are not treated. Moreover, the only known therapeutic effect of thrombolytic drugs that is now known is lysis of thrombi. In all studies the success of reperfusion highly correlates with outcome. These studies can define the rate of acute successful recanalization.

To place the results of trials that did not define arterial lesions (NINDS *[4]*, ECASS 1 *[5]*, and ECASS 2 *[6]*) in context, it is important to review those studies in which the arterial lesions have been shown by angiography before intra-arterial and intravenous thrombolysis. These studies reveal important data about the effectiveness of the drug in producing recanalization, and the relation of recanalization to clinical outcome. They also indicate the risks of intracranial bleeding in patients with known occlusive lesions.

Intra-Arterial Thrombolytic Studies

Intra-arterial studies by definition have all been performed under angiographic control. After a diagnostic angiogram shows an acute vascular occlusion, a physician trained and experienced in interventional endovascular therapy introduces a catheter into a region near the thrombus and applies a thrombolytic drug at or near the proximal end of the clot. At times, physicians use the catheter to physically manipulate the clot to facilitate clot fragmentation and lysis. Table 1 lists data from various large published intra-arterial studies including drugs used, occluded arteries, frequency of successful reperfusion, presence of hemorrhagic complications, and outcomes *(7–24)*. The timing of treatment varied considerably in these studies but the agent was always given within 24 h. In one study, which included only patients treated with urokinase after middle cerebral artery (MCA) occlusions related to angiographic or endovascular procedures, the patients were all treated within 3 h *(18)*.

The presence and extent of reperfusion depended greatly on the pathophysiology of the stroke and the location of the occluded artery. Among the 469 patients treated in these 13 studies, about two-thirds had effective recanalization after therapy. In general, mainstem and divisional MCA occlusions responded best, intracranial carotid artery (ICA) occlusions responded less well. Distal MCA branch occlusions did not respond as well as more proximal MCA lesions. Sixty-nine percent of patients with basilar artery occlusion showed recanalization. Thrombolytic treatment of patients with occlusion of the ICA bifurcation (the carotid "T" portion) was almost invariably unsuccessful *(25)*. Embolic occlusions were generally more successfully recanalized than thrombosis engrafted upon *in situ* atherosclerosis *(26)*. In some patients transluminal angioplasty was needed after thrombolysis to keep the occluded artery open *(27)*. Recanalization was helped by mechanical clot disruption. This was especially important in patients with carotid artery thromboses in whom emboli originating

Table 1
Intra-arterial Thrombolytic Studies

Author	Drug	Total	Reperfusion of arteries			Hem	"Good outcome"
			ICA	MCA	Basilar		
del Zoppo (7)	U/S	19	7/8	9/11		4	17 (89%)
Hacke (8)	U/S	43			19/43	4	13 (30%)
Zeumer (9)	U/t-PA	59	29/31		28/28	8	17 (29%)
Mori (10)	U	22		8/22		4	11 (50%)
Mori (11)	U	44	1/8	13/31	2/5	10	16 (36%)
Mobius (12)	U/S	18			14/18		10 (56%)
Matsumoto (13)	U/t-PA	93	21/36	28/41	9/16	25	30 (32%)
Theron (14)	S/U	12	3/3	9/9		3	11 (92%)
Zeumer (15)	S	5			4/5		3 (60%)
Casto (16)	U	12		8/8	3/4	3	5 (42%)
Barnwell (17)	U	12	2/2	5/8	2/2	3	9 (75%)
Berg-Dammer (18)*	S/U	14		13/14			9 (64%)
Mitchell (19)	U	16			13/16	2	7 (44%)
Jansen (20)	U/tPA	16	2/16			3	1 (6%)
Becker (21)	U	12			10/13*	2	3 (25%)
Cross (23)	U	20			11/20	7	4 (20%)
Wijdicks (23)	U	9			7/9	1	5 (56%)
Gonner (24)	U	43	1/9	13/23	5/10	8	26 (60%)
Totals recanalized		469	37/82	106/167	127/189	87	197 (42%)
		299 (64%)	45%	62%	67%	18.5%	

U = Urokinase; S = Streptokinase; tPA, tissue plasminogen activator; Hem, hemorrhagic changes.
*13 occlusions/12 patients; 2 basilar, 10 bilat vertebral artery.

from the carotid thrombus had occluded the MCA. Penetration of the catheter through the clot in the neck allowed placement of the catheter at the MCA clot with subsequent successful recanalization. Hemorrhagic complications occurred in 18.5% of patients and 42% of the treated patients had a good outcome as judged by the authors of the reports (Table 1).

Intravenous Angiographic Studies Using rt-PA in Patients With Defined Vascular Lesions

In seven clinical studies, the vascular lesions were defined by angiography but the thrombolytic drug was delivered intravenously (25–31). In these studies, the angiographic catheters were left in situ so that angiography could be performed both before and after intravenous delivery of the drug. Table 2 outlines the results of these studies. Only two of these studies (25,27) included control patients that were not given a thrombolytic drug. In all of the series except one (30,31), rt-PA was given within 6 h, whereas in the other study there was an 8 h limit. Among the total of 370 patients treated with rt-PA, one-third of the arteries treated showed significant recanalization as compared to only 5% of 58 control arteries. MCA branch occlusions recanalized best followed by occlusions of the superior and inferior divisions of the MCA. Mainstem MCA occlusions recanalized less often than branch and division MCA lesions. ICA occlusions recanalized seldom and there were no recanalizations when both the ICA and MCA were occluded. Very few patients with documented basilar artery occlusions were given intravenous rt-PA and only one-sixth recanalized. Embolic occlusions recanalized more often than in situ thrombosis of atherostenotic arteries. Recanalization was better when there was angiographic evidence of good collateral circulation prior to administration of rt-PA. Both hemorrhagic infarction and parenchymatous hematomas were slightly more common after intravenous as compared to intraarterial delivery of the thrombolytic agents.

SOME PATIENTS THAT MEET PRESENT CRITERIA FOR USE OF THROMBOLYTIC DRUGS DO NOT HAVE OCCLUSIVE VASCULAR LESIONS

Clearly not all patients who come to doctors and hospital emergency rooms with a preliminary diagnosis of stroke have lesions treatable by thrombolytic drugs. Some patients have nonvascular conditions. Seizures and postictal neurological deficits are often difficult to distinguish from brain ischemia. Migraine with aura is another common stroke mimic. Some patients have nonorganic deficits. Some have peripheral disorders that produce weakness and other neurological signs. Patients with all of these situations usually have normal or nondiagnostic computed tomography (CT) scans. Differentiation of these various conditions from strokes is difficult especially within a short period of time.

Table 2
Intravenous rt-PA-Angiographic Studies

Author	Time	Total patients treated	Arteries recanalized/total			Hemorrhage	Outcome
			ICA	MCA	BA		
Yamaguchi (25)	<6 h	51 t-PA	10/47 t-PA		0	24 HI, 4 PH	37% good;
		47 control	2/46			22 HI, 5 PH	22% C good
Yamaguchi (26)	<6 h	121 t-PA	28/121			11 HI & PH	MCA>ICA
Mori (27)	<6 h	19 t-PA,	1/6	7/13	0	8 HI, 1 PH	t-PA>C
		12 control	0/4	1/8		4 HI, 1 PH	
von Kummer (28)	<6 h	32 t-PA	1/11	10/21	0	9 HI, 3 PH	44% good
von Kummer (29)	<6 h	27 t-PA	3/10	9/17	1/5	6 HI, 0 PH	44% good
Jansen@ (20)	<6 h	8 t-PA, 8U	2/16			1 PH	19% good
del Zoppo (30,31)	<8 h	104 (93*) tPA	2/23	12/34 mst 14/26M2 29/44 br	0/1	21 HI, 11 PH	no data
Totals		370	128/389 (33%) t-PA		16%	58 HI, 20 PH	
		59 Controls	3/58 (5%) Controls			26 HI, 6 PH	

*93 of the 104 completed rt-PA therapy according to protocol; recanalization data presented as arteries not as patients.

**Only patients with ICA/MCA emboli included.

HI = hemorrhagic infarct; PH = parenchymatous hemorrhage.

mst = mainstem MCA; M2 = MCA divisions; br = branch.

@ -Only intracranial ICA occlusions.

Table 3
Vascular Lesions Causing Ischemia Not Likely to Be Treatable
by Thrombolytic Drugs

Preocclusive atherostenosis
Vasoconstriction without superimposed thrombosis, e.g., related to migraine
Embolism of substances other than red erythrocyte-fibrin clots (such as cholesterol chrystals, atheromatous plaques, bacteria, myxoma material, fat, air, calcium fragments from plaques and valves, white platelet-fibrin thrombi

Table 4
Vascular Processes That Probably Will Not Respond
But Further Trials Are Needed

Emboli that have passed
Penetrating artery disease related brain infarcts

Following the recommendations for treatment within 3 h, clinical history, general and neurological examinations, blood drawing, CT scan, and discussions with family and patients must be completed within the time interval between arrival and 3 h in order for thrombolytic treatment to be used. This limits the thoroughness of the examinations even in the best of hands. Of course, the more experienced the clinician is with stroke patients and with neurological disorders, the more likely that stroke mimics will be identified. However, most patients in Europe and the US and throughout the world who have acute neurological symptoms are not seen by experienced neurologists or other stroke clinicians. Brain ischemia is caused by a variety of very different specific pathophysiologies. I have discussed arterial occlusive lesions in Chapter 2 of the first section of this book. Atherostenosis and thrombotic occlusion of large extracranial arteries, intrinsic atherothrombotic disease of large intracranial arteries, cardiogenic embolism, intra-arterial embolism from the aorta or from plaques in proximal arteries, arterial dissections, vasoconstriction, lipohyalinosis of penetrating small arteries, thrombosis related to abnormalities of blood coagulation represent the most common disorders. Large stroke registries such as the Harvard Stroke Registry *(32)*, the Stroke Data Bank *(33)*, and the Lausanne Stroke Registry *(34)* have shown convincingly that outcome depends heavily on stroke pathophysiological mechanisms. Optimal stroke treatment depends on recognition of stroke subtype and definition of the nature, location, and severity of the causative cardiac, hematological, and vascular lesions.

Among those patients who do have brain ischemia, many do not have arterial occlusions likely to respond to intravenously applied thrombolytic drugs. Table 3 lists the processes which would not be posited to respond to thrombolytic drugs and Table 4 lists conditions that are unlikely to respond but require further study.

Table 5
Vascular Occlusive Lesions Unlikely to Respond Well to Intravenous Therapy
But Might Respond Better to Intra-Arterial Therapy

ICA occlusions in the neck with embolism to the intracranial ICA or MCA
Intracranial ICA occlusions
Mainstem MCA occlusions near the origin
Basilar artery occlusion
Occlusion of the bilateral vertebral arteries
Extracranial vertebral artery occlusions with intracranial intra-arterial embolism

Some patients have occlusive lesions that preliminary data and knowledge of pathology would lead to the prediction that intra-arterial thrombolysis is likely to be better than intravenous. These occlusive lesions are enumerated in Table 5. There is little available data about thrombolytic treatment of vertebral artery occlusive lesions.

Modern technological advances now make it possible in the hands of experienced clinical stroke research teams to determine stroke subtype and vascular lesions quickly and safely. A decade ago, when the NINDS (4) and ECASS 1 (5) studies, were designed, angiography was the only well-accepted means of defining arterial lesions. Angiography took time to arrange and perform and had definite patient risks. During the past decade, concurrent with the trials of thrombolytic therapy, there has been a revolution in noninvasive technology that can yield rapid and accurate information about vascular lesions. Duplex, color-flow, and transcranial Doppler ultrasound can be performed quickly and are accurate in detecting vascular occlusions when performed by experienced technicians and physicians. Transcranial Doppler can be used at the bedside to monitor recanalization. CT angiography (CTA) can be performed at the same time as CT scan, does not greatly extend the time of imaging, and can also reliably image occlusions of large arteries (35,36). Magnetic resonance imaging (MRI) diffusion and perfusion imaging can be performed using echo planar equipment at the same time as MRI scans, and can give very important data about brain infarction and perfusion. Magnetic resonance angiography (MRA) can also be performed concurrently and can image occlusive lesions. All of the MR studies can be performed within a very few minutes using modern equipment. All of the thrombolytic protocols require brain imaging prior to infusion of drug. The addition of vascular imaging (CTA, MRA, ultrasound) can be done at well-equipped experienced centers without adding significant time. The suggested use of rt-PA without vascular imaging ignores the revolutionary technological progress of the last decades and is a step backwards in time. Studies have shown that ultrasound, MRA, and CTA are all reliable, specific, and sensitive to occlusions of the large arteries that supply the brain (37).

A thrombus will not be found at angiography or noninvasive studies if the embolus had broken up and passed, the process was atherosclerotic stenosis without thrombosis, the process is narrowing of penetrating arteries without thrombosis, and in vasospastic conditions. The safety and utility of thrombolytic drugs in the circumstance of a nonocclusive vascular study is unknown. I am opposed to exposing patients who probably have little or no likelihood of therapeutic efficacy to a drug that may have a 5–10% chance of causing brain hemorrhage. Some proponents of thrombolytic therapy argue that, even if an occlusive lesion is not shown (e.g., an embolus that has fragmented and passed on, or a lacunar infarct possibly caused by a micro-thrombus), there may be sufficient small thrombi in the microvascular bed so that thrombolysis would still be effective. Certainly this is a testable hypothesis that can be explored systematically at selected centers in patients who have been thoroughly evaluated clinically and by modern brain and vascular imaging tests.

ETHICAL CONSIDERATIONS

Can a physician in good conscience give a patient a potentially hazardous medication when that patient might not have the disorder that the medicine treats? Suppose it was well-documented that thrombolytic drugs were effective in treating 85 patients among a large group of 100 patients who had acute brain ischemia. However, that 100 patients contained 5 patients who might not have the disorder the drug treats effectively, resulting in needless harm to the 5. Would it be appropriate to give all 100 patients the drug, possibly sacrificing the 5 "innocent" individuals?

Using an analogy, suppose that radiation therapy was 85% effective in patients with undefined lumps that appeared as mass lesions on brain imaging scans, but 5% of the patients did not have tumors and would be harmed by the radiation? Would we radiate all 100 or instead insist on a definitive diagnosis of cancer before radiation?

Stroke is a cerebrovascular disease. Thrombolytic drugs have one known action—they lyse red thrombi within brain arteries. We have tests that are safe and can be done quickly that can screen patients presenting with symptoms that suggest brain ischemia that can reliably identify patients with occluded arteries. These tests can be done at the same time as brain imaging. All recommendations now already require brain imaging. Vascular imaging should also be a part of the suggested evaluation.

SUGGESTIONS FOR NEW RECOMMENDATIONS FOR THROMBOLYSIS

Who Should Treat?

Whenever possible, thrombolytic drugs should be given by physicians experienced in treating stroke patients. Optimally, the patient will be studied at a center that has a team of physicians trained and experienced in stroke care. The center should have modern brain and vascular imaging technology and have protocols for rapid examinations and imaging. Ordinarily the team will be led by a stroke neurologist, but emergency physicians and internists may be part of the team. Communities should devise schema to be able to deliver stroke patients to these centers just as trauma victims are now triaged.

When? With What Time Window?

Treatment should be given as early as possible. The aim of thrombolytic treatment is to reperfuse brain tissue beyond occluded arteries to prevent brain that is at-risk for further ischemia from becoming infarcted. The tissue at-risk is brain that is underperfused but not yet infarcted. Some modern imaging technologies, e.g., diffusion and perfusion weighted MRI performed with MRA and CT performed with CTA can yield information about tissue that is infarcted, tissue that is underperfused, and whether arteries are still blocked. This technology is especially useful when the time of onset of symptoms is unknown, e.g., in patients said to have awakened with symptoms. Some patients with considerable brain still at-risk for further ischemia should be offered treatment even if studied beyond the usual 3 h window. Patients with basilar artery occlusion have responded even after 12 h of ischemia. The time window should not be rigidly clock bound.

What Tests Should Be Performed Before Thrombolysis?

Brain imaging tests are mandatory to determine presence and size of infarcts and to exclude hemorrhages and nonvascular etiologies of symptoms. MRI can be substituted for CT scan if the available MRI technology has the capability of excluding recent bleeding (e.g., susceptibility scans). Whenever possible, vascular imaging (CTA or MRA, and/or ultrasound-extracranial and transcranial) should also be performed before thrombolysis.

Is Thrombolysis Now the Standard of Care and for What Patients Under What Circumstances?

Brain ischemia is complex. Many physicians and hospitals will not be equipped to use this treatment safely and judiciously. Thrombolysis is and in the near future should clearly not be considered standard of care. There is still far too much to learn. Trials are still needed to determine which patients with what vascular lesions with what severity of ischemia should be treated when and with what drugs at what dose and given by what route. If thrombolysis without vascular investigations is mandated the answers to these questions will never be learned and some patients will be needlessly harmed by the treatment.

REFERENCES

1. Adams HP, Brott TG, Furlan AJ, et al. Use of thrombolytic drugs. A supplement to the guidelines for the management of patients with acute ischemic stroke. A statement for Health Care Professionals from a special writing group of the Stroke Council American Heart Association. *Stroke* 1996; 27:1711–1718.

2. Quality Standards Subcommittee of the American Academy of Neurology, Practice advisory: Thrombolytic therapy for acute ischemic stroke—summary statement. *Neurology* 1996; 47:835–839.

3. The National Institute of Neurological Disorders and Stroke rt-PA Study Group. Tissue plasminogen activator for acute ischemic stroke. *N Engl J Med* 1995;333:1581–1587.

4. Caplan LR, Mohr JP, Kistler JP, Koroshetz W. Thrombolysis: Not a panacea for ischemic stroke. *N Eng J Med* 1997;337:1309–1310, 1313.

5. Hacke W, Kaste M, Fieschi C, et al. Intravenous thrombolysis with recombinant tissue plasminogen activator for acute hemispheric stroke. The European Cooperative Acute Stroke Study (ECASS). *JAMA* 1995;274:1017–1025.

6. Hacke W, Kaste M, Fieschi C, von Kummer R, Davalos A, Meier D, et al. Randomized double-blind placebo-controlled trial of thrombolytic therapy with intravenous alteplase in acute ischaemic stroke (ECASS II). Second European-Australasian Acute Stroke Study Investigators. *Lancet* 1998;352:1245–1251.

7. del Zoppo G, Ferbert A, Otis S, et al. Local intra-arterial fibrinolytic therapy in acute carotid territory stroke. A pilot study. *Stroke* 1988;19:307–313.

8. Hacke W, Zeumer H, Ferbert A, Bruckmann H, del Zoppo G. Intra-arterial thrombolytic therapy improves outcome in patients with acute vertebrobasilar occlusive disease. *Stroke* 1988;19:1216–1222.

9. Zeumer H, Freitag H-J, Zanella F, Thie A, Arning C. Local intra-arterial fibrinolytic therapy in patients with stroke: Urokinase versus recombinant tissue plasminogen activator (r-tPA). *Neuroradiology* 1993;35:159–162.

10. Mori E, Tabuchi M, Yoshida T, Yamadori A. Intracarotid urokinase with thromboembolic occlusion of the middle cerebral artery. *Stroke* 1988;19:808–812.

11. Mori E. Fibrinolytic recanalization therapy in acute cerebrovascular thromboembolism. In: *Thrombolytic Therapy in Acute Ischemic Stroke*, Hacke W, del Zoppo GJ, Hirschberg M, eds. Springer-Verlag: Heidelberg. 1991; pp. 137–145.

12. Mobius E, Berg-Dammer E, Kuhne D, Nahser HC. Local thrombolytic therapy in acute basilar artery occlusion. Experience with 18 patients. In Thrombolytic Therapy in Acute Ischemic Stroke, Hacke W, del Zoppo GJ, Hirschberg M (eds.), Springer-Verlag, Heidelberg, 1991, pp. 213–215.

13. Matsumoto K, Satoh K. Topical intraarterial urokinase infusion for acute stroke. In: *Thrombolytic Therapy in Acute Ischemic Stroke*, Hacke W, del Zoppo GJ, Hirshberg M, eds. Springer-Verlag: Heidelberg. 1991; pp. 207–212.

14. Theron J, Courtheoux P, Casasco A, et al. Local intraarterial fibrinolysis in the carotid territory. *AJNR* 1989;10:753–765.

15. Zeumer H, Hacke W, Ringelstein EB. Local intra-arterial thrombolysis in vertebrobasilar thromboembolic disease. *AJNR* 1983;4:401–404.

16. Casto L, Caverni L, Canerlingo M, et al. Intra-arterial thrombolysis in acute ischaemic stroke: Experience with a superselective catheter embedded in the clot. *J Neurol Neurosurg Psychiatry* 1996;60:667–670.

17. Barnwell SL, Clark WM, Nguyen, TT, et al. Safety and efficacy of delayed intra-arterial urokinase therapy with mechanical clot disruption for thromboembolic stroke. *AJNR* 1994;15:1817–1822.

18. Berg-Dammer E, Henkes H, Nahser HC, Kuhne D. Thromboembolic occlusion of the middle cerebral artery due to angiography and endovascular procedures: safety and efficacy of local intra-arterial fibrinolysis. *Cerebrovasc Dis* 1996;6:222–230.

19. Mitchell PJ, Gerraty RP, Donnan GA, et al. Thrombolysis in the vertebrobasilar circulation: the Australian Urokinase Stroke Trial. Cerebrovasc Dis 1997;7:94–99.

20. Jansen O, von Kummer R, Forsting M, Hacke W, Sartor K. Thrombolytic therapy in acute occlusion of the intracranial internal carotid artery bifurcation. *AJNR* 1995;16:1977–1986.

21. Becker KJ, Monsein LH, Ulatowski J, et al. Intra-arterial thrombolysis in vertebrobasilar occlusion. *AJNR* 1996;17:255–262.

22. Cross III, DT, Moran CJ, Akins PT, Angtuaco E, Diringer MN. Relationship between clot location and outcome after basilar artery thrombosis. *AJNR* 1997;18:1221–1228.

23. Wijdicks EFM, Nichols DA, Thielen KR, et al. Intra-arterial thrombolysis in acute basilar artery thromboembolism: the initial Mayo Clinic experience. *Mayo Clin Proc* 1997;72:1005–1013.

24. Gonner F, Remonda L, Mattle H, et al. Local intra-arterial thrombolysis in acute ischemic stroke. *Stroke* 1998;29:1894–1900.

25. Yamaguchi T, Hayakawa T, Kikuchi H for the Japanese Thrombolytic Study Group, Intravenous tissue plasminogen activator in acute thromboembolic stroke: a placebo-controlled double-blind trial. In: *Thrombolytic Therapy in Acute Ischemic Stroke II*, del Zoppo GJ, Mori E, Hacke W, eds. Springer-Verlag: Berlin. 1993; pp. 59–65.

26. Yamaguchi T, Kikuchi H, Hayakawa T, for the Japanese Thrombolysis Study Group. Clinical efficacy and safety of intravenous tissue plasminogen activator in acute embolic stroke: a randomized double-blind, dose-comparison study of duteplase. In: *Thrombolytic Therapy in Acute Ischemic Stroke III*, Yamaguchi T, Mori E, Minematsu K, del Zoppo GJ, eds. Springer-Verlag: Tokyo. 1995; pp. 223–229.

27. Mori E, Yoneda Y, Tabuchi M, et al. Intravenous recombinant tissue plasminogen activator in acute carotid artery territory stroke. *Neurology* 1992;42:976–982.

28. von Kummer R, Hacke W. Safety and efficacy of intravenous tissue plasminogen activator and heparin in acute middle cerebral artery stroke. *Stroke* 1992;23:646–652.

29. von Kummer R, Forsting M, Sartor K, Hacke W. Intravenous plasminogen activator in acute stroke. In: *Thrombolytic Therapy in Acute Ischemic Stroke*, Hacke W, del Zoppo GJ, Hirschberg M, eds. Springer-Verlag: Heidelberg. 1991; pp. 161–167.

30. del Zoppo GJ, Poeck K, Pessin MS, et al. Recombinant tissue plasminogen activator in acute thrombotic and embolic stroke. *Ann Neurol* 1992;32:78–86.

31. Wolpert SM, Bruckmann H, Greenlee R, Wechsler L, Pessin MS, del Zoppo GJ, and the rt-PA Acute Stroke Study Group, *AJNR* 1993;14:3–13.

32. Mohr JP, Caplan LR, Melski JW, et al. The Harvard Cooperative Stroke Registry: a prospective registry. *Neurology* 1978;28:754–762.

33. Foulkes MA, Wolf PA, Price TR, et al. The Stroke Data Bank: Design, methods, and baseline characteristics. *Stroke* 1988;19:547–554.

34. Bogousslavsky J, Melle GV, Regli F. The Lausanne Stroke Registry: an analysis of 1000 consecutive patients with first strokes. *Stroke* 1988; 19:1083–1092.

35. Knauth M, von Kummer R, Jansen O, et al. Potential of CT angiography in acute ischemic stroke. *AJNR* 1997;18:1001–1010.

36. Shrier DA, Tanaka H, Numaguchi Y, et al. CT angiography in the evaluation of acute stroke. *AJNR* 1997;18:1011–1020.

37. Yamaguchi T, Mori E, Minematsu K, del Zoppo GJ (eds.), Thrombolytic therapy in acute ischemic stroke III, Springer-Verlag: Tokyo. 1995.

14 How to Run a Code Stroke

Christopher Lewandowski, *MD*

CONTENTS

INTRODUCTION: THE TRAUMA SCENE
PARTNERS: THE STROKE TEAM
PREPARE: SYSTEM DEVELOPMENT
PERFORM: RUNNING THE CODE
REFERENCES

INTRODUCTION: THE TRAUMA SCENE

Southbound on I-75 on a clear Sunday morning, life would never be the same again for the elderly couple. Returning from a summer weekend trip at 70 mph they hit a bridge abutment. They lay motionless in the quiet morning until the first witnesses called 911. Within minutes the Emergency Medical Services (EMS) paramedics arrived as if from the forest in this relatively rural stretch accompanied by fire trucks and state police. Life support measures were started immediately through the shattered windows. Extrication proved difficult but the team was prepared. The Jaws of Life cut and peeled back the roof like a tin can. The state police closed the highway while the firefighters secured the scene from fire risk. Initial assessments were communicated to the trauma center. The helicopter was called in. With absolute minimal scene time the couple was extricated, stabilized, and transported to the waiting arms of the trauma team. The doctors, nurses, and technicians from the Emergency Department (ED), Surgery, Orthopedics, Neurosurgery, and Anesthesiology had been through this many times before. Radiology, blood bank, and the OR were standing by. They divided into two teams upon their arrival and systematically evaluated and treated the victims. The husband died in the resuscitation room, his wife was taken to the operating room and ultimately survived her numerous injuries.

This type of rapid response and treatment of trauma victims has not always been part of the healthcare landscape. Those of us interested in the care of trauma

From: *Thrombolytic Therapy for Stroke*
Edited by: P. D. Lyden © Humana Press Inc., Totowa, NJ

patients have learned over the past 30 years that this response is normal, expected, and routine. In previous times both patients would have died. As recently as the 1970s, it was said that life expectancy after injury was better in the fields of Vietnam than on the streets and highways at home *(1)*. The lessons learned from treating casualties during military conflicts, from the Civil War through Vietnam, have been applied to civilian trauma *(2)*. Only recently, however, have the lessons learned in the military been applied to stroke.

Field resuscitation with rapid evacuation to well-prepared facilities for early aggressive care has led to a progressive decline in the mortality rates among battle casualties. In World War I, the mortality for battle casualties was 8%. In World War II with evacuation times of 6–12 h, it was 5.8%. In Korea, the institution of field hospitals (MASH units) dropped the mortality of battle casualties to 2.5%, and in Vietnam it was 1.7% with the time from injury to definitive care reduced to 65–80 min *(3)*. For major trauma, a window of approx 1 h exists to get victims to definitive care, the Golden Hour.

A review of critical care and emergency medical services conducted in the 1960s by the National Academy of Science and the National Research Council ultimately led to the Emergency Medical Systems Act of 1973 *(4)*. Since then, an extensive system of coordinated care from the prehospital setting to the ED to the hospital has been implemented across the United States. In Orange County, California, a regionalized trauma system with this type of coordinated care led to a dramatic drop in preventable trauma deaths from 73% to 9% *(5)*. Trauma centers that emphasize a systems approach to trauma care can be certified by state agencies or the American College of Surgeons as Level 1 Trauma Centers *(6)*. These systems maintain a trauma registry that allows for continuous system improvement and monitoring of outcomes by measuring key performance indicators such as time to definitive treatment.

These same systems have been adapted for rapid cardiac care and resuscitation. Cardiac arrest, most often precipitated by focal cardiac ischemia, causes global myocardial and cerebral ischemia. For victims of cardiac arrest the window of opportunity is much shorter, literally minutes. The brain can tolerate only a few minutes of global cerebral ischemia before permanent damage occurs; even the best EMS response times may be too long. A system of bystander initiated CPR, which has been taught successfully to the general public, is needed to initiate and facilitate the resuscitation effort *(7)*. In Seattle, high rates of citizen training in Basic Life Support (BLS) and rapid EMS response times have led to very high rates of successful resuscitation from out-of-hospital cardiac arrest *(8)*. The basic principles include recognition, activating 911, initiating CPR, and establishing the chain of survival *(9)*.

Acute myocardial infarction (AMI), or focal cardiac ischemia, often presents with chest pain. The public has been educated that chest pain may signify a heart attack and requires rapid evaluation; therefore, the 911 system should be activated. Many different strategies have been investigated in an effort to minimize the time to treatment of patients with chest pain and an acute myocardial infarction (MI), including prehospital 12 lead electrocardiograms (EKGs) and intravenous thrombolysis. An ED "door-to-drug" time of 30 min has been established as a nationwide goal by the National Heart Attack Alert Program *(10)*. Optimal time for treatment and reestablishment of reperfusion is within 4 h, though up to 12 h treatment may still be beneficial. Rapid recanalization and reperfusion, whether established using medical means or mechanical techniques, is the goal.

Stroke, or focal cerebral ischemia, requires a resuscitation effort similar to that carried out for other types of tissue ischemia and injury that have a time-limited therapeutic window. Because stroke is the leading cause of adult disability and the third leading cause of death in the United States *(11)*, a trauma-like approach to emergency brain resuscitation is just as important as medical or trauma resuscitations, though the systems are not yet as well-organized and executed. A general lack of understanding about stroke is an immense barrier to early presentation and treatment. More subtle and less painful presentations of acute stroke falsely lead patients to believe that the urgency and need for treatment is low. Unlike chest pain, there is no single cardinal warning sign that precipitates rapid and urgent action. This is particularly detrimental since we now know that treatment of stroke, like the treatment of a heart attack, is very time sensitive. In the NINDS recombinant tissue-plasminogen activator (rt-PA) Stroke Trial, further subanalysis of the time from the onset of symptoms to treatment with intravenous rt-PA showed that the sooner the patient is treated the better the chances for favorable outcome *(12)*. Those treated within 1 h of symptoms onset were over four times more likely to have full resolution of their symptoms as compared to those treated at the 3-h mark. It is helpful to think of stroke in the same light as a heart attack or as "Brain Attack" as this concept does underscore the need for speed *(13)*.

As in trauma, a significant amount of information needs to be collected in order to provide the opportunity for maximal benefit. This evaluation should occur in an organized manner within the context of a system that allows for process evaluation and improvement. This chapter focuses on the methods of organizing and carrying out a "Code Stroke" in order to provide this opportunity to as many patients as possible. In order to run an efficient Code Stroke one must create the context in which this task is to be carried out. Consequently, one needs to partner with colleagues in order to plan and prepare a Code Stroke system that needs to be practiced, performed, and perfected in a systematic manner, and ultimately perpetuated into routine practice.

PARTNERS: THE STROKE TEAM

The Stroke Team is a core component of an efficient and well-organized Code Stroke system. Teams have been made up of specifically identified individuals that respond to stroke alerts *(14,15)*. Typically, this response team includes those involved in acute stroke therapy such as neurologists, neurosurgeons, and stroke nurses, but should also include emergency physicians and nurses, paramedics, pharmacists, and other interested parties. Hospital and prehospital leadership EMS directors, chief of staff, department chairpeople, medical directors, and nursing directors should assist in identifying those who would best fit the role of champion in their institution. These "champions" should be very visible in educational and organizational efforts. They must be able to effectively communicate the goals of acute stroke care to all involved. In addition, they need sufficient conviction, commitment, and energy to overcome any nihilistic inertia that may exist in current practice. At least one person should be identified from the prehospital system (EMS), the ED, the hospital staff of stroke experts, and the department of nursing to form a core group or team. A detailed understanding of each level of care at a nuts-and-bolts level is important and open communication and feedback from those who will be actually implementing the process should be fostered. These individuals must work together in the development of systems to manage stroke patients efficiently across the various phases of care *(16)*.

The definition of the team may vary based on the human resources available. Usually, stroke team members are available for the evaluation, treatment, and management of every identified stroke patient *(17)*. They are generally available 24 h a day through a system of pagers that are activated through a single beeper number that can be accessed by EMS, dispatchers, physicians, or nurses that encounter acute stroke patients. This core team would train the prehospital, emergency, and hospital personnel to rapidly identify, screen, and support stroke patients. In its broadest sense, the team should include all individuals who participate in the direct and indirect care of the acute stroke patient. Each person that fulfills a specific role should be trained to complete his or her task and receive feedback on performance as well as patient outcome.

The duty of the stroke team is to develop and implement a system of care for the acute stroke patient. This would include assessing available resources, organizing the system, developing documentation forms, treating patients, maintaining a registry, and providing feedback and ongoing education.

PREPARE: SYSTEM DEVELOPMENT

The first task of the team should be to analyze their current system of acute stroke care while identifying the resources needed to care for patients in the desired manner. Analyzing the three phases of care from the patient's point of view helps to create a system that is smooth and efficient.

Some participating centers in the NINDS rt-PA Stroke Study used flow charting to gain a clear and detailed understanding of the processes involved in the care of stroke patients *(18)*. This process identified treatment delays as well as opportunities to improve efficiency. Detailed flowcharting identifies key personnel that participate in the processes (such as nurses, unit clerks, laboratory technicians, computed tomography [CT] technicians, dispatchers, pharmacists, paramedics, and various physicians) who may be added to the team to assist in process modification, educational efforts, and subsequent stroke patient care. Therefore, process problems are identified and modified by involving those that carry out the actual process before any patients are ever treated. The care plan developed should be easy to use, simple, and not unduly burden the patient care systems that are already in place for stroke or other diseases *(19)*. Furthermore, they should be designed to function under the most difficult situations such as ED overcrowding or multicasualty incidents. Patients who suffer their stroke while on an inpatient unit or in a catheterization lab need to be included in the system. These patients are frequently discovered late into the 3-h window, but may have a great deal of necessary information already available.

Individualized analysis and process development is necessary at each location. As acute stroke treatment can be carried out in a wide variety of settings, it is unlikely that any two systems will be identical. The exact type of response will depend on the resources of the individual institution. Common characteristics of all methods include parameters that can be timed, monitored, evaluated, and improved. These common parameters have been established at the NINDS Consensus Conference as goals for the evaluation of potential thrombolytic candidates *(20)* (*see* Chapter 16).

This system should provide a streamlined process that will reliably supply the necessary information to treat patients rapidly. The information needed is relatively straightforward (*see* Chapter 17). It includes (1) the history and physical examination (including the time of onset of symptoms, the past medical history, the National Institute of Health Stroke Scale Score [NIH-SSS], and the patient's weight), (2) basic laboratory data (CBC with platelet count, electrolytes and glucose, prothrombin [PT] and partial thromboplastin time [PTT]), and (3) head CT scan results (the EKG and chest X-ray are not required for treatment). Obtaining this information in a timely fashion may impact numerous processes (outlined in Table 1) that involve many health care workers and need to be clearly worked out in advance.

A practical approach to developing these systems is to analyze them from the inside out, that is, work backward, starting with the hospital phase, proceeding to the emergency phase, and finally moving outward to the prehospital phase. Understanding the patients' and caregivers' needs in the subsequent phase of care allows for anticipation and facilitation of these needs. For example, it is important for the ED to understand how and when to access intensive care beds for patients with stroke. Likewise, if EMS can transport a family member or a witness with the patient, it allows for more accurate and rapid determination of the time of onset of stroke symptoms during emergency care. This will create a greater understanding of the needs of each component, and opportunities to meet the needs of the ensuing phase will not be missed.

Table 1
Processes That Impact Rapid Care of the Stroke Patient

Prehospital
EMS response
Field Management
Transport protocol
Communication/prenotification
Stroke team activation

Emergency Department
Rapid triage and stroke team activation
Primary patient assessment and management responsibilities
Blood pressure management
CT availability and reading
Blood testing process
Drug preparation and administration
Adverse event management
Inpatient admission process

Hospital Phase
Inpatient management responsibilities
Monitoring process
Adverse event management

Documentation procedures should also be incorporated that permit system analysis, feedback, and the evaluation of quality indicators such as time to treatment. A flowsheet for documentation of patient care helps keep track of patient information and facilitates communication as the patient moves through the system (*see* Chapter 16). It serves as an excellent quality assurance document that can record all of the relevant time points, lab data, and monitoring parameters as well as a billing document.

Education is the next step after the system is in place. Personnel need the knowledge to have a positive impact on these patients. Determine the focus of the educational effort by reviewing the flowsheet to include all those that interface with stroke patients. They need to know about stroke in general, how to access the system and why their role is of vital importance. All team members must have a clear understanding of their role and its urgency especially since a stroke can have a very nonemergent feel because of a tradition of nihilism.

Once the team has been assembled, the patient management systems are in place, and all involved have been trained, a series of practice cases or patient simulations should be instituted. This will expose previously unrecognized obstacles to rapid and efficient care. All efforts should be made to ensure a smooth functioning system prior to treatment of the first case so that chances of a good outcome and a positive experience are maximized. Initial success in patient management is critical to the development of team pride and sense of accomplishment. As this grows, acute stroke care principles and methods will be incorporated into the practice patterns of the health care workers involved as a part of their daily and routine duties. As this develops, maintaining the educational level will be more a matter of updates than total reeducation.

If the on-call Stroke Team is not actively involved in patient care, they may be in an excellent position to participate in research protocols. Like AMI there are many unanswered questions on treatment of acute stroke and intracranial hemorrhage (ICH) patients. Consortiums with local academic institutions can be developed to incorporate many different practice environments in these efforts.

Evolution of the Team

This model is extremely useful in initially developing systems, educating colleagues (including providing clinical experience in acute stroke patient management), providing patient care, and facilitating stroke research. Ultimately, this model for a team of individuals is extremely labor intensive and can be difficult to sustain if only a limited number are involved. Therefore this primary stroke team may evolve after sufficient clinical experience and education to create long-term sustainable teams that are based upon the specific roles rather than specific individuals. The transitional team may eventually evolve into a coordinating, consultative, and steering role. A broad, role-based team is similar to the way trauma and cardiac resuscitation teams are currently organized. Ultimately, the general public behaves as key team members for cardiac resuscitation, and need to be educated to fulfill a role involving stroke recognition and system activation using the 911 system. The challenge in sustaining role-based teams is commitment to ongoing education, monitoring, and feedback. Ultimately, as in cardiac ischemia, this will become part of the general practice of medicine.

PERFORM: RUNNING THE CODE

The American Heart Association has developed the idea of the "Stroke Chain of Survival and Recovery" that refers to the Prehospital and ED phase of acute stroke care. It consists of the seven "Ds" or steps that are involved in the management of acute stroke patients: detection, dispatch, delivery, door, data, decision, and drug *(21)*. The initial three involve prehospital care and the remaining four refer to ED care. The hospital or inpatient phase, of course, follows this process.

Detection

Potential patients, their families, caretakers, and even bystanders need to know the signs and symptoms of stroke and activate the 911 system so those patients can be evaluated within the time frame for treatment.

Dispatch

Not only does the EMS or 911 system require immediate activation, but also a proper EMS response must be triggered. Dispatchers need education to be able to recognize a potential stroke victim, dispatch the proper personnel, and provide instructions to those on the scene.

Delivery

Once on the scene, the EMS needs to be able to quickly assess the patient. Simplified prehospital stroke scales have been developed in order to facilitate the evaluation. The Cincinnati Prehospital Stroke Scale focuses upon the testing of speech, arm drift, and facial asymmetry. Comprehensive EMS educational programs have been developed so that responders understand the principles of prehospital evaluation, treatment, and transport. The EMS provides essential supportive care, may be able to start an intravenous line, and check for hypoglycemia. They should avoid giving the patient hypotonic fluids and glucose unless hypoglycemia is documented. The EMS is critical in establishing the onset time of symptoms. A family member should come with the EMS to the hospital in order to discuss treatment options and verify the time of onset. EMS should establish radio contact and notify the receiving ED as soon as possible so that the necessary preparations can be made. These preparations may include stroke team activation, alerting the technicians in the lab and CT suite, notifying the pharmacy, or preparing an ICU bed.

Door

The ED phase begins with patient arrival. Even though the activities in the ED are described in a linear fashion they actually should be carried out simultaneously. Upon arrival to the ED, the patient must be met with an appropriate response. If not, the opportunity to treat will be lost and the EMS team will be discouraged from providing efficient care in the future. Stroke Team activation for "false alarms" presents an opportunity to teach and positively reinforce the patient care efforts. A single Code leader should be identified from the beginning to ensure all the data are reviewed prior to treatment and to avoid confusion in decision making.

Basic emergent supportive care should be instituted for all patients with stroke to ensure maximal perfusion and oxygenation of the brain regardless of the underlying pathology (subarachnoid hemorrhage, intracerebral hemorrhage, or ischemic stroke). Supportive care should commence before the clinical assessment and the diagnostic studies for stroke are completed. The basic measures are the "ABCs" of airway, breathing, and circulation taught in the Advanced Cardiac Life Support and Advanced Trauma Life Support courses (21).

Airway management is always the first step. The initial evaluation is aimed at ensuring upper airway patency. Assessment of the level of consciousness, which can be performed quickly simply by asking the patient "How are you?" (or using the level of consciousness questions and commands from the NIHSS) will provide information on mentation and speech as well as airway control. The oropharynx should be inspected for loose dentures, food, or other foreign bodies. An evaluation should be made of the patient's gag reflex, and the ability to control the tongue and secretions. Basic airway management includes foreign body removal, suctioning, and proper patient positioning using the chin lift or jaw thrust techniques. If these maneuvers fail to maintain a patent airway, most commonly due to a depressed level of consciousness, the patient may require a nasal airway (nasal trumpet) or even an oral airway. Patients tolerate oral airways poorly unless they are obtunded because of the gag reflex. If the patient has a depressed level of consciousness and is unable to manage secretions or maintain a patent airway, intubation with mechanical ventilation is indicated.

Once the airway is secure, breathing (ventilation and oxygenation) needs to be evaluated. If the patient does not have any respiratory effort, support should be instituted with a bag-valve-mask device or, if the patient is already intubated, assisted with a bag-valve until placement on a ventilator is accomplished. Respirations should be evaluated for rate and depth. Paradoxical respirations, a sign of impending respiratory failure, occur when the chest normally expands during inspiration and the abdomen abnormally contracts. This indicates that the diaphragm is no longer functioning and is being pulled into the chest, therefore, preparations should be made to support the patient with advanced airway techniques.

Pulse oximetry will reveal the percent oxygen saturation of hemoglobin. Supplemental oxygen should be applied to ensure oxygen saturations of 95% or greater. False readings on the pulse oximeter may occur in cases of peripheral vascular occlusive disease, hypotension with peripheral vasoconstriction, or carbon monoxide poisoning. Pulse oximetry does not evaluate ventilation, though capnography (a noninvasive measure of expired carbon dioxide) or arterial blood gas measurement will. Owing to the possibility of thrombolysis, blood for arterial blood gas studies should not be drawn routinely during Code Stroke unless indicated by other signs of respiratory failure.

The initial evaluation of the circulation is aimed at ensuring adequate organ perfusion. Circulation has multiple components including pulse, heart rate, and blood pressure. Pulses should be present and symmetric in all four extremities. Blood pressure measurement should be done in both arms because vascular emergencies, such as aortic dissections, can present as acute neurologic events. While the pulse and blood pressure are being checked, the patient should be placed on a cardiac monitor and an EKG obtained. EKG changes, such as T-wave inversions, occur frequently in acute stroke patients (22–24). They are most commonly associated with subarachnoid and intracerebral hemorrhages. Cardiac rhythm and function can be affected by an acute stroke when catecholamines are released from the brain, precipitating EKG changes but also arrhythmias, congestive heart failure, and even AMIs. Treatment of arrhythmias should be instituted if there is any hemodynamic compromise or the possibility thereof.

Blood pressure and pulse should be monitored at least every 15 min in the acute setting. Hypertension is common in acute stroke and should be treated judiciously (25,26). Hemodynamic compromise or hypotension can dramatically decrease the cerebral perfusion pressure and cerebral blood flow, extending the area of infarction. Hypotension should be viewed in the context of the past medical history, understanding that in patients with long-standing hypertension, the autoregulatory curve is shifted to the right. Autoregulation is a physiologic mechanism that maintains constant cerebral blood flow across a wide range of mean arterial blood pressure. During an acute stroke, ischemic brain tissue may lose autoregulatory function, and blood flow is directly related to the mean arterial pressure. "Normal" blood pressures can be relatively hypotensive in those with a history of hypertension. Hypotension should be evaluated and treated aggressively in order to prevent extension of the infarct.

In most cases, high blood pressure should not be treated during the acute phase of a stroke (26,27). Exceptions include certain patients with intracranial hemorrhage and when hypertension develops during or soon after rt-PA administration for ischemic stroke. Hypertension, if extreme, may also be deleterious, especially for patients with intracerebral hemorrhage or subarachnoid hemorrhage. For patients with ischemic strokes undergoing evaluation for thrombolysis, the American Heart Association guidelines recommend that the blood pressure not exceed 185/110 mm Hg at the time of treatment. The blood pressure should not be aggressively treated in order to bring patients into the normal range, but mild forms of drug therapy are acceptable (Table 2). Simple maneuvers such as elevation of the head of the bed may help control hypertension by increasing the cerebral venous drainage, this maneuver will also ease dyspnea and anxiety in patients with congestive heart failure. Euvolemia or slight hypervolemia may improve cerebral blood flow unless clinically contraindicated by heart failure or renal insufficiency. This is important in elderly patients who are prone to dehydration or may present with unknown down times. Hypotonic fluid (D5W) should be avoided as it may contribute to cerebral edema.

A trauma examination should be performed in all patients without good historical details to rule out cranial or cervical injury that could either mimic a stroke or occur from a fall or seizure associated with a stroke. Vascular access should be obtained in all stroke patients. Two intravenous catheters may be placed, one connected to normal saline and the other capped and flushed with saline to provide access for future blood draws, but line placement should not delay other tests. Intravenous fluids should not include glucose, as hyperglycemia is associated with worse neurologic outcomes. In fact, severe hyperglycemia may worsen stroke outcome, and should be treated (28,29). Any degree of fever should be aggressively treated with antipyretics

Table 2
Blood Pressure Guidelines

Pretreatment Blood Pressure Guidelines

If the blood pressure is over 185/110, the blood pressure may be treated with nitroglycerine paste or 1 to 2 doses of iv labetalol 10 to 20 mg each. If these do not reduce the blood pressure (bp) below 185/110 over 1 h, the patient should not be treated with rt-PA.

During and Posttreatment

For systolic bp 180–230 mm Hg or diastolic bp 105–120 mm Hg on 2 readings 5–10 min a part use:

1. Labetalol 10 mg iv over 1–2 min, repeat or double every 10–20 min, total maximum dose 150 mg.
2. Monitor BP every 15 min.

For systolic bp >230 mm Hg or diastolic 121–140 mm Hg for 2 or more readings, for at least 2 readings 5–10 min a part.

1. Use labetalol 10 mg iv over 1–2 min, repeat or double every 10 min to a maximum of 150 mg.
2. Monitor BP every 15 min.
3. If response unsatisfactory, use sodium nitroprusside with continuous blood pressure monitoring.

For diastolic bp >140 for 2 or more readings, 5–10 min a part use.

1. Sodium nitroprusside.
2. Monitor blood pressure every 15 min.

(e.g., acetaminophen), and its cause should be immediately sought out, as hyperthermia has also been associated with worse neurologic outcome *(30–32)*.

Data

Additional studies are required to complete the initial evaluation of the acute stroke patient, help discern the differential diagnoses as well as define some of the potential risks of thrombolysis. The CT scan of the head (*see* Chapter 14) is the most urgent study, though the blood tests can be obtained quickly during the initial exam at the time vascular access is acquired. The EKG and chest X-ray is important but is not mandatory prior to initiation of thrombolytic therapy unless specifically indicated in an individual patient. The utility of new magnetic resonance modalities such as diffusion-weighted and perfusion imaging is being actively investigated, and may ultimately help guide selection of patients for acute treatment with thrombolysis or neuroprotective agents.

The neurologic exam is the cornerstone of detecting a focal neurologic deficit in a characteristic vascular distribution. It should include an evaluation of the patient's mental status, cranial nerve function, motor strength, sensory function (including double simultaneous stimulation), coordination, and reflexes. This

Table 3
Current Form of the NIHSS

Item	Name	Response
1a.	Level of consciousness	0 = Alert
		1 = not alert, arousable
		2 = not alert, obtunded
		3 = unresponsive
1b.	Questions	0 = answers both correctly
		1 = answers one correctly
		2 = answers neither correctly
1c.	Commands	0 = performs both tasks correctly
		1 = performs one task correctly
		2 = performs neither task
2.	Gaze	0 = normal
		1 = partial gaze palsy
		2 = total gaze palsy
3.	Visual Fields	0 = no visual loss
		1 = partial hemianopsia
		2 = complete hemianopsia
		3 = bilateral hemianopsia
4.	Facial Palsy	0 = normal
		1 = minor paralysis
		2 = partial paralysis
		3 = complete paralysis
5a.	Left Motor Arm	0 = no drift
		1 = drift before 10 s
		2 = falls before 10 s
		3 = no effort against gravity
		4 = no movement
5b.	Right Motor Arm	0 = no drift
		1 = drift before 10 s
		2 = falls before 10 s
		3 = no effort against gravity
		4 = no movement
6a.	Left Motor Leg	0 = no drift
		1 = drift before 5 s
		2 = falls before 5 s
		3 = no effort against gravity
		4 = no movement
6b.	Right Motor Leg	0 = no drift
		1 = drift before 5 s
		2 = falls before 5 s
		3 = no effort against gravity
		4 = no movement

Table 3 *(continued)*

Item	Name	Response
7.	Ataxia	0 = absent
		1 = one limb
		2 = two limbs
8.	Sensory	0 = normal
		1 = mild loss
		2 = severe loss
9.	Language	0 = normal
		1 = mild aphasia
		2 = severe aphasia
		3 = mute or global aphasia
10.	Dysarthria	0 = normal
		1 = mild
		2 = severe
11.	Extinction/Inattention	0 = normal
		1 = mild
		2 = severe

assessment will provide the examiner with an understanding of the location of the lesion as well as the severity of the stroke. In order to provide for uniform assessments that are consistent and reproducible between examiners, various stroke severity scales have been developed. The NIHSS (Table 3) is a 42-point standardized scale that was developed for the NINDS rt-PA Stroke Trial *(33)* and is currently in common use as an indicator of the severity of neurologic dysfunction. Total NIHSS scores of 0 or 1 indicate a normal or near normal exam. Total scores of 1 to 4 indicate minor strokes though certain syndromes (such as global aphasia) may be severely disabling while having a low NIH-SS score. Total scores of 5–15 generally indicate a moderate stroke, 15–20 a moderately severe stroke, and >20 a severe stroke. The use of this scale should be encouraged as it provides for a reliable, valid method of communication between health care workers of all levels, and allows for accurate documentation of stroke severity that facilitates the analysis of outcomes, and allows comparison of therapeutic interventions. It does not replace the detailed conventional neurologic exam.

The differential diagnosis of acute ischemic stroke includes hemorrhagic stroke as well as numerous other maladies that can cause neurologic deficits (*see* Table 4). The characteristic feature of a stroke is the history of a sudden onset with a focal neurologic deficit in a specific vascular territory. The history, physical exam, CT scan of the head, and blood tests are used to differentiate mimics of acute stroke. These include intracerebral hemorrhage, seizures, trauma, tumors, abscess, vascular catastrophes, metabolic derangement, infections, and other neurologic conditions such as complex migraines.

Table 4
Some Stroke Mimics

Seizures
Trauma
Tumors/ Abscess
Complex migraines
Peripheral neuropathies
Hypertensive encephalopathy
Vascular catastrophes
Cerebral Venous or Sinus Thrombosis
Metabolic
Infections

Decision

Prior to making the decision to treat a patient with thrombolytics, specific information must be collected in a systematic fashion to determine patient eligibility. The most difficult piece of information to reliably obtain is the time of onset of symptoms. If a patient awakens with symptoms of an acute stroke, then the time of onset is considered the time he went to sleep. A baseline NIH stroke scale score needs to be obtained on all patients, as well as specific blood tests (platelet count, PT, PTT, glucose), and a noncontrast CT scan of the brain.

The decision to treat a specific patient with thrombolytics should be based on the risk and benefits of treating as compared to the risks and benefits of not treating. Clearly, those patients that do not meet the inclusion and exclusion criteria should not be treated (*see* Chapter 17). Patients who are treated outside the currently established parameters have been shown to have higher complication rates. Patients with high baseline NIH stroke scales (>20) may be at relatively higher risk of bleeding and higher risk for a poor outcome, but do benefit from therapy *(34)*. Patients with extensive early ischemic signs on the baseline CT scan are also at increased risk of ICH but also respond well to treatment (*see* Chapter 15). No subgroup of patients has been identified that does not benefit from treatment.

Drug

The only FDA-approved drug for acute treatment of ischemic stroke is t-PA. Recent trials have shown that two other drugs are also effective in acute therapy (*see* Chapter 12). Ancrod, a fibrinolytic drug (made from snake venom) and recombinant pro-urokinase, given intra-arterially within 6 h to selected patients. Heparin and low molecular weight heparin have not been shown to improve outcomes. Aspirin does reduce the risk of recurrent stroke over the first few weeks after stroke, but may be withheld safely for 24 h after giving thrombolytics.

After receiving thrombolysis, patients need to be admitted to a facility where intensive monitoring and care can be provided for the initial 24–36 h. This included frequent monitoring of vital signs and neurochecks (*see* Protocol in Chapter 17). If necessary, after treatment, patients can be transferred to a regional institution that may be more familiar with this level of care. A neurosurgeon should be available for consultation in the event of an ICH, but does not need to be physically available for two reasons. First, immediate evacuation of cerebral hematoma has not been proven to help patients. Second, the types of hemorrhages seen after thrombolytic therapy are not usually amenable to surgical therapy: the blood is usually intermixed with normal brain (hemorrhagic infarction). A discrete cerebral hematoma, which are very easy to remove surgically, even stereotactically, do not occur very often, if at all, after thrombolysis.

In summary, the Code Stroke should run as efficiently as those for trauma or cardiac arrest. An organized team must prepare a system to provide the context for a Code Stroke that can be reviewed and improved in order to obtain the greatest benefit and limit disability among stroke patients. This means that the time goals should be analyzed and those who are actually implementing the system should be interviewed to understand the obstructions that they may face. Not every environment can have all of the components described above; each system is different and is specifically designed based on the resources available. Irrespective of these limitations, a team can always start small and build with experience. There is no better way to generate enthusiasm for this effort than to successfully run a Code Stroke that results in a dramatic patient improvement.

REFERENCES

1. Boyd DR. The History of Emergency Medical services (EMS) in the United States of America. In: *Systems Approach to Emergency Medical Care*, Boyd DR, Edlich RF, Micik, SH, eds. Appleton-Century-Crofts: Norwalk, Conn. 1983; Chapter 1, pp. 3.
2. Boyd DR. The History of Emergency Medical services (EMS) in the United States of America. In: *Systems Approach to Emergency Medical Care*, Boyd DR, Edlich RF, Micik, SH, eds. Appleton-Century-Crofts: Norwalk, Conn. 1983; Chapter 1, pp. 2.
3. Barsan, W. Acute Medical care in the United States. In: *National Institute of Neurological Disorders and Stroke, Proceedings of a National Symposium on Rapid Identification and Treatment of Acute Stroke*, Marler JR, Winters-Jones P, Emr M, eds. National Institutes of Health: Bethesda, Maryland. 1997, 97–4239, pp. 11–16.
4. *Emergency Medical Services Systems Act of 1973*. 93rd Congress, Public Law 93–154: Washington, D.C. 1973.
5. West JG, Cales R, Gazzaniga A. Impact of regionalization: The Orange County Experience. *Arch Surg* 1983; 118:740.
6. *Advanced Trauma Life Support Program for Doctors*. 6th ed. American College of Surgeons: Chicago, IL. 1997.
7. *Basic Life Support for Healthcare Providers*. American Heart Association: Chandra, NC, Hazinski, MF, eds. Dallas, TX. 1997.
8. Eisenberg MS, Cummins RO, Larsen MP. Numerators, denominators, and survival rates: reporting survival from out-of-hospital cardiac arrests. *Am J Emerg Med* 1991;9:544–546.

9. Cummins RO. Emergency medical services and sudden cardiac arrest: The "chain of survival" concept. *Annu Rev Public Health* 1993;14:313–333.

10. National Heart Attack Alert Program Coordinating Committee, 60 Minutes to Treatment Working Group. Emergency Department: Rapid identification and treatment of patients with acute infarction. *Ann Emerg Med* 1994;23:311–329.

11. American Heart Association. 1998 Heart and Stroke Statistical Update. Dallas, TX: *American Heart Association*, 1997, 13–14.

12. Marler JR, Tilley BC, Lu M, Brott T, Lyden P, Broderick JP, et al, the NINDS rt-PA Stroke Study Group. Earlier treatment associated with better outcome in the NINDS t-PA stroke study. *Stroke* 1999;30:244(abstr).

13. Camarata P, Heros RC, Latchaw RE. Brain Attack: The rationale for treating stroke as a medical emergency. *Neurosurg* 1994;34:144–157.

14. Lyden PD, Rapp K, Babcock T, Rothrock J. Ultra-rapid identification, triage, and enrollment of stroke patients into clinical trials. *J Stroke Cerebrovasc Dis* 1994;4:106–113.

15. Bratina P, Greenberg L, Pasteur W, Grotta J. Current emergency department management of stroke in Houston, Texas. *Stroke* 1995;26:409–414.

16. Lewandowski, C. Developing Leadership and Systems Analysis. *National Institute of Neurological Disorders and Stroke, Proceedings of a National Symposium on Rapid Identification and Treatment of Acute Stroke*, Marler JR, Winters-Jones P, Emr M, eds. National Institutes of Health: Bethesda, Maryland. 1997, 97–4239, pp. 103–107.

17. Zweifler RM, Drinkard R, Cunningham S, Brody ML, Rothrock JF, Implementation of a stroke code system in Mobile, Alabama. Diagnostic and therapeutic yield. *Stroke* 1997;28:981–983.

18. Tilley BC, Lyden PD, Brott TG, Lu M, Levine SR, Welch KMA, and the NINDS rt-PA Stroke Study Group. Total quality improvement methodology reduces delays between emergency department admission and treatment of acute ischemic stroke. *Arch Neurol* 1997;54:1466–1474.

19. The NINDS rt-PA Stroke Study Group: A systems approach to immediate evaluation and management of hyperacute stroke: Experience at 8 centers and implications for community practice and patient care. *Stroke* 1997;28:1530–1540.

20. Recommendations. *National Institute of Neurological Disorders and Stroke, Proceedings of a National Symposium on Rapid Identification and Treatment of Acute Stroke*, Marler JR, Winters-Jones P, Emr M, eds. National Institutes of Health: Bethesda, Maryland. 1997, 97–4239, pp. 147–165.

21. Kothari R. *Textbook of Advanced Cardiac Life Support*, 4th ed. In Cummins RO, ed. American Heart Association: Dallas, TX. 1997; Chapter 10.

22. Komrad MS, Coffey CE, Coffey KS, McKinnis R, Massey EW, Califf RM. Myocardial infarction and stroke. *Neurology* 1984;34:1403–1409.

23. Myers MG, Norris JW, Hachinski VC, Weingert ME, Sole MJ. Cardiac sequelae of acute stroke. *Stroke* 1982;13:838–842.

24. Dimant J, Grob D. Electrocardiographic changes and myocardial damage in patients with acute cerebrovascular accidents. *Stroke* 1977;4:448–455.

25. Powers WJ. Acute hypertension after stroke: The scientific basis for treatment decisions. *Neurology* 1993;43:461–467.

26. Britton M, Carlsson A, de Faire U. Blood pressure course in patients with acute stroke and matched controls. *Stroke* 1986;17:861–864.

27. Yatsu FM, Zivin JA. Hypertension in acute ischemic strokes: Not to treat. *Arch Neurol* 1985;42:999,1000.

28. Auer RN. Insulin, blood glucose levels, and ischemic brain damage. *Neurology* 1998; 51:S39–S43.

29. Bruno A, Biller J, Adams HP, Clarke WR, Woolson RF, Williams LS, Hansen MD, TOAST Investigators. Acute blood glucose level and outcome from ischemic stroke. *Neurology* 999;52:280–284.
30. Busto R, Dietrich W, Mordecai G. Small differences in intraischemic brain temperature critically determines the extent of neuronal injury. *J Cereb Blood Flow Metab* 1987;7:729–738.
31. Castillo J, Martinez F, Leira R, Prieto JM, Lema M, Noya M. Mortality and morbidity of acute cerebral infarction related to temperature and basal analytic parameters. *Cerebrovasc Dis* 1994;4:66–71.
32. Ginsberg MD, Busto R. Combating Hyperthermia in Acute Stroke A Significant Clinical Concern. *Stroke* 1998;29:529–534.
33. Lyden P, Brott T, Tilley B, Welch KMA, Mascha EJ, Levine S, et al., NINDS TPA Stroke Study Group. Improved reliability of the NIH stroke scale using video training. *Stroke* 1994;25:2220–2226.
34. NINDS TPA Stroke Study Group. Generalized Efficacy of t-PA for Acute Stroke. *Stroke* 1997;28:2119–2125.
35. Adams HP, Brott TG, Furlan AJ, Gomez CR, Grotta J, Helgason CM, et al. Guidelines for thrombolytic therapy for acute stroke: a supplement to the guidelines for the management of patients with acute ischemic stroke. *Circulation* 1996;94:1167–1174.
36. The National Institute of Neurologic Disorders and Stroke rt-PA Stroke Study Group. Tissue plasminogen activator for acute ischemic stroke. *N Engl J Med* 1995;333:1581–1587.

15 Interpretation of CT Scans for Acute Stroke

Rüdiger von Kummer

CONTENTS

INTRODUCTION: IMAGING IN ACUTE STROKE
BASIC PRINCIPLES FOR THE INTERPRETATION
  OF CT IN ACUTE STROKE
TECHNICAL NOTE: HOW TO PERFORM CT IN ACUTE STROKE
TYPICAL CT FINDINGS WITHIN THE FIRST SIX HOURS
  OF STROKE ONSET
CONSEQUENCES OF CT FINDINGS FOR THROMBOLYTIC THERAPY
CONCLUSIONS
REFERENCES

INTRODUCTION: IMAGING IN ACUTE STROKE

The term "stroke" stands for a syndrome of sudden cerebral dysfunction caused by vascular diseases and representing different pathophysiological states of brain tissue including irreversible damage. Neurological examination can usually pinpoint the region of impairment and can even yield information about the amount of tissue affected, but it tells little about the exact type of process occurring. When a patient presents with acute focal cerebral dysfunction, focal cerebral ischemia is the most probable explanation, but ruling out the presence of intracranial hemorrhage (ICH) and other intracranial abnormalities including tumor, vascular malformation, encephalitis, or demyelinating disease remains the first consideration in order to initiate treatment. Imaging in acute stroke has, therefore, two objectives: 1) to assess the immediate pathophysiological state of the cerebral circulation and tissue, and 2) to assess the underlying disease. Assessment of the brain's current pathophysiological state is a prerequisite to choosing proper treatment for the prevention of permanent functional disturbance.

From: *Thrombolytic Therapy for Stroke*
Edited by: P. D. Lyden © Humana Press Inc., Totowa, NJ

Diagnosis of the underlying disease will help in the choice of proper secondary prophylaxis and is the less urgent of the two objectives. The imaging tool must be available and employed promptly within the first hours of stroke onset. The imaging modality should reliably differentiate cerebral ischemia from other causes of a sudden central nervous deficit and should additionally be able to differentiate early on normal brain tissue from tissue at risk and from tissue already irreversibly damaged.

Computed tomography (CT) and magnetic resonance imaging (MRI) are most promising for meeting these objectives in the clinical setting of acute stroke. Both imaging modalities can early detect ischemic edema. Moreover, both modalities offer the opportunity to image brain perfusion and brain vessels. Although CT is considered relatively insensitive in acute ischemic stroke by some authors, all major clinical trials on stroke treatment are using CT before the randomization of patients. The vast availability and high practicability of CT explain this. This chapter will focus on CT and discuss whether CT can distinguish the reversible ischemic from the irreversible injured tissue in order to define patients most likely to benefit from thrombolysis.

BASIC PRINCIPLES FOR THE INTERPRETATION OF CT IN ACUTE STROKE

The image provided by CT consists of a limited number of volume units (voxels). A typical matrix has 256×256 voxels or 512×512 voxels. The matrix and the slice thickness determine spatial resolution. The X-ray attenuation of each voxel is electronically detected, grouped in relative attenuation values = Hounsfield Units (HU) between -1000 and $+1000$ in relation to the attenuation of water (HU = 0), and translated into 20 levels of a gray scale, which can be distinguished by the human eye. To enhance contrast resolution, the entire gray scale is used to represent the attenuation of the brain, which normally varies between 0 and 50 HU (Table 1). Another section ("window") of the entire HU scale is used if structures with different attenuation, e.g., the temporal bone, are examined. A typical CT window for the brain has a width of 80 HU. The mean value of such CT-windows is called "level" and is responsible for the brightness of the image. X-ray attenuation below the range of the CT window appears as black on the image, above this range as white. A broader window diminishes the contrast between gray and white matter and impairs the detection of subtle changes in X-ray attenuation. If a CT window of 80 HU is used, each gray level represents 4 HU. The contrast resolution is thus limited to 4 HU and could be enhanced by a reduction of the window width. A smaller window will, however, reduce the signal/noise ratio (Fig. 1).

Table 1 presents normal and pathological values of x-ray attenuation in unenhanced cranial CT.

Table 1
X-Ray Attenuation in Cranial CT

	X-ray attenuation (HU)
Gray matter	35–45
White matter	20–30
Cerebro-spinal-fluid	4–8
Skull	100–1000
Large vessels	40–50
Tissue calcification	80–150
Bloodclot	70–90
Fat	−70–−60
Air	−1000

The electron densities of the substrate under study attenuate X-rays (1). In biological tissue, X-ray attenuation is directly correlated with its specific gravity (2). The different electron densities of gray and white matter, brain vessels, cerebro-spinal fluid (CSF), and skull allow differentiation of these structures on CT and recognition of pathological alterations.

Pathological findings on CT in acute stroke may be ischemic edema, thromboembolic occlusion of large vessels, focal brain tissue swelling caused by vasodilatation, intracranial hemorrhage, or tumor-like lesions. CT identifies these findings by detecting a change in X-ray attenuation of normal brain structures or a shift or replacement of brain structures by pathological substrates. A pathological increase in X-ray attenuation is called "hyperdensity," a pathological decrease "hypodensity." These terms are somewhat confusing because they do not define a fixed degree of X-ray attenuation. They are commonly used to characterize the attenuation of a structure in comparison to other tissue, e.g., a parenchymal hematoma is identified by its hyperdensity if compared with gray matter. They are best used, however, to characterize a change in X-ray attenuation by comparing the "density" of an affected structure to its normal "density." The symmetry of the brain structures in transaxial planes facilitates this comparison. For example, the putamen is best evaluated by comparing its attenuation to that of the contralateral putamen and to that of the head of the caudate nucleus, because the caudate nucleus and the putamen are portions of the same anatomical structure, the striatum (Fig. 2). It is obvious that low technical quality of the scan (motion artifacts, wrong window or level) and, in particular, any obliquity of the scan impair the recognition of real changes in X-ray attenuation (Fig. 3).

Cerebral artery occlusion causes the brain tissue to immediately take up water, if the perfusion falls below 12 mL/100g × min (3,4). In experimental animals, tissue water concentration increased steadily from 80.7% to 83% at 4 h after middle cerebral artery (MCA) occlusion (3). A 1% increase in tissue water con-

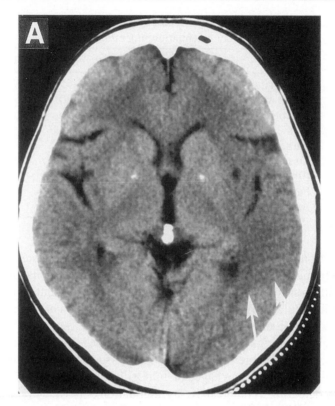

Fig. 1. Two documentations of the identical section of a CT in a patient with acute stroke. Both sections are documented with the same level, but with a different window. With a window of 80 HU (**A**) the contrast between normal cortical density and cortical hypodensity is less than with a window of 31 HU, (**B**). The area of hypodensity covers partially the temporal lobe, the entire insular cortex, and the lateral rim of the putamen and is better outlined with the small CT window (arrows). Note however the increase of noise in B.

tent causes a 2 to 3 HU decrease of X-ray attentuation *(5)*. In our own experiments, X-ray attenuation declined by 7.5 ± 1.6 HU within 4 h of MCA occlusion and hypodensity became visible in the MCA territory of 2 of 10 animals within 2 h after MCA occlusion. Hypodensity could be differentiated from normal brain parenchyma in all 10 animals at 3 h after MCA occlusion *(6)*. The decline in attenuation by 7.5 ± 1.6 HU corresponded to a 2.5% to 3.8% increase in brain tissue water content, in good agreement with the observations by Schuier and Hossmann *(3)*. Using a CT window of 80 HU or less, however, the contrast resolution is 4 HU or less which corresponds to an increase in brain tissue water content of <1.3%–2%. In consequence to this experimental data, the first stage of the developing ischemic edema during the first 2 to 3 h cannot be recognized

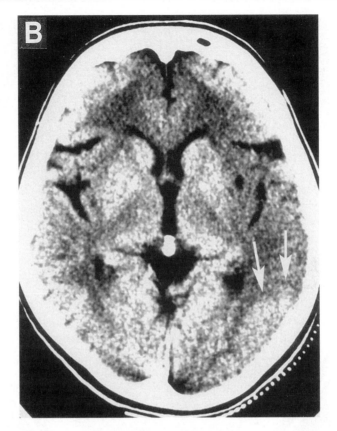

Fig. 1. (B).

on CT because the attenuation decline has not reached the contrast resolution of 4 HU. In other words: when the brain parenchyma becomes hypodense on CT after arterial occlusion, the difference between normal and hypodense tissue is ≥4 HU, and the occlusion has occurred 2 to 3 h earlier. Hypodensity of gray matter causes a diminished contrast to adjacent white matter and thus a loss of anatomical margins. Gray matter hypodensity explains negative phenomena like "obscuration of lentiform nucleus" *(7)* and "loss of the insular ribbon" *(8)*, so called "early infarct signs" (Figs. 2,4). Gray matter hypodensity in its early stage causes a loss in anatomical information, which may explain why this finding is easily missed.

The delayed detection of parenchymal hypodensity after arterial occlusion has another important consequence: the CT finding of parenchymal hypodensity is highly specific for irreversible tissue damages, because ischemic edema probably becomes irreversible after about 2 h *(3,9)* and indicates irreversibly damaged brain tissue *(4)*. A CT without hypodensity, however, means that no or a

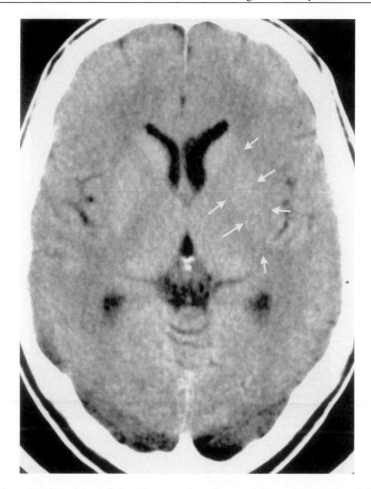

Fig. 2. Hypodensity of the left lentiform nucleus (arrows). X-ray attenuation is here less in comparison to the right lentiform nucleus, and attenuation of the left putamen is less than the attenuation of the left head of caudate nucleus. With further decline in attenuation, the lentiform nucleus cannot be distinguished from the internal and external capsule; it will be obscured.

still-reversible ischemic edema may be present, and an irreversible ischemic tissue damage has not developed so far.

Partial volume artifacts may mimic parenchymal hypodensity. These artifacts occur if the CT section is parallel to the brain's surface and includes parenchyma and CSF in same voxels. A typical location for this artifact is the temporal lobe (Fig. 5B).

Thrombo-embolic occlusion of large brain arteries may result in a segmental hyperdensity (Fig. 5A). This finding is called the hyperdense artery sign and is highly specific for the obstruction of this artery if "hyperdensity" is defined as an increased X-ray attenuation of one arterial segment in comparison to other portions of the same artery or its contralateral counterpart *(10)*. A hyperdense MCA trunk was observed on CT in 48% of patients with angiographically proven MCA trunk occlusion *(11)*. It is unclear why some arterial obstructions do not cause intraluminal hyperdensity. A hyperdense artery is not an "infarct sign," because arteries can occlude without a subsequent or immediate brain infarct if there is adequate collateral blood supply. A hyperdense MCA trunk in association with normal tissue density may indicate a large tissue volume at risk from hypoperfusion, but no irreversible damage so far. Nevertheless, a hyperdense MCA trunk is often associated with a severe stroke and large infarct *(12–14)*. It is, therefore, prudent to carefully examine the territory of a hyperdense artery for parenchymal hypodensity.

Ischemic edema and vasodilatation can cause swelling of the brain parenchyma. Ischemic edema means net uptake of water into brain tissue and is thus associated with a decline in X-ray attenuation. It develops immediately, if cerebral blood flow (CBF) falls below 12 mL/100g × min, and its extent depends on the volume of the affected brain tissue with such low CBF *(4)*. Brain swelling due to vasodilatation can develop under two conditions: 1) with low perfusion pressure, but intact cerebrovascular autoregulatory capacity, and 2) with venous obstruction *(15,16)*. This type of brain tissue is not associated with hypodensity, but can be associated with hyperdensity because of the increase in regional cerebral blood volume (CBV). As explained above, brain swelling with hypodensity means irreversible tissue damage. Brain swelling with iso—or hyperdensity is, however, reversible, if the arterial or venous obstruction is successfully treated.

Early brain swelling is not reliably detected by CT. Enlargement of brain tissue causes compression of the CSF space. Because of the natural asymmetry of cerebral sulci, cisterns, and ventricles, it could be hard to decide whether the CSF space is unilaterally compressed or contralaterally enlarged. Clearer signs are the regional effacement of sulci, compression of the entire lateral ventricle, and the combination of both (Fig. 6).

In acute stroke, blood may be present in one or more of the cerebral compartments: brain parenchyma, ventricles, subarachnoid space, and subdural or epidural space. Clinically, an acute parenchymal hemorrhage cannot be reliably distinguished from ischemic stroke. After acute hemorrhage, blood appears on CT as a hyperattenuated, often space-occupying mass (Fig. 7). The degree of hyperdensity depends on the amount of blood, whether it is clotted or not, and whether the blood is intermixed with CSF or brain tissue. Hemorrhages related to coagulopathies or treatment with anticoagulants or thrombolytics are often inhomogeneous with fluid levels. (Fig. 8) Sensitivity of CT for detection of parenchymal hemorrhage is nearly 100%, but small hemorrhages into the brain

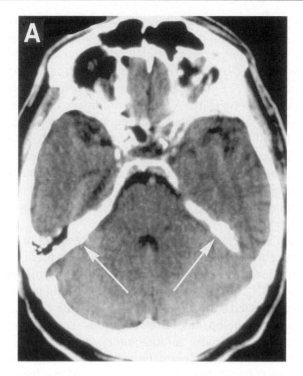

Fig. 3. *(continued on opposite page)* The obliquity of a CT scan can be recognized by comparing the upper rim of both pyramids **(A)**. In consequence of this obliquity, the right lentiform nucleus appeared less dense in one section **(B)**, and the left putamen appeared less dense in the adjacent upper section when compared to the contralateral side **(C)**.

parenchyma or subarachnoid space can be overlooked (Fig. 9). The investigators of the European Cooperative Acute Stroke Studies (ECASS I and II) missed two small parenchymal hemorrhages and one subarachnoid hemorrhage (SAH) in 1420 patients (0.1%) *(17,18)*. The location of the hematoma often provides clues about its underlying etiology (Table 2).

Acute hemorrhages usually show hyperattenuation without surrounding edema. If marked edema is present under those circumstances, underlying neoplasm should be suspected. Multiple hemorrhagic lesions should suggest metastatic disease, coagulopathy, or cerebral amyloid angiopathy. CT is 90% sensitive for detection of SAH within the first 24 h of bleeding. When blood later intermixes with cerebrospinal fluid, the density will be similar to the adjacent brain and difficult to visualize. If the hemorrhage is small, it may be missed entirely by the scan, necessitating lumbar puncture for definitive diagnosis in patients with a syndrome highly suspicious for SAH. The sensitivity of CT in detecting subarachnoid blood declines to approx 50% at 1 wk after SAH *(19)*.

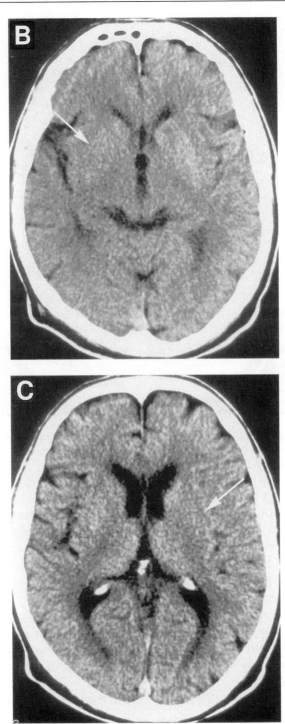

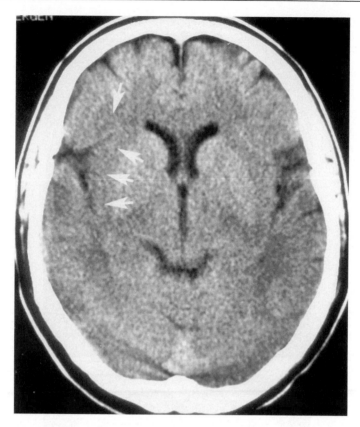

Fig. 4. CT obtained 32 min after a stroke with left-sided hemiparesis in a 35-yr-old man. The entire right insular cortex (arrows) is hypodense to such an extent that it is obscured. Compare with the left insular cortex.

Calcification of the basal ganglia can occasionally be mistaken for deep intraparenchymal hemorrhage. It has a similar degree of attenuation as acute blood, but may be distinguished by its characteristic location and tendency to be bilateral. Brain tumors and tumor-like lesions, e.g., acute focal demyelinations in multiple sclerosis, can cause a stroke syndrome. The characteristics of these lesions on CT are the space occupying effect on the surrounding structures, caused by cell neoplasia and/or reactive edema, and the replacement of normal anatomy by structures showing a mixture of attenuation values. <u>Hypo</u>density in this regard can be attributed to necrosis, cysts, or edema. An increased neoplastic or inflammatory cell density causes <u>hyper</u>density of these lesions on the unenhanced CT.

An approach to the interpretation of CT in the setting of acute stroke is presented in Table 3.

TECHNICAL NOTE:
HOW TO PERFORM CT IN ACUTE STROKE

If the imaging facility is informed in advance, the scanner can be kept free for the patient with acute stroke. Emergent life support should be continued during the patient's imaging test if necessary. Although a detailed neurologic examination is not needed before the brain imaging is done, localizing the stroke to the posterior fossa or the cerebral hemisphere will assist in tailoring the imaging techniques.

CT should be performed with a rapid scan time to reduce motion artifact. Contrast is not necessary and would prolong the procedure needlessly. A correct head position is crucial to avoid obliquity of the sections. If necessary, specific section cuts can be repeated. The high density of bone often causes an artifact, which may impair visualization of the lower part of the brain stem in the posterior fossa. Thin (<5 mm) transaxial sections from the posterior fossa and the base of the cerebral hemispheres and a broader CT window can minimize this artifact. The rest of the brain is best examined with 8 or 10-mm sections. Image windows should be adjusted so that gray and white matter can be easily distinguished and subtle hypodensities detected. A close communication between the stroke physician and the radiologist or technician will enhance the information gained from CT. The image should be optimized for spatial and contrast resolution in the region of interest. Additional bone window views can be performed if head trauma is a possibility to search for skull fractures, subdural air or blood, or effusions on the nasal sinuses and the middle ear. A contrast-enhanced scan should be obtained later if there is suspicion for neoplasm or localized infection and no MRI available.

Advanced CT technology provides the opportunity for CT angiography (CTA) and CT perfusion imaging *(20,21)*. A CTA is performed after bolus injection of 130 mL nonionic contrast (injection rate: 4–5 mL/s) with a spiral scan of the brain base and 3-dimensional reconstruction of the Circle of Willis on a workstation *(20)*. Perfusion imaging with CT requires repeated imaging of one or more sections to measure the contrast uptake and clearance curve in each voxel. Parameter images are then calculated for CBV, mean transit times, CBF, or time intervals to the peaks of contrast enhancement. These techniques are not yet widely available.

TYPICAL CT FINDINGS WITHIN THE FIRST SIX HOURS OF STROKE ONSET

The most relevant and highly underestimated finding in patients with acute stroke is a normal CT. Figure 10 shows the CT and the diffusion weighted MRI of a man with a rightsided hemiparesis for 2 d. This patient had a severe stenosis of his left internal carotid artery. The symptoms resolved completely after the patient was operated on 4 d after stroke onset. Many physicians still think that a

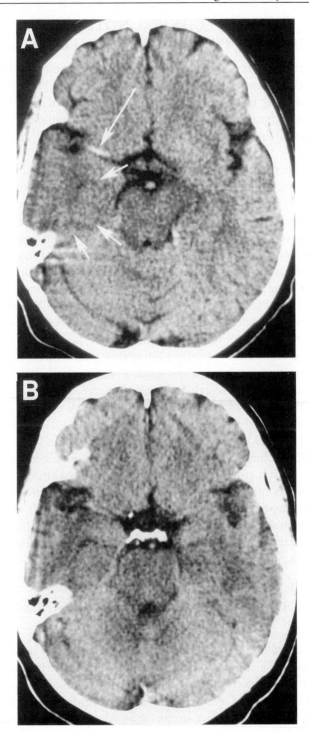

lack of pathological imaging findings in patients with acute stroke reflects a poor sensitivity. It is widely overlooked that the sensitivity of CT cannot be measured with the gold standard "stroke syndrome" because the stroke syndrome itself is highly unspecific for the underlying pathophysiology. As mentioned previously, CT detects ischemic edema and other pathologies, which may not be present in patients with acute stroke, but will develop later or will never develop. Moreover, it is highly relevant for the management of stroke patients if the CT shows that ischemic edema has not developed and clinical recovery is consequently still possible if blood flow is restored to the functionally disturbed brain.

The prejudice that CT is negative within the first 24 to 48 h after stroke is still handed down in review articles *(22)* although many studies have described positive findings even within the first 6 h of stroke onset: Tomura et al. *(7)* studied 25 patients with embolic cerebral infarction between 40 and 340 min after the onset of symptoms. Twenty-three CT scans (92%) were positive with "obscuration of the lentiform nucleus" caused by hypodensity. Bozzao et al. *(23)* observed parenchymal hypodensity in 25 of 36 patients (69%). A "loss of the insular ribbon" was reported in 23 of 27 (85%) patients *(8)*. Horowitz et al. *(24)* reported on hypodensity and mass effect in 56% of 50 scans. When comparing MR vs CT imaging in identical patients within 3 h of symptom onset, CT was positive in 19 patients (53%) and MRI in 18 (50%) patients with hemispheric stroke *(25)*. We reported 17 positive CT scans (68%) performed in a series of 25 patients with MCA trunk occlusion during the first 2 h after symptom onset.

The incidence of positive CT findings increased to 89% in the third hour and to 100% thereafter *(11)*. In another series of patients with hemispheric stroke, the incidence of early CT signs of infarction was 82% *(26)*. In patients selected for thrombolytic therapy, 12 of 23 patients (52%) had a parenchymal hypodensity on the CT performed within 3 h of stroke onset *(27)*. In a series of 100 consecutive patients with MCA infarction, CT detected hypodensity of the lentiform nucleus in 48% and of the insular cortex in 59% of the patients within 14 h of stroke onset *(28)*. In the NINDS t-PA for Acute Stroke Study 53/616 (27%) showed loss of gray-white matter distinction, and 17/616 (9%) showed hypodensity (unpublished data).

To our knowledge, the incidence of early CT findings in stroke was never assessed in an unselected population of stroke patients. Patient selection and the capability to recognize ischemic edema on CT may be responsible for the obser-

---

Fig. 5. *(opposite page)* Oblique CT in a patient with acute stroke (<6 h). **(A)** The segmental tubular shaped hyperattenuation (long arrow) indicates thrombo-embolic occlusion of the right middle cerebral artery (hyperdense artery sign). The "hypodensity" of the right lower temporal lobe (short arrows) is owing to a partial volume artifact (mixture of fluid and tissue in voxels at the lower surface of the temporal lobe), **(B)** Twenty-four hours later, the follow-up CT confirmed an intact temporal lobe. Note the normal attenuation of the right MCA trunk after treatment with 1.1 mg rt-PA/kg IV.

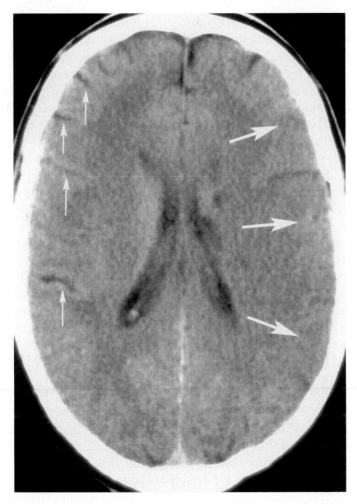

Fig. 6. Stroke with severe right-sided hemiparesis in a 40-yr-old man. Effacement of the left cortical sulci in addition to hypodensity (large arrows). For comparison, note the sulci of the right cerebral hemisphere (small arrows).

vation that the incidence of findings varies among studies. The detection of parenchymal hypodensity in patients with acute stroke by neuroradiologists is possible with moderate to good interrater reliability (28–30). Moreover, it was shown that special training of nonradiologists can enhance the proportion of CT findings and improve the estimation of the extent of early ischemic edema (31).

The incidence of early CT findings varies among the large studies on thrombolytic therapy (Table 4). In ECASS II, a panel of three neuroradiologists prospectively evaluated all CT scans using predefined categories blinded to clinical

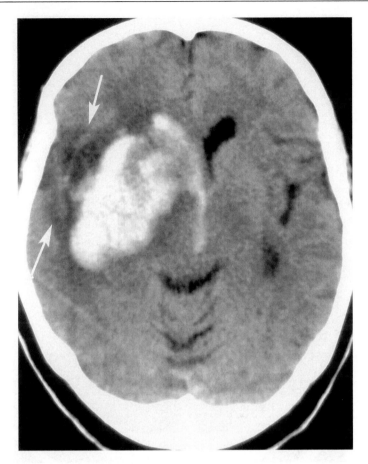

Fig. 7. Parenchymal hematoma of the right basal ganglia and intraventricular hemorrhage. The wedge shaped hypodensity lateral of the hematoma (arrows) is suspicious for an underlying ischemic infarction.

outcome and follow-up CT. This panel categorized the extent of hypodensities on baseline CT scans: normal, hypodensity of the MCA territory 33% or >33%, and hypodensity outside the MCA territory. These data offer the opportunity to study the clinical relevance and prospective value of 792 early CT findings with the limitation that the ECASS II investigators tried to exclude patients with MCA territory hypodensity >33%. Only 37 (4.6%) of these patients were randomized.

The ECASS II investigators randomized 800 patients. Eight baseline CT (1%) got lost for the evaluation by the CT panel owing to technical and logistic problems. No hypodensity was seen in 341 (43%) patients. Parenchymal hypodensities were associated with tissue swelling in 50% of the patients. Only one patient showed focal tissue swelling, but no hypodensity on the baseline CT. This patient

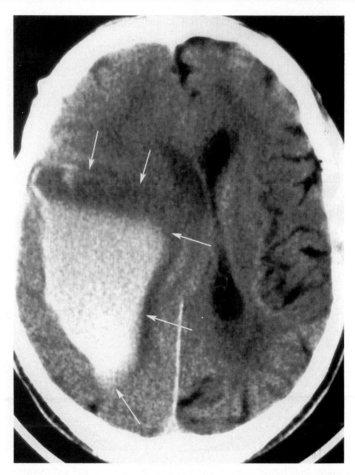

Fig. 8. Parenchymal hemorrhage after myocardial infarction (MI) and thrombolysis. Signs of unclotted blood: The upper portion is free of cells and hypodense. Increasing density in the lower portion owing to sedimentation of cellular elements (arrows).

was randomized to recombinant tissue plasminogen activator (rt-PA), developed a small infarct, and had an excellent clinical outcome without functional disturbance at 90 d after stroke. Four hundred three patients (50%) had a hypodensity ≤33% MCA territory, and 11 patients (1.4%) had a hypodensity outside the MCA territory. The National Institute of Health Stroke Score (NIHSS) at baseline—applied without the score for distal motor function—was different among these groups: Patients with a normal CT or a hypodensity outside the MCA territory had a mean NIHSS of 9.5 ± 5.1, patients with ≤33% hypodensity had a NIHSS of 13.3 ± 6.0, and patients with larger hypodensity a NIHSS of 17.1 ± 6.9 ($p < 0.0001$, Bonferroni-Dunn). Table 5 presents the association between the extent of hypodensity at baseline and the clinical follow-up in placebo-treated patients.

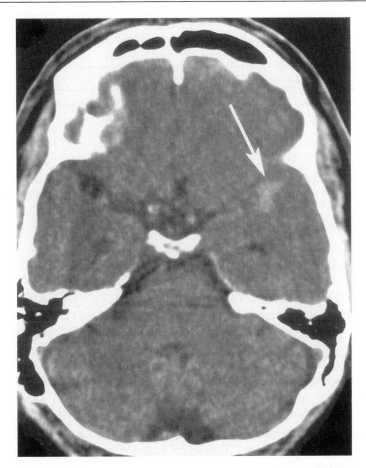

Fig. 9. Small hyperattenuated area in the left anterior Sylvian fissure (arrow). Low contrast because of broad window of 160 HU. The subarachnoid hemorrhage was overlooked, and the patient was randomized to rt-PA. The hemorrhage was confirmed by the follow-up CT. The patient had an excellent clinical outcome.

The incidence of positive CT findings varied during the time between symptom onset and CT scan (Fig. 11). CT was positive in 18 of 36 patients (50%) who underwent CT within 1 h of symptom onset. The first positive CT was obtained at 22 min after witnessed symptom onset (Fig. 12). This observation suggests that the ischemic edema may develop faster in humans than in experimental animals. The proportion of positive findings increased only slightly up to 60% after the first hour, and declined remarkably in the 6 h after stroke onset. The late decline in positive CT findings is best explained by a selection bias: relatively lately recruited patients were clinically less severely affected and developed smaller infarcts.

Table 2
Common Causes of Spontaneous Cerebral Hemorrhage
and their Typical Locations

Cause	Location
Hypertension	Basal ganglia (usually putamen)
	Thalamus
	Pons
	Cerebellum
	External Capsule
Vascular Malformation	All intracranial locations possible
Cerebral Amyloid Angiopathy	Adjacent to the brain surface
	Lobar
Bleeding Diathesis	Lobar
	Multiple locations

If one takes a well-demarcated infarct on CT one day after stroke as the gold standard for a permanent ischemic lesion, the predictive values of the baseline CT can be calculated (Table 6). In ECASS II, the baseline CT was highly predictive and specific for ischemic lesions. Eleven findings in the placebo group and four findings in the group treated with rt-PA were falsely judged as early infarct, but could retrospectively be identified as artifacts. Remarkably, no hypodense ischemic lesion on baseline CT became normal, even after rt-PA treatment. The sensitivity of early CT for permanent ischemic lesions was 66% in the placebo group and 65% in the rt-PA group: one-third of permanent ischemic lesions developed after the baseline CT was performed whether the patient was treated with placebo or rt-PA.

CONSEQUENCES OF CT FINDINGS
FOR THROMBOLYTIC THERAPY

The CT data of ECASS II suggest that parenchymal hypodensity on CT within 6 h of symptom onset represents an ischemic lesion which cannot be reversed or diminished by treatment with IV 0.9 mg/kg rt-PA. Moreover, rt-PA treatment in this study did not prevent delayed infarction in one-third of the patients. If this is true, treatment with rt-PA may be beneficial if only a minor proportion of an arterial territory is hypodense when treatment is initiated. When designing their trials, the ECASS investigators followed the hypothesis that treatment with rt-PA will be ineffective and probably risky in patients with large ischemic edema already present at randomization. "Large" ischemic edema was artificially defined as a volume of hypodense brain tissue exceeding one-third of the MCA territory. This definition was based on the consideration that patients with

Table 3
Important Questions for the Interpretation of CT in Acute Stroke

	Characteristics of CT Findings			
Normal	*Tissue hypodensity*	*Hyperdensity*	*Tissue swelling*	*Arterial hyperdensity*
No subtle hypodensity or swelling in the region suspicious from the clinical findings? How severe is the stroke syndrome? Brain stem infarction?	No artifact? Extent and shape? Correspondence to arterial territory? Which artery? If no correspondence: venous infarction, astrocytoma, encephalitis?	Blood or calcification? If blood: Location? Mass effect? Blockage of CSF pathways? Edema already? Abnormal vessels? Tumor?	Is it real? With hypodensity? Extent? Corresponding to arterial territory? Direct signs of vascular obstruction?	Which segment of which artery? Associated tissue hypodensity or swelling?

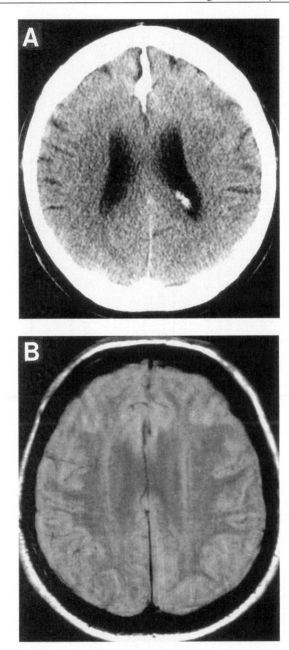

Fig. 10. (**A**) CT of a 72-yr-old man with right-sided hemiparesis since 2 d. The diffusion weighted MRI was obtained on the same day as the CT, (**B**). Both examinations did not show any abnormality. A severe stenosis of the left internal carotid artery was detected by Doppler ultrasound and confirmed by angiogram. The symptoms resolved completely after endarterectomy 4 d after symptom onset.

Table 4
Positive CT Findings in Trials on Thrombolytic Therapy

Study	Time interval	Findings (%)	Extent of ischemic edema
ECASS I	6 h	54	yes
ECASS II	6 h	66	yes
MAST-I	6 h	12	no
MAST-E	6 h	68	no
PROACT II	6 h	83	yes
NINDS	3 h	10	no

ECASS, European Cooperative Acute Stroke Study *(17,18)*; MAST-I, Multicentre Acute Stroke Trial–Italy Group *(33)*; The Multicentre Acute Stroke Trial–Europe Study Group *(34)*; PROACT, Prolyse in Acute Cerebral Thromboembolism Trial *(35)*.

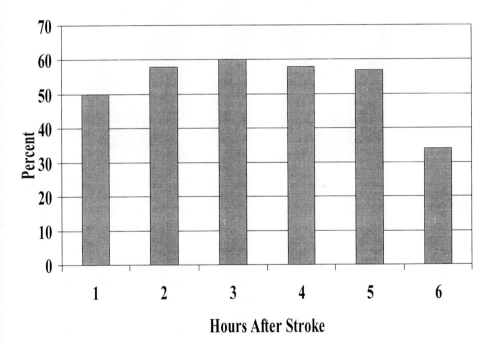

Fig. 11. Incidence of hypodensities on CT at various intervals after symptom onset in ECASS II. The decline in the 6th hour reflects an increased proportion of patients with small subcortical infarcts.

such large edema have only minor chances to recover *(11)* and that they may have an increased risk for cerebral hemorrhage after thrombolysis. On the other hand, more subtle findings such as sulcal effacement, loss of the insular ribbon did not predict whether rt-PA treatment might be successful.

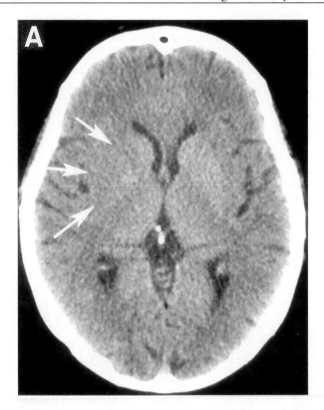

Fig. 12. *(continued on opposite page)* Hypodensity of the right putamen detected 22 min after the onset of left hemiparesis in a 79-yr-old woman **(A)**. NIH Stroke Score at baseline: 11. The ischemic lesion is confirmed by the follow-up CT 26 h later **(B)**. The patient was randomized to rt-PA and had an excellent outcome without functional disturbance.

In ECASS I and II, 9 of 51 patients with a MCA territory hypodensity >33% died from cerebral hemorrhages after rt-PA treatment, but none after placebo ($p < 0.01$, chi square). The absolute risk increase for fatal cerebral hemorrhage was 17.6% in these patients and only 3.3% in patients with normal CT and 1.4% in patients with small hypodensity (Table 7). The risk to die from large ischemic edema with mass effect was clearly associated with the extent of hypodense tissue on baseline CT in both treatment groups ($p < 0.0001$, chi square) and appeared slightly reduced after treatment with rt-PA (n.s.). Some of these large ischemic edemas were presumably transformed into hemorrhages and patients died then from "cerebral hemorrhage" because the hemorrhage was more obvious on follow-up CT than the ischemic changes, but the patient was destined to die anyway.

This risk increase for fatal hemorrhages in patients with large volumes of hypodense brain tissue on baseline CT does not clearly influence the overall

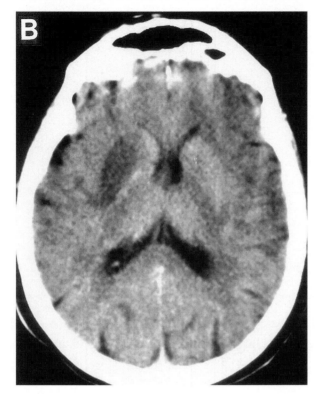

Fig. 12. (B).

Table 5
Extent of MCA Territory Hypodensity on Baseline CT, Baseline Characteristics, NIHSS at Baseline and Follow-up, Symptomatic Hemorrhage, Disability, and Death in the ECASS II Placebo Group (N = 391)

	Hypodensity of MCA Territory			
	No	*≤33%*	*>33%*	p
Age (years)	67 ± 11	65 ± 11	63 ± 14	0.168 #
Male (%)	55	59	41	0.327 §
NIHSS				
Baseline	9.6 ± 5.2	13.5 ± 6.6	15.1 ± 5.5	<0.0001 #
24 hours	7.8 ± 6.6	12.5 ± 8.7	16.5 ± 9.6	<0.0001 #
3 months	6.4 ± 11.8	10.4 ± 13.3	19.4 ± 17.6	<0.0001 #
Sympt. Hemorrhage (%)	3.0	8.8	0	0.072 §
Disability/Death (%)	44	60	82	0.002 §
(Rankin >2)				
Death (%)	7.9	11.3	35.3	0.005 §

MCA, middle cerebral artery; NIHSS, National Institute of Health Stroke Score; #, ANOVA; § chi square test.

Table 6
Predictive Values of Baseline CT for Ischemic Infarcts on Follow-up CT in ECASS II

	Placebo			rt-PA			All		
	N	%	95% CI	N	%	95% CI	N	%	95% CI
Sensitivity	213/331	64	59–69	220/344	64	59–69	433/675	64	60–68
Specificity	39/50	78	65–87	56/61	92	82–96	95/111	86	78–91
PPV	213/224	95	91–97	220/225	98	95–99	433/449	96	94–98
NPV	39/157	25	19–32	56/180	31	25–38	95/337	28	24–33
Accuracy	252/381	66	61–71	276/405	68	63–72	528/786	67	64–70

rt-PA, recombinant tissue plasminogen activator; 95% CI, 95% confidence interval; PPV, positive predictive value; NPV, negative predictive value.

Table 7

ECASS I and II: Parenchymal Hypodensity of the MCA Territory on Baseline CT and Response to Treatment with rt-PA

Outcome Events	No Hypodensity n = 688				Hypodensity 33% MCA Territory n = 618				Hypodensity >33% MCA Territory n = 89			
	rt-PA n = 354	Placebo n = 334	Difference %	OR 95% CI	rt-PA n = 304	Placebo n = 314	Difference %	OR 95% CI	rt-PA n = 51	Placebo n = 38	Difference %	OR 95% CI
Rankin: 0–1	170 (48.0)	144 (43.1)	5.9	1.22 0.90–1.65	97 (31.9)	75 (23.9)	8.0	1.49 1.05–2.13	6 (11.8)	6 (15.8)	-4.0	0.71 0.21–2.41
Fatal Edema	3 (0.8)	4 (1.2)	-0.4	0.71 0.16–3.17	15 (4.9)	18 (5.7)	-0.8	0.85 0.42–1.73	11 (21.6)	10 (26.3)	-4.7	0.77 0.28–2.06
Fatal Hemorrhage	16 (4.5)	4 (1.2)	3.3	3.91 1.29–11.80	11 (3.6)	7 (2.2)	1.4	1.65 0.63–4.30	9 (17.6)	0 (0)	17.6	–

outcome analysis. The results of ECASS I and II could not prove so far that the response to 1.1 mg/kg or 0.9 mg/kg rt-PA IV is different if the patients have no, small, or large hypodensities on the baseline CT. Table 7 presents outcome data of both studies after stratification according to the baseline CT: a significant beneficial effect of rt-PA is seen only in patients with MCA territory hypodensity ≤33%, and patients with >33% hypodensity show a trend for deterioration with rt-PA *(32)*. The 95% confidence intervals of the 3 subgroups overlap each other, however, so that any difference among them could be caused by chance. In the NINDS t-PA for Stroke Trial, the role of hypodensity suggested in ECASS could not be confirmed. For example, the odds ratio for symptomatic hemorrhage after t-PA therapy in a patient with MCA hypodensity >33% was 1.5 (95% CL 0.3, 7.2; data unpublished). Extensive analyses of the NINDS dataset for other signs or early ischemia have failed to yield data to support the hypotheses generated by the ECASS data.

CONCLUSIONS

After arterial occlusion, CT detects ischemic edema if the tissue water content has increased by about 2%. Focal brain tissue hypoattenuation, or hypodensity, is highly specific for a permanent ischemic lesion, which cannot be diminished by thrombolysis.

The ECASS results suggest that patients with hypodensity exceeding one-third of the MCA territory do not benefit from treatment with rt-PA and have a higher risk for symptomatic cerebral hemorrhage, but this was not confirmed by the NINDS data. The number of patients with large hypodensity studied so far is rather small, however, and no definite conclusions can be drawn for other types of stroke treatment. In patients with acute stroke and no or only small volumes of hypodensity, additional information is needed to find out whether an arterial obstruction and relevant hypoperfusion is present when treatment is initiated.

REFERENCES

1. Brooks RA. A quantitative theory of the Hounsfield unit and its application of dual energy scanning. *J Comput Assist Tomogr* 1977;1:487–493.
2. Rieth KG, Fujiwara K, Di Chiro G, Klatzo I, Brooks RA, Johnston GS, et al. Serial measurements of CT attenuation and specific gravity in experimental cerebral edema. *Radiology* 1980;135:343–348.
3. Schuier FJ, Hossmann KA. Experimental brain infarcts in cats. II. Ischemic brain edema. *Stroke* 1980;11:593–601.
4. Hossmann KA. Viability thresholds and the penumbra of focal ischemia. *Ann Neurol* 1994;36:557–565.
5. Unger E, Littlefield J, Gado M. Water content and water structure in CT and MR signal changes: Possible influence in detection of early stroke. *AJNR* 1988;9:687–691.
6. von Kummer R, Weber J. Brain and vascular imaging in acute ischemic stroke: The potential of computed tomography. *Neurology* 1997;49(Suppl 4),S52–S55.

7. Tomura N, Uemura K, Inugami A, Fujita H, Higano S, Shishido F. Early CT finding in cerebral infarction. *Radiology* 1988;168:463–467.
8. Truwit CL, Barkovich AJ, Gean-Marton A, Hibri N, Norman D. Loss of the insular ribbon: Another early CT sign of acute middle cerebral artery infarction. *Radiology* 1990;176: 801–806.
9. Ianotti F, Hoff J. Ischemic brain edema with and without reperfusion: An experimental study in gerbils. *Stroke* 1983;14:562–567.
10. Tomsick TA. Commentary. Sensitivity and prognostic value of early CT in occlusion of the middle cerebral artery trunk. *AJNR* 1994;15:16–18.
11. von Kummer R, Meyding-Lamadé U, Forsting M, Rosin L, Rieke K, Hacke W, Sartor K. Sensitivity and prognostic value of early computed tomography in middle cerebral artery trunk occlusion. *AJNR* 1994;15:9–15.
12. Launes J, Ketonen L. Dense middle cerebral artery sign: an indicator of poor outcome in middle cerebral artery infarction. *J Neurol Neurosurg Psychiatry* 1987;50:1550–1552.
13. Leys D, Pruvo JP, Godefroy O, Rondepierre P, Leclerc X. Prevalence and significance of hyperdense middle cerebral artery in acute stroke. *Stroke* 1992;23:317–324.
14. Tomsick TA, Brott TG, Olinger CP, Barsan W, Spilker J, Eberle R, Adams H. Hyperdense middle cerebral artery: incidence and quantitative significance. *Neuroradiology* 1989;31: 312–315.
15. Gibbs JM, Wise RJS, Leenders KL, Jones T Evaluation of cerebral perfusion reserve in patients with carotid-artery occlusion. *Lancet* 1984;8372:310–314.
16. Yuh WTC, Simonson T, Wang A, Koci TM, Tali ET, Fisher DJ, et al. Venous sinus occlusive Disease: MR Findings. *AJNR* 1994;15:309–316.
17. Hacke W, Kaste M, Fieschi C, Toni D, Lesaffre E, von Kummer R, et al., for the ECASS Study Group. Intravenous thrombolysis with recombinant tissue plasminogen activator for treatment of acute hemispheric stroke: The European cooperative acute stroke study (ECASS). *JAMA* 1995;274:1017–1025.
18. Hacke W, Kaste M, Fieschi C, von Kummer R, Davalos A, Meier D, et al. Randomised double-blind placebo-controlled trial of thrombolytic therapy with intravenous alteplase in acute ischaemic stroke (ECASS II). *Lancet* 1998;352:1245–1251.
19. Schievink W. Intracranial aneurysms. *New Engl J Med* 1997;336:28–40.
20. Knauth M, von Kummer R, Jansen O, Hähnel S, Dörfler A, Sartor K. Potential of CT angiography in acute ischemic stroke. *AJNR* 1997;18:1001–1010.
21. Koenig M, Klotz E, Luka B, Venderink D, Spittler J, Heuser L. Perfusion CT of the brain: Diagnostic approach for early detection of ischemic stroke. *Radiology* 1998;209:85–93.
22. Gilman S. Imaging of the brain. N Engl J Med 1998;338:812–820.
23. Bozzao L, Bastianello S, Fantozzi LM, Angeloni U, Argentino C, Fieschi C. Correlation of angiographic and sequential CT findings in patients with evolving cerebral infarction. *AJNR* 1989;10:1215–1222.
24. Horowitz SH, Zito JL, Donnarumma R, Patel M, Alvir J. Computed tomographic—angiographic findings within the first five hours of cerebral infarction. *Stroke* 1991;22: 1245–1253.
25. Mohr JP, Biller J, Hilal SK, Yuh WTC, Tatemichi TK, Hedges S, et al. Magnetic resonance versus computed tomographic imaging in acute stroke. *Stroke* 1995;26:807–812.
26. von Kummer R, Nolte PN, Schnittger H, Thron A, Ringelstein EB. Detectability of hemispheric ischemic infarction by computed tomography within 6 hours after stroke. *Neuroradiology* 1996;38:31–33.
27. Grond M, von Kummer R, Sobesky J, Schmülling S, Heiss W-D. Relevance of early CT abnormalities in acute stroke. *Lancet* 1997;350:1595–1596.

28. Moulin T, Cattin F, Crépin-Leblond T, Tatu L, Chavot D, Piotin M, et al. Early CT signs in acute middle cerebral artery infarction: Predictive value for subsequent infarct locations and outcome. *Neurology* 1996;47:366–375.
29. von Kummer R, Holle R, Grzyska U, Hofmann E, Jansen O, Petersen D, et al. Interobserver agreement in assessing early CT signs of middle cerebral artery infarction. *AJNR* 1996; 17:1743–1748.
30. Marks MP, Holmgren EB, Fox AJ, Patel S, von Kummer R, Froehlich J. Evaluation of early computed tomographic findings in acute ischemic stroke. *Stroke* 1999;30:389–392.
31. von Kummer R. Effect of training in reading CT scans on patient selection for ECASS II. *Neurology* 1998;51(Suppl 3),S50–S52.
32. von Kummer R, Allen KL, Holle R, Bozzao L, Bastianello S, Manelfe C, et al. Acute stroke: usefulness of early CT findings before thrombolytic therapy. *Radiology* 1997;205:327–333.
33. Multicentre Acute Stroke Trial–Italy (MAST–I) Group. Randomised controlled trial of streptokinase, aspirin, and combination of both in treatment of acute ischaemic stroke. *Lancet* 1995;346:1509–1514.
34. The Multicentre Acute Stroke Trial–Europe Study Group. Thrombolytic therapy with streptokinase in acute ischemic stroke. *N Engl J Med* 1996;335:145–150.
35. Furlan AJ, Higashida R, Wechsler L, Schulz G, PROACT II Investigators. PROACT II: Recombinant prourokinase (r-ProUK) in acute cerebral thromboembolism. Initial trial results. *Stroke* 1999;30:234.

16
Identifying and Overcoming Obstacles to Acute Stroke Treatment with rt-PA
Establishing Hospital and EMS Protocols

Karen Rapp, RN, BSN
and Patti Bratina, RN, BSN

CONTENTS

INTRODUCTION
PUBLIC AWARENESS
EMERGENCY MEDICAL SERVICES
THE 911 SYSTEM
PREHOSPITAL CARE: FIRST RESPONDERS
EMERGENCY TRIAGE
TIME OF ONSET DETERMINATION
ED TOOLS AND PROCEDURES
INITIATION OF TREATMENT
IDENTIFYING OBSTACLES AND TRACKING IMPROVEMENT
REFERENCES

INTRODUCTION

Obstacles exist in rapidly treating stroke victims. The public is generally unaware of the warning signs of stroke and the urgency of treatment. The Emergency Medical Services (EMS) has traditionally not viewed stroke as an emergent medical condition requiring hyperacute care. Healthcare professionals, having no acute treatment options available in the past, may continue to triage and treat stroke as nonurgent. The public, EMS, and healthcare professionals

From: *Thrombolytic Therapy for Stroke*
Edited by: P. D. Lyden © Humana Press Inc., Totowa, NJ

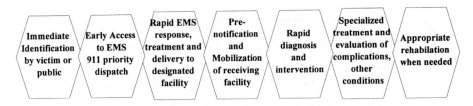

Fig. 1. Chain of recovery for acute ischemic stroke patients key links.

must change their perception of stroke from an emphasis on rehabilitation to a focus on emergency treatment.

PUBLIC AWARENESS

Public awareness of stroke is extremely poor. Although stroke is the nation's third leading cause of death, over half of stroke victims interviewed after their arrival to the Emergency Department (ED) did not perceive their event as a potentially life threatening emergency *(1)*. Stroke victims who immediately access the 911 system arrive at emergency rooms on average within 70 min from their onset of stroke. Those who call their personal physician or go to the hospital bypassing the 911 system decrease the likelihood of recombinant tissue-plasminogen activator (rt-PA) treatment. Median arrival time for these patients increases to approx 4 h, which is beyond the therapeutic treatment window *(1,2)*.

Interviewing the public at large about their knowledge of stroke signs and symptoms reveals a severe lack of awareness. According to a large national survey conducted by the National Stroke Association (NSA), 42% of those interviewed did not know that weakness and numbness are stroke symptoms, 60% would not call 911 immediately, and only 33% knew that there is a limited time window in which treatment for stroke will be effective *(3)*.

The ultimate result of this lack of public knowledge is that few patients arrive at a healthcare provider soon enough to be eligible for t-PA. Educating the public on recognizing the signs and symptoms of stroke and also of its emergency nature is a key link to successful treatment (Fig. 1) *(4,5)*.

Following the FDA approval of rt-PA in 1996, several public awareness campaigns have been implemented. Operation Stroke is a grass roots program funded by the American Stroke Association in 40 key cities in the United States. Their primary mission is to raise public and professional awareness. The NSA funds local chapters around the country in an effort to promote stroke signs and symptoms, prevention, treatment and coordinates stroke survivor groups. The NSA designates May as their annual stroke awareness month and supports hospitals, clinics, and stroke support groups on educating the public on the warning signs of stroke.

EMERGENCY MEDICAL SERVICES

Because of the approval of rt-PA for acute ischemic stroke, EMS must reevaluate the way stroke victims are triaged, transported, and treated. EMS is comprised of 911 dispatchers, first responders, and ED personnel of the receiving facility in most areas of the United States. Each of these components requires reassessment of educational materials, stroke guidelines, and stroke protocols in order to meet the tight therapeutic treatment window for rt-PA. Stroke care mandates the same emergency response as with cardiac arrest or acute trauma. The concept of Code Stroke is useful in this regard *(6)*.

THE 911 SYSTEM

A Code Stroke Protocol begins when 911 is called or a patient arrives at the emergency department. In the NINDS rt-PA Stroke Trial, approx 76% of treated patients activated 911 as their first point of contact, suggesting early identification in the prehospital arena is a crucial link in providing rapid transport, triage, and treatment to stroke victims *(4,7)*. Unfortunately, one study reported that 911 dispatchers identified only 52% of calls correctly as stroke *(8)*. This fact illustrates the need for additional education of 911 dispatchers. Education should be provided regarding rt-PA as a potential stroke treatment as well as the narrow window of opportunity, in order for the 911 dispatchers to expedite handling of the stroke call. Protocols used by 911 emergency dispatchers should be examined to assure that all patients who have a potential diagnosis of stroke are given high priority and expeditious care.

PREHOSPITAL CARE: FIRST RESPONDERS

Emergency response protocols for stroke victims also require review and possible revision to expedite identification and transport of stroke victims. On arrival to the scene, first responders initially address the fundamental ABCs of emergency care (airway; breathing; and circulation). The next step is the rapid assessment of the patient's neurologic condition. EMS curriculum must teach both the various presentations of stroke as well as the quick assessment tools designed to select appropriate patients. The Cincinnati Prehospital Stroke Screen (CPSS) (Table 1) is one tool that can assist personnel at the scene in quickly identifying potential t-PA candidates. This tool assesses the patient on three items taken from the National Institutes of Health Stroke Scale (NIHSS): facial droop, motor drift, and speech. An abnormality found on any one of these three items would qualify as a positive screen. This screen has been shown to have good reliability and validity *(9,10)*.

Once stroke symptoms are identified, time of stroke onset must be determined. Time of onset is an important factor in treating patients safely with rt-PA. Onset

Table 1
Cincinnati Prehospital Stroke Screen (CPSS) *(9,10)*

Facial Droop (have patient show teeth or smile)
- Normal–both sides of face move equally well
- Abnormal–one side of face does not move as well as the other side

Arm Drift (patient closes eyes and holds both arms out)
- Normal–both arms move the same or both arms do not move at all (other findings, such as pronator grip, may be helpful)
- Abnormal–one arm does not move or one arm drifts down compared with the other

Speech (have the patient say "you can't teach an old dog new tricks")
- Normal–patient uses correct words with no slurring
- Abnormal–patient slurs words, uses inappropriate words or is unable to speak

time should be determined by prehospital personnel if possible, but never delay transport of the patient. All patients who fall within the time window of less than 3 h from onset and screen positive for the CPSS are potential t-PA candidates. The EMS then prenotifies the receiving hospital from the field that a potential t-PA patient is enroute. Prenotification provides time for the receiving facility to mobilize the physicians, nurses, and technicians to assemble and prepare for the patient's arrival *(4,6)*.

The next priority for first responders is to immediately transport to the closest facility experienced with acute stroke thrombolysis, or even better, a facility designated as an Acute Stroke Treatment Center. During transport, several procedures can be performed to prepare the patient for treatment. Intravenous access should be obtained. One intravenous line is all that is needed for treatment, however, two intravenous lines are preferred. Excessive fluid administration should be avoided unless medically indicated. Oxygen should be administered if needed. Collection of blood samples for laboratory chemistry, hematology, and coagulation in the prehospital setting can save time if feasible. Once the patient arrives at the ED, these specimens are ready for immediate delivery and processing at the hospital laboratory. Glucose is checked by fingerstick to rule out or treat hypoglycemia. Although these procedures help facilitate the possibility of rapid treatment, transport to the ED should never be delayed in order to initiate additional IV lines or the collection of lab samples in the prehospital setting. Every minute saved in the field increases the opportunity for t-PA treatment *(4,6)*.

EMERGENCY TRIAGE

Stroke screening tools can assist triage nurses in identifying potential thrombolysis candidates *(6,9–12)*. Patients who arrive and have a positive stroke screen or show signs of a focal neurologic deficit on arrival should have a Code Stroke activated and be treated emergently until it is determined that rt-PA is contraindicated. In order to provide these patients with the appropriate level of resources in the least amount of time, these patients should be placed in a high acuity bed (e.g., resuscitation room, cardiac or intensive care bed) within the ED throughout the Code Stroke process *(6)*.

Code Strokes help by streamlining acute stroke care *(11,13)*. This process varies from institution to institution and may consist of activating personnel from EMS, ED, neurology, radiology, pharmacy, and/or laboratory. Each of these departments is responsible for establishing a plan on how to respond to the acute stroke patient in order to facilitate early treatment. The process used to activate a Code Stroke by ED personnel should be quick and simple. In many institutions, a Code Stroke is set up like all other hospital emergencies (e.g., Code Blue or cardiac arrest; Code Red or fire alarm) using a designated emergency telephone line for the hospital. The operator is then responsible for immediately paging the Stroke Team members and/or notifying key departments to prepare for and respond to the stroke patient. Mechanisms should exist at every facility that allow Code Strokes to be activated by incoming EMS, ED personnel, and all patient care units. Strokes that occur in hospitalized patients should access the system in the same manner as those who arrive via the emergency department. Regardless of the point of entry, quick and prompt notification of the personnel involved which results in rapid treatment remains the goal.

TIME OF ONSET DETERMINATION

One obstacle after the patient arrives in the ED is to determine or reverify the time of stroke onset. Determining or reverifying the time of stroke onset requires skills similar to a police detective, the only difference being there is usually less than 1 h to solve the mystery. The investigation must also occur simultaneously with all other required procedures prior to initiation of treatment and the 3-h time window expiring (e.g., lab work, CT scan).

The stroke patient, a witness at the time of the event, time anchors, and EMS are all sources that can help establish onset time. Many stroke victims are unreliable when it comes to the onset of their symptoms because of an altered level of consciousness or symptoms of neglect. The best way to determine onset time is to question the family member or witness who was with the patient when the symptoms began. In many cases, the stroke has occurred without the presence of a witness. For these patients the stroke onset time is better identified as the last time the patient was seen to be normal, even though the stroke may have started at a later, unwitnessed time. Instead of asking *"What time did the stroke symptoms start?"* the question needs to be rephrased to *"When was the patient last seen normal?"*

Most patients who awaken with stroke symptoms in the morning will not be eligible for rt-PA because the time of onset is unknown and the last time they were seen normal is usually greater than 3 h. However, numerous elderly patients arise several times in the night. If the patient or family member can report the time they got up, and also report they were normal, the clock can be reset using this as the time of onset.

Another useful technique is the concept of time anchors. Time anchors are routine occurrences that happen consistently at the same time each day. This might include the time one leaves for work each day, walk the dog, eat dinner, or watch a particular television show. If a patient can report what he or she was doing at the time symptoms began, and this activity can be associated with a routine time anchor, it is then possible to estimate the time elapsed between stroke onset and their anchor point. Consider this: the patient always takes a morning walk at 9:00 AM, and sometime during the walk collapses. A neighbor finds the patient at 10:00 AM. The exact time of onset is unknown. However, the patient reports he or she was feeling fine when he or she left the house around 9:00 AM. This time anchor could be used to document the last time the patient was normal, i.e., 9:00 AM.

Another valuable and concrete method is the dispatch time or the actual time that the call to 911 was made. This information can usually be obtained from paramedics or the 911 central dispatch office. If the dispatch time is known, the patient, family or witness of the stroke can report how long it took them to call 911 after the first symptoms occurred. Fairly accurate times of onset can be calculated with this information.

Once determined, the onset time should be clearly documented on the patient's hospital record.

ED TOOLS AND PROCEDURES

Standing orders and treatment pathways are the most efficient process to move the patient rapidly through the system (Tables 2 and 3 and Fig. 2). An Acute Code Stroke Box is utilized at many facilities, which is simply a tackle box that contains all the necessary tools and supplies needed for stroke thrombolysis (Table 4).

After an initial assessment of the ABCs and vital signs, a baseline neurologic exam should be obtained using the National Institutes of Health Stroke Scale (NIHSS). The NIHSS is a quick, easy, and highly reproducible neurologic scale that can be performed by both physicians and nurses *(14,15,16)*. In addition, patients should be thoughtfully evaluated to ensure the accuracy of the diagnosis. The most common false positive diagnoses in patients who presented with stroke-like symptoms are unrecognized seizures with post-ictal deficits, systemic infections, brain tumors, and toxic-metabolic disturbances.

Table 2
Code Stroke Standing Orders *(6)*

Date	*Physician's Order*

1. Activate Stroke Code
2. Record time of stroke onset
3. Complete vital signs once, then check blood pressure every 15 minutes
4. Continuous cardiac monitoring
5. STAT noncontrast computerized tomography scan of head
6. STAT Blood draw for:
   Complete blood count with platelet count
   Fibrinogen
   Protime/Partial Thromboplastin Time
   Glucose (can be done by fingerstick)
7. Intravenous access: normal saline at 50cc/h
8. No heparin, warfarin, or aspirin

IS PATIENT AN APPROPRIATE t-PA CANDIDATE?
_____ NO (STOP HERE and document reason in chart)
_____ YES (Continue with orders below)

1. Second intravenous access: Saline lock with normal saline flush in opposite arm.
2. Record results of head computerized tomography, and all laboratory values.
3. Calculate TOTAL dose (0.9 mg/kg t-PA)
   0.9 mg. × _____ (pt's wt in kg) = _____ mg (total dose)
   NOTE: Maximum dose = 90 mg
4. Give 10% of total dose as an intravenous bolus over 1 min followed by an immediate continuous infusion of the remaining volume over 60 min.
5. Vital signs and neuro checks every 15 min.
6. No heparin, warfarin, or aspirin for 24 h from the start of the t-PA.
7. Transfer to an acute stroke or intensive care unit for monitoring.

Adapted from The NINDS TPA Stroke Study Group Protocol Guidelines.

The likelihood of a false positive diagnosis increases with decreased level of consciousness and normal eye movements upon first evaluation. Conversely, presenting with stroke symptoms and a history of angina is highly predictive of an actual stroke event *(17)*.

Although obtaining the neurologic exam, a head computerized tomography (CT) scan without contrast is ordered, one or two IV access lines are placed and blood specimens are collected for hematology, chemistry, and coagulation if not already performed in the field. These laboratory tests are performed immediately to detect bleeding disorders or other stroke mimicking conditions (e.g., hypoglycemia, hyperglycemia, hyponatremia, hepatic encephalopathy) *(17)*. Owing to the potential bleeding complications associated with thrombolytic therapy, multiple venipunctures and invasive lines and procedures should be avoided when possible.

Table 3

Acute Ischemic Stroke

Pretreatment Clinical Pathway for rt-PA Use

Time of Arrival to ED_____.	Patient Sticker

Time Labs sent_____.Results reviewed_____.
Time of CT Scan_____.
Time of Neuro Exam_____.
Time of t-PA treatment_____.
Time patient D/C from ED_____D/C to_____.
Reason patient did not receive t-PA_____.

Care Element	Triage	0 - 10 Minutes	10 - 25 Minutes	25 - 60 Minutes	1- 3 Hours*
Consults	Activate Code Stroke	ED Physician	Stroke Team		
Diagnostics	NA	Order CT scan of head without contrast; Draw CBC, PLT, Chemistry, PT/PTT send STAT; fingersitick; pregnancy test STAT if child bearing potential; continuous cardiac monitoring	CT scan completed; 12 lead EKG	CT scan reading available	CT scan reading available
Treatments	NA	IV access (preferably two)	Review t-PA inclusion and exclusion criteria; consider t-PA treatment	Consider t-PA treatment	Consider t-PA treatment
Assessments	Assess for neuro deficit, symptom onset time, ask for EMS dispatch time	VS, neuro exam (NIHSS), establish onset time (document on chart)	VS, neuro exam, current medications, estimate patient's weight	VS q 15", neuro exam, review lab results	VS q 15", neuro exam
Activity	Place patient in high acuity area; instruct family to stay in ED	bedrest	bedrest	bedrest/transfer to ICU after initiation of treatment	bedrest/transfer to ICU after initiation of treatment
Nutrition	NPO	NPO	NPO	NPO	NPO

*Patients are eligible for t-PA treatment if the time of the onset of their symptoms to the time of treatment is 3 hours or less.

Pathway adapted with permission from the Univ. of Texas, Houston, Dept. of Neurology Stroke Team; Published in the Journal of Neuroscience Nursing special supplement.

Obtaining the noncontrast head CT scan is a high priority. However, if there is a delay in the CT being ready, an electrocardiogram should be performed. This test is not an absolute prerequisite to treatment and should never delay the head CT scan. With early notification via the Code Stroke, the CT scan department should be scanning the patient within 25 min or less of hospital arrival (18). Other, nonemergent CT scans should be postponed until after the suspected stroke patient's scan is completed. Images of the brain are obtained using 10-mm slices to save time. The head CT scan is primarily performed to rule out hemorrhagic stroke, so thinner slices are unnecessary. This scan is not obtained to

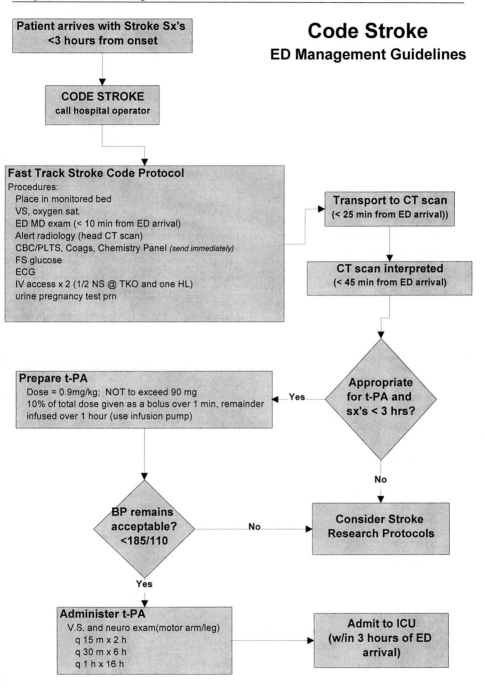

Fig. 2. Clinical pathway for code stroke.

Table 4
Stroke Code Box Contents

General Supplies	*Medications*
0.45 Normal saline	t-PA 50 mg
Normal Saline	t-PA 100 mg
IV tubing and ext. tubing	Labetolol
angioneedles/heplocks	NTG Paste
butterfly needles	Nitroprusside (used only after tpa initiated)
needles	
syringes 10cc/20cc	*Reference Materials*
alcohol wipes/tape/cotton	Patient selection criteria
vacutainer	BP Management Guidelines
tourniquets	NIHSS
lab tubes/requisitions	AHA Guidelines for t-PA and acute stroke
Urine pregnancy kit	weight dosing chart
hemocult slides	calculator
penlight	ICH Algorithm
safety pins/Q-tips	
Dextrose sticks	
Dextrose 50%	
prepacked lab tubes	
& requisitions	

diagnose or define the location of the stroke and any early changes suggestive of ischemia on CT scan should prompt the team to be suspicious of the accuracy of the symptom onset time, and requestion the patient or witnesses about the temporal sequence.

A quick yet thorough medical history should be acquired to rule out contraindications to treatment. Eligibility criteria used in the NINDS rt-PA Stroke Trial and the contraindications to treatment are listed in Chapter 17. The three most frequent reasons for patient ineligibility in the NINDS rt-PA Stroke Trial were time (onset more than 3 h) (50%), rapidly resolving symptoms (transient ischemic attack [TIA]) (10%) and intracranial hemorrhage (ICH) (8%) *(7)*. This underscores the importance of a solid history of the stroke event to confirm concrete time of onset, quick neurologic exam upon arrival and just prior to drug administration to eliminate patients with TIA, and an accurate and qualified reading of the head CT scan to rule out hemorrhagic stroke.

Hypertension and current anticoagulant therapy are two other important factors that may exclude a patient from receiving rt-PA treatment and often become obstacles to treatment. Vital signs should be obtained at least every 15 min in the pretreatment setting. If hypertension is present, the blood pressure should be gently lowered to less than 185/110 *(7)*. However, caution and judgment must be exercised; lowering the blood pressure too rapidly or too far may have a deleterious effect on the already ischemic brain by further lowering the cerebral perfusion pressure. Therefore, no aggressive treatment of blood pressure should occur. Intravenous drips such as nitroprusside were considered aggressive in the NINDS rt-PA Stroke Trial and are not recommended in the pretreatment setting. Low doses of intravenous labetalol (≤20 mg) were occasionally used to lower the blood pressure to a more acceptable range. Chapter 14 outlines the management guidelines used in the NINDS rt-PA Stroke Trial to control blood pressure in the pretreatment and posttreatment setting. Patients with sustained hypertension who do not respond to antihypertensive treatment should not be considered for rt-PA therapy. Prothrombin (PT) and/or partial thromboplastin time (PTT) results are necessary for patients currently prescribed coumadin or who have received heparin in the previous 48 h. Those with prolonged coagulation times would be ineligible owing to a presumed increased risk of bleeding complications *(7)*.

INITIATION OF TREATMENT

Treatment should begin immediately once the patient is determined to be an appropriate rt-PA candidate. An acute ischemic stroke patient is deemed appropriate when the laboratory values are acceptable, neurologic exam is consistent with a stroke, medical history is complete and free of any contraindications to treatment, a head CT scan is negative for hemorrhage or other lesion that would preclude treatment (tumor, and so on) and rt-PA therapy can begin within 3 h of symptom onset. If the head CT scan is the last piece of data to determine the patient's eligibility, and is without a lesion contraindicating therapy, the bolus of rt-PA should be immediately pushed in the CT scan department followed by the continuous infusion. Time and more importantly brain cells should not be sacrificed in order to transport the patient back to the ED or intensive care unit prior to drug initiation.

Just prior to dosing, the blood pressure should be rechecked as well as a quick neurologic exam to once again reverify the appropriateness of initiating treatment. The dosage of rt-PA is 0.9 mg/kg and is calculated using the patient's estimated body weight (Table 2). It is not often feasible to obtain the actual body weight owing to the patient's physical disability or aphasia, so body weight is estimated by asking the patient, family member, or lastly by estimation. Once reconstituted, the drug should be gently swirled to dissolve any remaining powder. ED personnel mixing the drug should allow a minimum of 6 min to reconstitute and prepare the drug. The exact time the treatment begins should be documented and should be no more than 3 h from the beginning of the patient's symptoms. After the infusion is completed, the IV tubing should be flushed with normal saline to insure the total dose was delivered.

Table 5
Acute Stroke Management Goals

Time From ED Arrival to:	
ED Doctor	10 min
CT Scan	25 min
CT Reading	45 min
Drug Initiated	60 min*
Monitored Bed	3 h

*80% success target.
Recommendations–Acute Hospital Care Panel. *National Institute of Neurological Disorders and Stroke, Proceedings of a National Symposium on Rapid Identification and Treatment of Acute Stroke*, Marler JR, Winters-Jones P, Emr M, eds. National Institutes of Heath: Bethesda, Maryland. 1997; NIH Publication No. 97-4239, pp. 157–158.

IDENTIFYING OBSTACLES AND TRACKING IMPROVEMENT

A symposium sponsored by NINDS published acute stroke management time goals for emergency departments treating acute stroke patients that identifies acceptable time intervals for the necessary tests and procedures once the patient arrives in the ED *(11)* (Table 5). These practice goals are ideal for Continuously Quality Improvement (CQI) projects for ED staff. Collecting time data as a patient moves through the system can help identify bottlenecks and pinpoint delays. CQI tracking forms (Fig. 2) can be attached to the patient's record upon arrival so data can be collected simultaneous to performing procedures. Data that illustrates how poorly patients are treated are very persuasive to management and staff that are resistant to change. Many stroke experts believe that stroke patients should only be transported to centers with documented track records demonstrating rapid evaluation and treatment. Similar to the Trauma Center model, this documentation would likely be a requirement for Stroke Center designation.

EDs need to evaluate their current system and track door (hospital arrival time) to lab, neurologic exam, head CT, and drug initiation times. EDs and EMS will need to develop a coordinated and organized system to expedite the identification, triage and treatment of acute stroke victims. Failure to implement a process to treat stroke acutely may cause unnecessary delays and missed opportunities to treat patients. Refining the system, identifying the obstacles and minimizing them, is an ongoing process that will benefit all stroke patients who seek treatment.

Continuous Quality Improvement

STROKE CODE

To be completed on every patient who presents with
stroke symptoms (i.e. weakness or numbness on one side
of the body, aphasia, slurred speech, difficulty
swallowing, visual difficulties, dizziness, or loss of
balance).

Addressograph

Date of ED arrival:

Time of ED arrival:

Stroke Code activated? ☐ No ☐ Yes

if yes time:

Did the patient arrive via EMS? ☐ Yes ☐ No

Suspected date/time of stroke symptom onset: OR ☐ unknown

Record the following times:

ED physician initial exam: Target: w/in 10 min

Neurology initial exam:

CT scan performed: Target: w/in 25 min

CT read by neurology
or radiology : Target: w/in 45 min

Stroke Code canceled? ☐ No ☐ Yes, if yes time:

New diagnosis/reason:_____
   (i.e. seizure, migraine, tumor, hypoglycemia)

Time treatment order given:

Treatment Given:
☐ t-PA; Time given : Target: w/in 60 min
☐ Refused t-PA; or delay by pt/family
☐ General Work up
☐ Research Protocol 1st dose given at:

Patient Disposition:
☐ Admitted; Time of admission: Target: w/in 3 hours
☐ Discharged to home
☐ Other_____

Fig. 3. Data collection form for Code Stroke Process Measurement and Improvement.

ACKNOWLEDGMENT

Portions of this manuscript have appeared previously in: Rapp K, Bratina P, et al. Code Stroke: Rapid Transport, Triage and Treatment Using rt-PA Therapy J Neurosci Nurs 1997;29:361–366.

REFERENCES

1. Feldmann E, Gordon N, Brooks JM, et al. Factors associated with early presentation of acute stroke. *Stroke* 1993;24:1805–1810.

2. Barsan WG, Brott TG, Broderick JP, Haley EC, Jr., Levy DE, Marler JR. Urgent therapy for acute stroke effects of a stroke trial on untreated patients. *Stroke* 1994;25:2132–2137.
3. 1996 *Gallup NSA Survey of Stroke Awareness in America*. Englewood, CO: National Stroke Association; 1996.
4. Pepe, P. The Initial Links in the Chain of Recovery for Brain Attack–Access, Prehospital Care, Notification, and Transport. In: *National Institute of Neurological Disorders and Stroke, Proceedings of a National Symposium on Rapid Identification and Treatment of Acute Stroke*, Marler JR, Winters-Jones P, Emr M, eds. National Institutes of Heath: Bethesda, Maryland. 1997; 97-4239: pp. 17–28, 147–165.
5. Alberts MJ, Perry A, Dawson, DV, et al. Effects of public and professional education on reducing the delay time in presentation and referral of stroke patients. *Stroke* 1992;23: 352–356.
6. Rapp K, Bratina P, Barch C et al. Code Stroke: Rapid Transport, Triage and Treatment Using rt-PA Therapy. *J Neurosci Nurs* 1997;29:361–366.
7. NINDS rt-PA Stroke Study Group. Tissue plasminogen activator for acute ischemic stroke. *N Engl J Med* 1995;333:1581–1587
8. Kothari R, Barsan W, Brott T, Broderick J, Ashbrock S. Frequency and accuracy of prehospital diagnosis of acute stroke. *Stroke* 1993;26:937–941.
9. Kothari RU, Pancioli A, Liu T, Brott TG, Broderick JP. Cincinnati Prehospital Stroke Scale: Reproducibility and Validity. *Annals of Emerg Med* 1999;4:373–378.
10. Kothari R, Hall K, Broderick J, Brott T. Early stroke recognition: developing an out-of-hospital stroke scale. *Acad Emerg Med* 1997;4:986–990.
11. Recommendations–Acute Hospital Care Panel. In: *National Institute of Neurological Disorders and Stroke, Proceedings of a National Symposium on Rapid Identification and Treatment of Acute Stroke*, Marler JR, Winters-Jones P, Emr M, eds. National Institutes of Heath: Bethesda, Maryland. 1997; 97-4239, pp. 157–158.
12. Lyden PD, Rapp K, Babcock T, Rothrock J. Ultra-rapid identification, triage, and enrollment of stroke patients into clinical trials. *J Stroke Cerebrovasc Dis* 1994;4:106–113.
13. Bratina P, Greenberg L, Pasteur W, Grotta JC. Current emergency department management of stroke in Houston, Texas. *Stroke* 1995;26:409–414.
14. Spilker J, Kongable G, Barch C, et al. Using the NIH Stroke Scale to assess stroke patients. *J Neurosci Nurs* 1997;29:384–392.
15. Lyden P, Brott T, Tilley B, et al. Improved reliability of the NIH stroke scale using video training. *Stroke* 1994;25:2220–2226.
16. Brott T. Utility of the NIH Stroke Scale. *Cerebrovascular Dis* 1992;2:241–242
17. Libman RB, Wirkowski E, Alvir J, Roa TH. Conditions that mimic stroke in the emergency department: implications for acute stroke trials. *Arch Neurol* 1995;52:1119–1122.
18. Bock B: Response System for Patients Presenting with Acute Stroke. In: *National Institute of Neurological Disorders and Stroke, Proceedings of a National Symposium on Rapid Identification and Treatment of Acute Stroke*, Marler JR, Winters-Jones P, Emr M, eds. National Institutes of Heath: Bethesda, Maryland. 1997; 97-4239, pp. 55–56.

17

The NINDS t-PA for Acute Stroke Protocol

John Marler, MD
and Patrick D. Lyden, MD

CONTENTS

INTRODUCTION
HISTORY AND RATIONALE
  FOR THROMBOLYTIC STROKE THERAPY PROTOCOLS
PATIENT SELECTION AND PROTOCOL
NONSPECIFIC THERAPY
FUTURE STRATEGIES
REFERENCES

INTRODUCTION

To successfully identify, triage, diagnose, and treat an acute stroke victim in time requires a coordinated, multidisciplinary effort that is organized around a predefined protocol. The protocol assures that all needed action will occur in a timely fashion. Also, the ratio of stroke to stroke-mimics may be 1 to 4 or 5, which mandates the presence of an efficient, skilled procedure for eliminating the mimics, e.g., Todd's paralysis, transient ischemic attack (TIA), hysteria, migraine, and carpal tunnel syndrome. Stroke patients must be stabilized according to basic protocols (airway, breathing, circulation) before the neurologic evaluation begins; this process should require no more than a minute or two (Chapter 14). Stroke management then includes diagnosis and possibly treatment. All of the above is best accomplished with an institutionalized Stroke Team, comparable to a Code Blue team that rehearses, monitors performance, and uses feedback to continually improve care (Chapter 16).

From: *Thrombolytic Therapy for Stroke*
Edited by: P. D. Lyden © Humana Press Inc., Totowa, NJ

HISTORY AND RATIONALE
FOR THROMBOLYTIC STROKE THERAPY PROTOCOLS

The current tissue-plasminogen activator (t-PA) for acute stroke protocol reflects considerable development efforts. Departing for this protocol is unwise, as has been confirmed in several studies. The published guidelines grew slowly over the course of several National Institute of Neurological Disorders (NINDS) sponsored trials (1–8). At each step in the development of the protocol, a team of investigators evaluated the clinical utility of each item in the protocol. Specific trials were done to determine the best, safest dose of t-PA (see Chapters 7–9). The final version of the protocol is contained in the FDA-approved package insert, based on the definitive US trial.

The NINDS Stroke Trial investigators published the US study of thrombolysis for stroke in December of 1995 (5). Patients received 0.9 mg/kg of t-PA within 3 h of stroke symptoms beginning. There was scrupulous attention to blood pressure management prior to thrombolysis: patients were not treated if their blood pressure remained elevated above 185/110 after gentle antihypertensive treatment. After thrombolysis, patients received sufficient blood pressure management to maintain their blood pressure below those limits. Subsequent analysis of the NINDS data revealed that all subgroups of patients responded to t-PA including patients with different subtypes of stroke, patients with a range of stroke severities and patients of all ages (7). As a result of this success, the research protocol developed for these trials has become the approved protocol for clinical use of t-PA.

PATIENT SELECTION AND PROTOCOL

Shortly after the publication of the NINDS study, practice guidelines for the use of t-PA in stroke patients were promulgated by the American Academy of Neurology, and the American Heart Association (9,10). Any physician contemplating thrombolytic stroke therapy should study these guidelines carefully, and a continuing medical education course may be helpful as well. A plethora of vital information, including protocols, guidelines, sample orders, and relevant summaries are available on the Web to any physician. Table 1 lists three starting pages. In addition, many stroke research centers have published websites containing their orders and protocols. These sites can generally be accessed via one of the sites listed in Table 1. Prior to the first use of any thrombolytic drug, physicians should rehearse the Code Stroke with a team consisting of, at a minimum, an emergency department nurse, and a radiologist. Health care systems may need to be changed to allow rapid identification, triage and treatment of acute stroke patients, and guidelines for this are available (11,12).

Potential stroke victims must be identified as early as possible. Ideally, bystanders and witnesses will learn to recognize strokes, and the American Stroke

Table 1
Important Web Sites Containing Useful Stroke Therapy Protocols

Site	Sponsor	Contents	Links to other sites?
Stroke-site.org	NINDS Stroke Division	Protocols, Scales, Guidelines, Sample Orders, Consensus Statements	Yes; very complete, very simple to use
Stroke.org	National Stroke Association	Protocols, Consensus	Yes, but commercial
Americanheart.org	American Stroke Association	Consensus Statements	No

Association's initiative, Operation Stroke, targets such public awareness. It is unlikely, however, that the complexity of stroke presentation will ever be fully appreciated by the lay public. There are simplified lists of stroke warning signs that may assist in this process.

Patients may be examined first by prehospital providers (Paramedics and Emergency Medical Technicians), and considerable advance work should be done by them (see Chapters 14 and 16). Patients will arrive in the hospital Emergency Department (ED) by ambulance, or as a walk-in. By whichever route, the next step should be activation of the Code Stroke system. In some communities, this could include radio activation of the Stroke Team by medics in the field. The Stroke Team must be prepared at all times to respond immediately to the ED. In busy Neurology practices, this preparedness will mandate an on-call schedule with reduced clinic schedules to facilitate immediate response. In medical centers with hospitalists, it may be better for the Neurologists to train Emergency Department or Hospitalist physicians to handle the early phases of the Code Stroke. Prior to arrival of the Code Team, the ED staff should begin the Code Stroke protocol. This process is facilitated by standing orders that can be initiated by ED nursing staff without MD authorization.

The first step is to establish the time of onset of the stroke. This is critical because thrombolysis for stroke must begin within 3 to 6 h of the stroke beginning. The physician should be suspicious of any second-hand estimates of onset time; it is critical to obtain corroboration from other witnesses. In many cases, the Code Team physician should telephone the home or scene and try to obtain information from a direct witness. When did this happen? What did you first notice? If you returned from an errand to find the victim symptomatic, when was the last time you knew the victim was symptom-free? Often using a "time anchor," a term coined by the Cincinnati Stroke Team, is useful: find an event with a known time, such as a television program or the time the call was made to 911, and relate the stroke onset to that event. If the patient awoke with symptoms, the onset time is pushed back to the bedtime or last time the victim was known to be at baseline.

Although it is important to carefully set the onset time, there is a risk in overemphasizing some statements from well-meaning friends and family. It is human nature to revisit memory, and try to "explain" a tragedy: often witnesses will embellish with statements like "Well, now that you mention it, he was feeling poorly last evening." We have frequently encountered a version of "She seemed different last night." These statements must be vigorously pursued: Was there weakness? Was there speech or language deficits? Unless a relatively clear-cut description of definite neurologic impairments can be elicited, such vague statements should not be used to set the onset time.

After setting the onset time, a brief past medical history is needed. A thorough history and review-of-symptoms will be obtained after the Code is over; at this point the focus is on stroke risk factors, emphasizing potential sources of cardiac embolism. Knowledge of the medications is essential, especially antithrombotics such as Coumadin and aspirin. Next, a brief but thorough examination must be done to elicit focal neurologic findings consistent with acute stroke. Until later, one avoids time consuming assessments such as a detailed mental status assessment or prolonged sensory battery. At this point, the sole purpose is to confirm the presence of focal findings and perform enough examination to preliminarily localize the occluded artery.

Next, specific laboratory studies must be drawn to search for conditions that mimic stroke, such as hypoglycemia, or that may confound therapy, such as a prolonged prothrombin time. The full list of tests is included in the standard orders, Tables 2–4. A 12 lead electrocardiogram (EKG) must be done to rule out a simultaneous myocardial infarction, which is present in about 5% of all stroke patients. Finally, the patient must be taken to radiology for a brain computer tomography (CT) scan to rule out hemorrhage.

Since time is critical, the above sequence must be amended as needed to maintain speed. The physician in charge of the Code Stroke must ask for status updates, and amend the sequence of events accordingly. For example, if the CT scanner is ready for the patient, but the EKG has not been done, it would be better to go to the scanner first and get the EKG upon returning from CT. A frequent source of delay is the transportation of the specimens or the patient. Neurologists are not generally accustomed to worrying about such details, but in the course of analyzing stroke teams at many medical centers, we have found this area problematic. The physician must specify that the STAT specimens from the Code Stroke must be walked over the laboratory specifically, even in hospitals that have an established Code Stroke system. Similarly, medical center policy usually mandates the use of escorts to physically transport a patient to radiology for a brain CT scan; this delays the scan. In our experience, quicker results will be obtained if the Stroke Team moves the patient personally.

Table 2

Sample Physician's Order for the Preliminary Evaluation
of a Stroke Patient After the Stroke Patient has been Brought
to the Emergency Department and While rt-PA Treatment is Being Considered

Date	Physician's order
	1. Record time of stroke onset (last time patient seen without stroke symptoms).
	2. Activate stroke response system.
	3. Complete vital signs once, then blood pressure every 15 min.
	4. STAT noncontrast CT scan of head.
	5. STAT blood draw for:
	a.) CBC with platelet count.
	b.) PT and aPTT.
	c.) Glucose (can be done by fingerstick).
	6. IV Access: NS or 0.45 NS keep open at 50 cc/h.
	7. No heparin, warfarin, or aspirin.

Physician Signature

These orders are available for public copying from the NINDS Stroke Division website at www.stroke-site.org.

Prior to administration of thrombolytics, blood pressure must be less than 185/110. A gentle antihypertensive, such as labetolol, may be used but if this fails then the patient must not receive thrombolysis. After thrombolysis, however, aggressive therapy must be used, if needed, to keep the pressure below those limits. Detailed laboratory studies confirmed that elevations of blood pressure predispose to hemorrhage after thrombolysis (13–16). Analysis of the patients in the NINDS study for deleterious effects of antihypertensive therapy revealed none (17). The patient should be admitted to an observation area where frequent vital signs and neuro checks can be performed.

The selection criteria for thrombolytic stroke therapy are listed in Table 5. These selection criteria are based on the NINDS Trial, and are listed here with minor modification. The criteria reflects primarily a concern for patient safety; therefore, some of the restrictions may seem over-cautious. Current studies will evaluate some of the more restrictive criteria, such as the prohibition of heparin for 24 h following thrombolysis. Physicians who depart from the guidelines should do so only after careful consideration and discussion with the patient and family. Clear documentation should detail the reasons for departing from the criteria. For example, a physician may judge that a patient with a platelet count of 95,000 could safely be treated. Such a decision is well within the purview of an individual physician's judgment, but the thoughts and decision-making process should be well-documented. Also, the physician should document concur-

Table 3
Sample Physician's Order for Treatment of Acute Ischemic Stroke
With rt-PA After Preliminary Evaluation

Date	Physician's order

1. Second IV Access: Saline Lock with NS flush in opposite arm.
2. Record results for CT scan, CBC, platelet count, glucose.
3. If patient has been on warfarin or heparin, record results for PT or PTT.
4. Give tissue plasminogen activator _____ mg. IV over 1 min as a 10% bolus followed immediately by _____ mg IV by continuous infusion over 60 min for a total dose of _____ mg. Dose calculation:
   Choose the smallest of the following two total stroke treatment doses:
   a) Maximum total dose 90 milligrams
   b) Estimated patient weight in kilograms _____ × 0.9 mg/kg. = _____ mg
   c) Loading dose = Total dose × 10% = _____ mg.
   d) Remainder (_____ mg) infused over one hour.
5. Vital signs and neuro checks q 15 min for 2 h after start of rt-PA infusion.
6. No heparin, warfarin, or aspirin for 24 h from start of rt-PA infusion.
7. Maintain systolic BP <185 and diastolic BP <110 as per protocol.
8. Transfer to Acute Stroke or Intensive Care Unit for monitoring.

Physician Signature

These orders represent only one potential approach to the management of patients with ischemic stroke. For each patient, physicians and institutions must determine treatment appropriate for their own situation. These orders are available for public copying from the NINDS Stroke Division website at www.stroke-site.org.

rence of the patient and family, and their understanding of increased risks with protocol deviations.

There are no special subgroups of patients that are particularly likely to respond to t-PA. A complete discussion of targeting subgroups for thrombolytic therapy is presented in Chapter 9. As presented there, extensive analysis failed to identify subgroups that fail to respond to thrombolysis or are particularly likely to hemorrhage (7,8). Thus, the criteria listed in Table 5 are the best guide to patient selection.

The t-PA is administered as an intravenous infusion of 0.9 mg/kg; a 10% bolus is given over 1 min and the remainder is infused over 60 min. The laboratory values may be checked after the bolus; that is, the bolus should not be delayed pending the laboratory results unless the patient is known to be taking Coumadin or is at risk for thrombocytopenia. During the infusion, blood pressure must be carefully maintained below 185/95; serial neuro checks are used to assess the patient's progress. During this hour, a more detailed history and neurologic

Table 4
Sample Physician's Order for Treatment of Acute Ischemic Stroke
in Acute Care Unit After Infusion of rt-PA

Date	Physician's order

1. Continue Emergency Department orders for rt-PA infusion and monitoring vital signs and neuro checks until 2 h after start of rt-PA infusion
2. Vital signs (BP, P, R) and neuro checks (LOC and arm/leg weakness) q 30 min for 6 h, then q 60 min for 16 h after start of rt-PA.
3. Bleeding precautions: check puncture sites for bleeding or hematomas. Apply digital pressure or pressure dressing to active compressible bleeding sites. Evaluate urine, stool, emesis, or other secretions for blood. Perform Hemoccult testing if there is evidence of bleeding.
4. Call Dr._____, pager #_____ immediately for evidence of bleeding, neurologic deterioration, or vital signs outside the following parameters:
   a) Systolic BP >185 or Systolic BP <110.
   b) Diastolic BP >105 or Diastolic BP <60.
   c) Pulse <50.
   d) Respirations >24.
   e) Decline in neurological status or worsening of stroke signs.
5. 0.45NS or NS IV to keep open at 50 cc/hr × 24 h.
6. O_2 at 2 l/min by nasal cannula (if needed).
7. Continuous cardiac monitoring (if needed).
8. I's and O's.
9. Diet: NPO except meds for 24 h.
10. Bed rest.
11. Medications: Acetaminophen 650 mg p.o. or p.r. PRN for pain q 4 to 6 h.
12. (Patient's regular medications previously prescribed, if appropriate.)
13. No heparin, warfarin, or aspirin for 24 h.
14. After 24 h: CT to exclude intracranial hemorrhage before any anticoagulants.

Physician Signature

These orders represent only one potential approach to the management of patients with ischemic stroke. For each patient, physicians and institutions must determine treatment appropriate for their own situation. These orders are available for public copying from the NINDS Stroke Division website at www.stroke-site.org.

examination are performed, noting any risk factors that may indicate etiology for the stroke. Ancillary investigations, including carotid ultrasound or cardiac echocardiography are considered. After the infusion is ended, the patient should be observed for evidence of response to therapy, or complications, in an observation or intensive care unit.

A number of research groups have now published data showing that community-based neurologists can deliver the drug with statistics that mirror the origi-

Table 5
Selection Criteria for Thrombolytic Therapy for Stroke

Patient Selection

Patients must be treated within 3 h of ischemic stroke symptom onset

Obtain baseline CT to rule out intracranial hemorrhage (ICH), subarachnoid hemorrhage (SAH)

Contraindications

Greater than 3 h from acute ischemic stroke symptom onset

Rapidly improving minor or major stroke (i.e., TIA)

ICH on CT or by history

Suspicion of SAH despite negative head CT

Recent intracranial surgery or serious head trauma or recent previous stroke (in last 3 mo)

Uncontrolled HTN at time of treatment (e.g., >185 mm Hg systolic or >105 mm Hg diastolic)

Seizure at the onset of stroke

Active internal bleeding (e.g., GI, urinary) within 21 d

Intracranial neoplasm, AVM, aneurysm

Glucose <50 or >400 mg/dL

Lumbar Puncture within 7 d, major surgery within 14 d

Arterial puncture at noncompressible site

Acute myocardial infarction or post MI pericarditis

Known bleeding diathesis, including but not limited to:

Current use of oral anticoagulants (e.g., warafin sodium) with prothrombin time >15 s

Administration of heparin within 48 h preceding the onset of stroke
   and have an elevated activated partial thromboplastin time (aPTT) at presentation

Platelet count <100,000/mm3

Warning: Carefully consider patients with major early infarct signs on a CT scan (e.g., substantial edema, mass effect, or midline shift)

Warning: Carefully consider risks/benefits in patients with severe neurological deficit (e.g., NIH Stroke Scale >22) at presentation. An increased risk of ICH may exist.

Adapted from the NINDS t-PA Stroke Trial Protocol and the Activase Package Insert, Genentech, South San Francisco. Patients may be considered for treatment up to 6h—see text.

nal study. For example, in Houston, Chiu and colleagues *(18)* found a hemorrhage rate of 7% in two community hospitals and one University hospital. Full recovery was seen in 37%, mirroring the data seen in the original study. Time to treatment (door-to-needle) was about 100 min, and there was no significant difference between the community and university settings. Similar results have been reported from a study of community hospitals in Cologne, Germany, where the symptomatic hemorrhage rate was 5% and the favorable response rate was 40 to 53% *(19)*. In a very large survey of 389 successfully treated patients, the rate of good outcomes was the same as in the NINDS trial, and the hemorrhage rate was lower *(20)*. This survey included patients from 57 medical centers, of which only 24 were academic. However, in a retrospective collection of cases, a hemorrhage rate of 16% and a protocol deviation rate of 50% were seen *(21)*.

All of these reports of community experiences are limited by the unavoidable fact that they cannot be blinded or placebo-controlled. Also, unless cases are collected prospectively, there is the risk of biased case selection. At this time, however, it is fair to conclude that if the NINDS protocol is followed scrupulously, then outcome results identical to the original study can be obtained in community hospitals.

NONSPECIFIC THERAPY

Simple measures may affect outcome in stroke patients, although none have been subjected to a rigorous clinical trial. Nevertheless, in the absence of any known side effects, clinicians may wish to consider nonspecific measures. The deleterious effect of hyperthermia upon stroke outcome is well-described in experimental subjects (22–25). There is minimal evidence for this in humans, but many stroke patients do suffer transient elevations of core temperature. Some clinicians routinely prescribe 650 mg acetaminophen orally or per rectum in stroke patients with temperature greater than 38°C. Hyperglycemia is also known to adversely effect outcome in experimental subjects (26–28). Most clinicians attempt to maintain serum glucose below 300 mg/dL after stroke, and some try for even lower levels. The risk of overshooting and causing hypoglycemia is real, and should be carefully considered. All stroke patients should be well-hydrated and provided supplemental oxygen if necessary. It should be borne in mind, though, that ischemia causes reactive oxygen free radicals, and supplemental oxygen should not be routinely ordered in all stroke patients regardless of need.

FUTURE STRATEGIES

Alternatives to thrombolysis will be necessary for a variety of reasons. Only half of all evaluated patients presented within 3 h of stroke symptoms beginning in the NINDS stroke trial. Few patients present to the hospital within 3 h because witnesses and patients do not recognize the warning signs of stroke (29). Delay in seeking care is attributable to the attitudes of patients, witnesses, and the healthcare system (30,31). Organizing community stroke networks, including stroke teams, may help in this regard (32–34). The success of public education efforts cannot be predicted, so it must be assumed that there will be many acute stroke patients who present beyond the time window needed for t-PA treatment. Neuroprotection may provide an alternative for reducing damage after stroke (35). Additionally, neuroprotection may prolong the window for safe use of thrombolysis (see Chapter 3). The pathophysiology of brain hemorrhage after thrombolysis is not clearly known, but it appears related to the volume of brain damage that occurs (36). If this is true, and if the volume of brain damage can be limited with a neuroprotectant, then it is reasonable to think that the time window for thrombolysis could be extended. Thus if paramedics were summoned to evaluate a patient, and it did not appear that there was time to get to the hospital for thrombolysis, then a neuroprotectant could be given in the field which might salvage enough brain that thrombolysis could be given at a later time point.

Without doubt, stroke treatment in the future will involve combination chemotherapy *(37)*. No one drug is likely to be successful in all patients and for all strokes. The challenge is to determine which drugs to use in what doses in the combination. An important limitation in this area is that combination trials are difficult. Considerable work is needed in the laboratory to develop criteria for evaluating combination treatments. Also, a logical and efficient strategy is needed for there are an infinite variety of drugs and different doses to try in combination.

REFERENCES

1. Brott T, Haley EC, Levy DE, Barsan WG, Reed RL, Olinger CP, Marler JR. Very early therapy for cerebral infarction with tissue plasminogen activator (tPA). *Stroke* 1988;19:8.
2. Brott TG, Haley EC Jr, Levy DE, Barsan W, Broderick J, Sheppard GL, et al. Urgent therapy for stroke: Part 1. Pilot study of tissue plasminogen activator administered within 90 minutes. *Stroke* 1992;23:632–640.
3. Haley EC Jr, Levy DE, Brott TG, Sheppard GL, Wong MC, Kongable GL, et al. Urgent therapy for stroke. Part II. Pilot study of tissue plasminogen activator administered 91–180 minutes from onset. *Stroke* 1992;23:641–645.
4. Haley EC, Brott TG, Sheppard GL, Barsan W, Broderick J, Marler JR, et al. Pilot randomized trial of tissue plasminogen activator in acute ischemic stroke. *Stroke* 1993;24:1000–1004.
5. NINDS rt-PA Stroke Study Group. Tissue plasminogen activator for acute ischemic stroke. *N Engl J Med* 1995;333:1581–1587.
6. Kwiatkowski TG, Libman RB, Frankel M, Tilley BC, Morgenstern LB, Lu M, et al., The National Institute of Neurological Disorders and Stroke rt-PA Stroke Study Group. Effects of tissue plasminogen activator for acute ischemic stroke at one year. *N Engl J Med* 1999;340:1781–1787.
7. NINDS TPA Stroke Study Group. Generalized Efficacy of t-PA for Acute Stroke. *Stroke* 1997;28:2119–2125.
8. NINDS TPA Stroke Study Group. Intracerebral Hemorrhage After Intravenous t-Pa Therapy for Ischemic Stroke. *Stroke* 1997;28:2109–2118.
9. Report of the Quality Standards Subcommittee of the American Academy of Neurology. Thrombolytic therapy for acute ischemic stroke—Summary Statement. *Neurology* 1996; 47:835–839.
10. Adams HP Jr, Brott TG, Furlan AJ, Gomez CR, Grotta J, Helgason CM, et al. Guidelines for thrombolytic therapy for acute stroke: A supplement to the guidelines for the management of patients with acute ischemic stroke. *Circulation* 1996;94:1167–1174.
11. Tilley BC, Lyden PD, Brott TG, Lu M, Levine SR, Welch KMA. Total quality improvement method for reduction of delays between emergency department admission and treatment of acute ischemic stroke. *Arch Neurol* 1997;54:1466–1474.
12. Lyden PD, Rapp K, Babcock T, Rothrock J. Ultra-rapid identification, triage, and enrollment of stroke patients into clinical trials. *J Stroke Cerebrovasc Dis* 1994;4:106–113.
13. Hårdemark H-G, Wesslén N, Persson L. Influence of clinical factors, CT findings and early management on outcome in supratentorial intracerebral hemorrhage. *Cerebrovasc Dis* 1999;9:10–21.

14. Levy DE, Brott TG, Haley EC Jr, Marler JR, Sheppard GP, Barsan W, Broderick JP. Factors related to intracranial hematoma formation in patients receiving tissue-type plasminogen activator for acute ischemic stroke. *Stroke* 1994;25:291–297.

15. Bowes MP, Zivin JA, Thomas GR, Thibodeaux H, Fagan SC. Acute hypertension, but not thrombolysis, increases the incidence and severity of hemorrhagic transformation following experimental stroke in rabbits. *Exp Neurol* 1996;141:40–46.

16. Fagan SC, Bowes MP, Lyden PD, Zivin JA. Acute hypertension promotes hemorrhagic transformation in a rabbit embolic stroke model: Effect of labetalol. *Exp Neurol* 1998;150:153–158.

17. Brott T, Lu M, Kothari R, Fagan SC, Frankel M, Grotta JC, et al. Hypertension and its treatment in the NINDS rt-PA stroke trial. *Stroke* 1998;29:1504–1509.

18. Chiu D, Krieger D, Villar-Cordova C, Kasner SE, Morgenstern LB, Bratina P, et al. Intravenous tissue plasminogen activator for acute ischemic stroke feasibility, safety, and efficacy in the first year of clinical practice. *Stroke* 1998;29:18–22.

19. Grond M, Rudolf J, Schmulling S, Stenzel C, Neveling M, Heiss WD. Early intravenous Thrombolysis with recombinant tissue-type plasminogen activator in vertebrobasilar ischemic stroke. *Arch Neurol* 1998;55:466–469.

20. Albers GW, Bates V, Clark W, Bell R, Verro P, Hamilton S. Intravenous tissue-type plasminogen activator for treatment of acute stroke: The standard treatment with alteplase to reverse stroke (STARS) Study (STARS). *JAMA* 2000;283:1145–1150.

21. Katzan I, Furlan A, Lloyd L, Frank J, Harper D, Hinchey J, Hammel J, Qu A, Sila C. Use of tissue-type plasminogen activator for acute ischemic stroke: The Cleveland area experience. *JAMA* 2000;283:1151–1158.

22. Chen H, Chopp M, Welch KMA. Effect of mild hyperthermia on the ischemic infarct volume after middle cerebral artery occlusion in the rat. *Neurology* 1991;41:1133–1135.

23. Dietrich WD, Busto R, Valdes I, Loor Y. Effects of normothermic versus mild hyperthemic forebrain ischemia in rats. *Stroke* 1990;21:1318–1325.

24. Ginsberg MD, Busto R. Combating Hyperthermia in Acute Stroke A Significant Clinical Concern. *Stroke* 1998;29:529–534.

25. Kuroiwa T, Bonnekoh P, Hossmann K-A. Prevention of postischemic hyperthermia prevents ischemic injury of CA_1 neurons in gerbils. *J Cereb Blood Flow and Metab* 1990; 10:550–556.

26. Candelise L, Landi G, Orazio EN, Boccardi E. Prognostic significance of hyperglycemia in acute stroke. *Arch Neurol* 1985;42:661–663.

27. Pulsinelli WA, Levy DE, Sigsbee B, Scherer P, Plum F. Increased damage after ischemic stroke in patients with hyperglycemia with or without established diabetes mellitus. *Am J Med* 1983;74:540–544.

28. Welsh FA, Ginsberg MD, Rieder W, Budd WW. Deleterious effect of glucose pretreatment on recovery from diffuse cerebral ischemia in the cat. Regional metabolite levels. *Stroke* 1980;11:355–363.

29. Feldmann E, Gordon N, Brooks JM, Brass LM, Fayad PB, Sawaya KL, et al. Factors associated with early presentation of acute stroke. *Stroke* 1993;24:1805–1810.

30. Harper GD, Haigh RA, Potter JF, Castleden CM. Factors delaying hospital admission after stroke in leicestershire. *Stroke* 1992;23:835–838.

31. Alberts MJ, Perry A, Dawson DV, Bertels C. Effects of public and professional education on reducing the delay in presentation and referral of stroke patients. *Stroke* 1992;23:352–356.

32. Andre C, Moraes-Neto J, Novis S. Experience with t-PA treatment in a large South American city. *J Stroke Cerebrovasc Dis* 1998;7:255–258.

33. Bratina P, Greenberg L, Pasteur W, Grotta JC. Current emergency department management of stroke in Houston, Texas. *Stroke* 1995;26:409–414.

34. Zweifler RM, Drinkard R, Cunningham S, Brody ML, Rothrock JF. Implementation of a stroke code system in Mobile, Alabama. Diagnostic and therapeutic yield. *Stroke* 1997;28:981–983.
35. Grotta J. The current status of neuronal protective therapy: Why have all neuronal protective drugs worked in animals but none so far in stroke patients? *Cerebrovasc Dis* 1994;4:115–120.
36. Lyden PD, Zivin JA. Hemorrhagic transformation after cerebral ischemia: Mechanisms and incidence. *Cerebrovasc Brain Met Rev* 1993;5:1–16.
37. Hallenbeck JM, Frerichs KU. Stroke therapy. It may be time for an integrated approach. *Arch Neurol* 1993;50:768–770.

18 Research Directions and the Future of Stroke Therapy

Patrick Lyden, MD

In this volume we have presented the data supporting the use of thrombolytic therapy for stroke, and reviewed the practical methods required to use thrombolysis safely. In addition, we presented a variety of methods and tools used to improve prehospital identification and transport of potential stroke victims. In the next section, we will present a variety of cases in tutorial format. These cases are designed to illustrate and emphasize the lessons presented elsewhere in the volume. After working the cases, the reader should feel reasonably confident in approaching a stroke patient and considering them for thrombolysis.

The approval of tissue-plasminogen activator (t-PA) as the first accepted treatment for acute stroke is only the beginning of a coming revolution in stroke therapy. Yet, too few patients present themselves early enough to receive thrombolysis. The first step toward improving stroke treatment lies in educating the general public and health care providers; educational projects are now underway at the National Stroke Association and the American Stroke Association. Stroke must be thought of as an emergency that requires immediate medical intervention, similar to heart attack or trauma. Most patients do not recognize the symptoms of stroke: it is crucial that the lay public learn to identify the warning signs of stroke and associate the signs with a "brain attack."

To fully extend the benefits of thrombolysis, however, we must create new ways of protecting the brain pending thrombolysis. Neuroprotection could benefit in two ways: first, neuroprotection could prolong the temporal window for thrombolysis. Second, neuroprotection might reduce the incidence of hemorrhagic transformation. A limiting step, however, is that neuroprotectants may not reach the brain until thrombolysis occurs. For this reason, some advocate hypothermia, a potent neuroprotective therapy that works in the absence of thrombolysis. To date, hypothermia has not proven feasible in humans, but new technology becomes available nearly daily.

From: *Thrombolytic Therapy for Stroke*
Edited by: P. D. Lyden © Humana Press Inc., Totowa, NJ

By attacking the mechanism of stroke at various sites, the likelihood of reducing the degree of deficits and improving the functional outcome is greater, hence it is likely that combination chemotherapy will prove beneficial for stroke patients. At the time of this writing (Fall 2000), however, the battlefield is littered with the remains of failed neuroprotectants. Pessimism for the future of neuroprotection increases with each additional failed clinical trial. We hope that from among the remaining players—GABA agonists, potassium maxi-channel drugs, and glycine-site antagonists—that a success may yet emerge. Once a winner is available, we may launch the arduous process of testing various combinations. It is unlikely that an agent with no neuroprotective effect alone will add much in combination with another drug. There are some agents, e.g., Citicholine, that exhibited some protective effects that were not powerful enough to emerge in stand-alone clinical trials. Perhaps a combination of such a drug with a proven winner may yield a more potent combination. Considerable research into trial methodology is needed, however, to facilitate studies of such combinations.

A compound that reduced the hemorrhage rate associated with thrombolysis could also rekindle enthusiasm, and potentially broaden the time spectrum for treatment. At the moment, no strategy has clearly proven effective. Several groups are actively looking at inhibitors of matrix metalloproteinases because these enzymes appear to play an essential role in mediating ischemic edema and hemorrhagic transformation. Such studies are difficult and time consuming, yet the progress so far is encouraging. Real progress in this area may have to wait for a clearer understanding of the basic biology of the ischemic blood brain barrier.

Mutant molecules, derived from t-PA and intended to offer advantages, have yet to prove their worth. The TNK variant has the advantage of single bolus therapy and greater fibrin specificity. In myocardial infarction trials, however, the molecule did not prove to be greatly superior. Stroke trials are underway.

Now is an exciting time to be in Neurology, and in Stroke particularly. We hope to have conveyed our enthusiasm for our research, and the results obtained so far. We look forward to furthering the revolution in Neurology, as we evolve from a diagnostic into an interventional specialty.

IV ILLUSTRATIVE CASES

Case 1

The patient is a 64-yr-old African-American who was brought to the emergency department by paramedics for the sudden onset of left-sided weakness and slurring of speech. At approx 9:00 AM, while walking, the patient noticed difficulty in the left upper and lower extremities. The patient was able to continue walking but went to a friend's house and called paramedics. The patient also had experienced chest pressure early that morning which he described as intensity of 5 out of 10. These episodes were relieved with sublingual nitroglycerin, which he took himself. He arrived in the Emergency Department at 1:00 PM.

His blood pressure was 128/80, pulse 92, respirations 20, temperature 98.1. Physical examination was pertinent for left hemiparesis including the left upper and lower extremities which were both essentially flaccid. The patient also had a mild left-sided facial droop with dysarthria. Sensory examination revealed decreased sensitivity to light touch, temperature, pinprick, and vibration on the left side of the body. CBC with differential, chemistry 20 and coag studies were all normal. EKG revealed normal sinus rhythm. A noncontrast CT scan was performed, which is shown on the next page.

At this point you decide to:

1. cancel the Code Stroke since he has presented too late,
2. cancel because his CT scan shows no lesion,
3. continue the Code Stroke and offer t-PA.

The baseline films, obtained 5 to 6 h after onset of stroke symptoms, show no findings. In particular, there is a normal external capsule and insular ribbon, and there are normal sulci bilaterally (Fig. 1A). Since the patient was symptomatic, and the CT scan showed no evidence of early lucency (*see* Chapter 15), the patient was offered t-PA. After a thorough discussion of risks and benefits, the patient consented to treatment and received 9 mg as a bolus, followed by 81 mg over 60 min. The left-sided numbness and weakness gradually improved over the course of admission. At the time of discharge, his hemisensory deficits were completely resolved and he was able to ambulate with the assistance of a walker demonstrating good strength and control of the walker with a slight dragging of the left lower extremity. A CT scan obtained on the second hospital day is shown in Fig. 1B.

From: *Thrombolytic Therapy for Stroke*
Edited by: P. D. Lyden © Humana Press Inc., Totowa, NJ

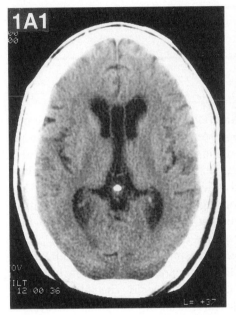

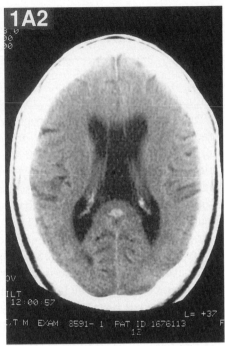

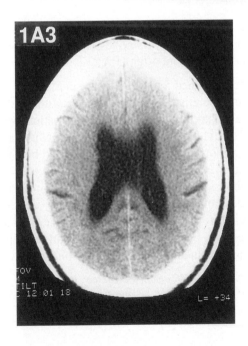

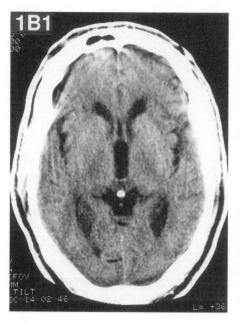

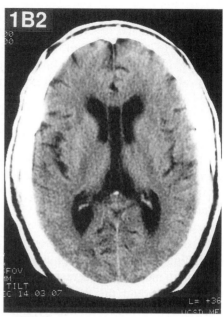

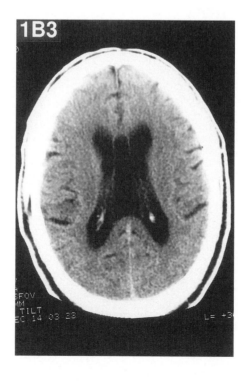

The films show no definite abnormalities. The official interpretation noted a faint hypodensity, less than 1.0 cm, in the white matter adjacent to the lateral ventricle (Fig. 1B3). A follow-up scan, obtained 3 mo later, did not reveal this finding, however. Thus, the faint lucency on the 24-h films may be artifact, or may reflect a transitory focal area of edema. In any event, the patient developed no visible signs of infarction.

COMMENT

This patient presented beyond the accepted 3-h time window for effective t-PA therapy. The decision was made to treat him with thrombolytic therapy anyway because his baseline CT scan was normal, and he was fairly young. Preliminary reports of the ATLANTIS and ECASS-2 trials have suggested safety when t-PA is given as late as 6 h following stroke (*see* Chapter 8). Weighing against these factors is the presence of a history of hypertension and diabetes. In weighing these risks, the physician should recall that no individual factor is proven to increase or decrease the risk of hemorrhage after thrombolytic stroke therapy; although this patient enjoyed a gratifying outcome, he could have suffered a hemorrhage. On balance, it seemed reasonable to proceed with therapy, and the patient and family agreed after a full discussion of all the risks and benefits.

Case 2

This 74-yr old woman started a nap at roughly 11:30 in the morning, after completing her usual morning routine with no problems. Upon awakening at 12:30 PM, the husband noted a complete right hemiparesis, right facial droop and apparent expressive aphasia. He called a local physician who instructed them to report immediately to the Emergency Room where they arrived at 1:00 PM. The patient entered the Code Stroke protocol: appropriate bloods were drawn, and she was sent for CT scan, which was completed by 2:00 PM. This scan is shown, and is notable for a lack of hemorrhagic abnormalities, early findings of cerebral ischemia, or hyperdense middle cerebral artery sign (Fig. 2A).

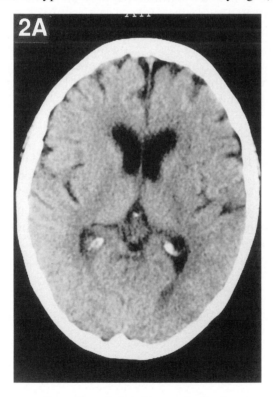

From: *Thrombolytic Therapy for Stroke*
Edited by: P. D. Lyden © Humana Press Inc., Totowa, NJ

After reviewing the images, decide if you would:

1. Exclude the patient from thrombolytic therapy because she is presenting too late,
2. Treat the patient, since thrombolytic therapy may be safe as late as 6 h after stroke onset,
3. Explain all of the risks and benefits to the patient and husband, and try to follow their wishes.

It was decided that, although the patient was beyond the 3-h time limit, t-PA would be given. This was primarily owing to a total absence of findings of early ischemia on her CT scan (*see* Chapter 15). The situation was explained to the patient, and it was specifically pointed out that this was a very uncertain situation, since she was beyond the 3-h time limit. Understanding the possible risks and benefits, the patient and family agreed to institute t-PA, which was started at 4:00 PM, about 4 1/2 h following onset of stroke, since the stroke occurred sometime during the patient's nap.

At 4:45 PM she exhibited dysarthria, but only minimal expressive problems and minimal word-finding problems. There was no apparent aphasia. A partial central-type right facial paresis was noted, but the visual field deficit was resolved. Right-sided strength was greatly improved. A previously noted left gaze preference was resolved. Sensory testing revealed a slight loss to light touch and pinprick over the entire right upper extremity. Twenty-four hours later, she was free of any discernible deficit.

COMMENT

The literature supports the use of thrombolysis beyond the 3-hr window (*see* Chapters 8 and 10). When used between 3 and 6 h of symptom onset, however, the family should be counseled that improvement is not expected. The safety profile is the same as when therapy is given under 3 h, so it may be worth taking the risk for an admittedly low chance of benefit. This decision is entirely within the judgment of the treating physician.

This case was kindly provided by Dr. Philip Ente, MD.

Case 3

This 70-yr-old patient was line dancing one evening; about 10:30 PM he fell over, with slurred speech, left-sided facial weakness, right-sided gaze preference, and dense left hemiparesis. There was no loss of consciousness. The patient had a previous history of transient ischemic attacks, but the details were poorly recalled by the patient and family. They did remember spells during which he had trouble focusing his vision. These occurred perhaps twice in the past 3 yr: none were recent.

The patient's previous risk factors for stroke included coronary artery disease and previous Doppler testing approx 4 yr ago that showed 20% stenosis bilaterally. The patient was evaluated for thrombolytic therapy at 11:30 PM. The CT scan is illustrated (Fig. 3A).

After reviewing the images, consider whether you would:

1. Discontinue the Code Stroke because he is too severe.
2. Discontinue because he is too mild.
3. Proceed with the evaluation and consider giving thrombolytic therapy.

The CT scan of the brain was reviewed with the radiologist on call. The physicians noted a hyperdense right MCA. This was followed by an immediate carotid Doppler that showed a total occlusion of the right carotid artery just above the bifurcation. The left artery was relatively intact, with minor stenosis.

With this information, decide if you would:

1. Discontinue the Code Stroke because the patient has an occluded ICA and intravenous thrombolytic therapy will not help.
2. Take the patient to angiography for intra-arterial imaging and possible thrombolysis.
3. Proceed with intravenous thrombolysis.

After full discussions with the patient's wife and daughter, with regards to benefits and risks, they elected to go ahead with t-PA treatment, understanding the risk of hemorrhage, and a possibility of improvement at 3 mo. Serial examinations at 2, 12, and 24 h showed no improvement, but no deterioration. A follow-up MRI scan is shown (Fig. 3B).

From: *Thrombolytic Therapy for Stroke*
Edited by: P. D. Lyden © Humana Press Inc., Totowa, NJ

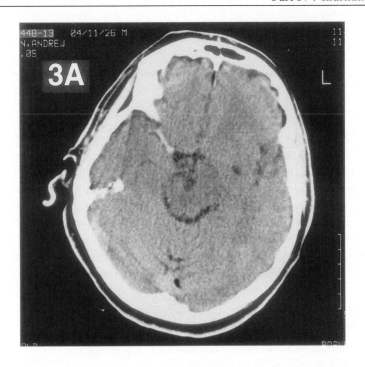

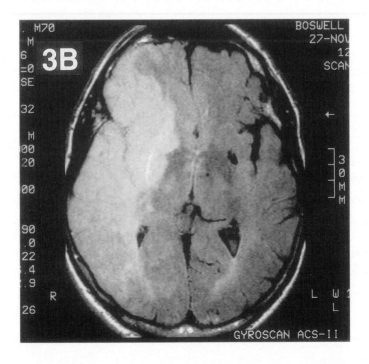

COMMENT

This case illustrates the argument for vascular imaging prior to undertaking thrombolysis (Chapter 13). There is no reported case of recanalization of an occluded ICA, and it seems doubtful that any amount of thrombolytic, IV or IA, would open up such a large amount of thrombus. On the other hand, many investigators have reported the so-called tandem pathology, in which the ICA is occluded, but there is a distal embolus to the MCA. In this setting, thrombolysis could be effective (*see* Chapters 8, 10, and 11). Since vascular imaging of the quality needed to rule out tandem pathology is time consuming, most authorities suggest treating with IV therapy in the 3-h time window. Some would then proceed to an angiogram to document the pathology. Whether IA therapy can work in this setting is not clear, and is the subject of ongoing studies. In the meantime, whether to use thrombolysis in this setting is up to the judgment of the individual treating physician. Intra-arterial therapy should be undertaken only in centers that have an organized team that is committed to interventional stroke therapy.

This case kindly provided by Dr. Kenneth Harris, MD.

Case 4

This 65-yr-old patient was suffering from an apparent right ear infection for 1 wk, consisting of ear pressure and fullness. The patient had a past medical history of hypertension. At roughly 1:00 PM, the patient noted the sudden onset of left hemisensory symptoms involving arm, face, and leg. She came to the Emergency Room immediately at which time she exhibited mild weakness in the left upper and lower extremity and sensory deficits. A CT scan was performed immediately. No early changes of ischemia were noted on the CT scan and there were also no signs of blood. It is now 3:15 PM.

At this point you decide to:

1. Terminate the Code Stroke because the symptoms are too mild,
2. Terminate the Code because it is almost 3 h after onset,
3. Continue.

Because of a persistent, moderate, weakness of the left side, it was recommended that t-PA be given. The risks and benefits were discussed with the family. Immediately prior to t-PA administration, the patient's blood pressure rose from her baseline of 170 to 200. 5mg of Labetalol were given, and blood pressure dropped to 150/90 roughly 10 min later. t-PA was then given, about 3 1/2 h after onset. Ten minutes after the t-PA bolus, there was improvement of left upper and lower extremity strength. Fifteen minutes later there was no appreciable weakness at left upper or lower extremities. The patient also reported disappearance of previous left subjective hemisensory phenomenon. Roughly 1 h after t-PA administration, the patient reported return of sensory disturbances over the left side of the face and then left arm. About 30 min later, her left upper extremity weakness returned. Weakness worsened to 0 out of 5 power at the left upper and lower extremities. An immediate CT scan was performed which did not show bleed. The patient was then rehydrated aggressively, since her blood pressure had dropped to 130/90. With rehydration, her left upper and left lower extremity strength again began to improve. On examination 3 mo later there was no discernible neurological deficit.

From: *Thrombolytic Therapy for Stroke*
Edited by: P. D. Lyden © Humana Press Inc., Totowa, NJ

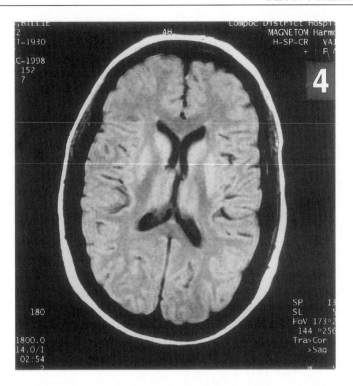

COMMENT

Patients with mild deficits tend to do well after stroke without treatment. Isolated sensory deficits, or isolated dysarthria, are examples of mild deficits. In this patient, there were motor and sensory findings in a large area of brain, as manifested by the weakness and numbness in the face, arm, and leg. Although it is possible that a small lesion in the internal capsule could be responsible for the presentation, there likely is a large amount of ischemic brain. The data show that therapy is of value in such patients.

After thrombolysis, it is critical to maintain blood pressure below certain limits (*see* Chapter 16). It was wise to delay therapy until labetolol had reduced the blood pressure to acceptable limits, even though this delay pushed the patient over the 3-h time limit. As shown by ECASS II, t-PA is still safe if used after 3 h, up to a max. of 6 h after stroke onset. The efficacy falls off as time goes by, but in this case there was only a delay of 30 min, a wise investment given the association of elevated blood pressure and hemorrhage (1–3).

This patient showed an immediate, dramatic response to t-PA with return of previous symptoms briefly. Whether or not fluid challenges caused resolution of this relapse is debatable. In any event, the patient recovered fully.

REFERENCES

1. Levy DE, Brott TG, Haley EC, Jr., Marler JR, Sheppard GP, Barsan W, Broderick JP. Factors related to intracranial hematoma formation in patients receiving tissue-type plasminogen activator for acute ischemic stroke. *Stroke* 1994; **25:** 291–297.
2. Bowes MP, Zivin JA, Thomas GR, Thibodeaux H, Fagan SC. Acute hypertension, but not thrombolysis, increases the incidence and severity of hemorrhagic transformation following experimental stroke in rabbits. *Exp. Neurol.* 1996; **141:** 40–46.
3. Fagan SC, Bowes MP, Lyden PD, Zivin JA. Acute hypertension promotes hemorrhagic transformation in a rabbit embolic stroke model: Effect of labetalol. *Exp. Neurol.* 1998; **150:** 153–158.

This case kindly provided by Dr. Phillip Ente, MD.

Case 5

This 85-yr-old retired nurse was living at a local chronic care facility. She was described as ambulatory, almost entirely self-sufficient, with intact higher cortical functions. She suffered from hypertension and was known to have exhibited equivocal EKG changes in the past. At 1:00 PM the patient suddenly developed a dense left hemiparesis. She was brought to the Emergency Room by Paramedics, an immediate CT brain scan was negative (Fig. 5A). Upon examination at 2:30 PM, the patient was noted to be fully alert but having some trouble with verbal expression. There was a dense right gaze preference, a complete, flaccid left hemiplegia and slight central type facial droop. There appeared to be a left hemisensory deficit but this was difficult to ascertain certainly. Reflexes were weak but symmetric at upper and lower extremities with absent ankle jerks. Toes were down going.

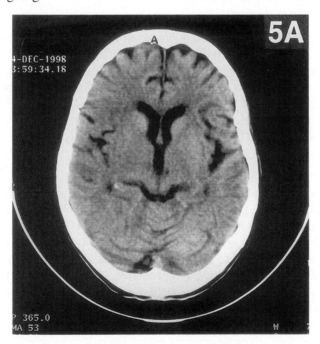

From: *Thrombolytic Therapy for Stroke*
Edited by: P. D. Lyden © Humana Press Inc., Totowa, NJ

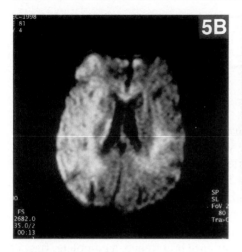

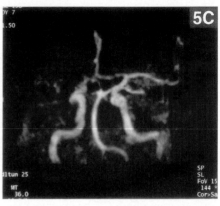

At this point you decide to:

1. Abort the Code Stroke because the patient is too old,
2. Abort because the patient's deficit is too severe,
3. Continue the evaluation.

It was decided to begin the t-PA protocol; the t-PA was started at roughly 3:00 PM after a full discussion of the potential risks and benefits. MRI results were available at roughly 3:15 PM and they showed significant area of changes throughout the entire distribution of the right middle cerebral artery on diffusion weighted images. At this point the t-PA drip was immediately discontinued. Further MRA studies showed a completely occluded right middle cerebral artery. The patient was seen at 8:00 PM at which time she was clinically unchanged.

COMMENT

Neither age nor deficit severity, alone, are contraindications to thrombolysis. Together, however, the two factors predict a lower likelihood of success. In a *post-hoc* analysis of the NINDS t-PA data set, age and severity were found to interact, and to adversely affect outcome *(1)*. The two factors had no influence on the potential to respond to t-PA, however. That is, even though older, more severe patients are less likely to be symptom free 3 mo after stroke, they do better if given t-PA. In this subgroup in particular, there were fewer patients severely disabled, and more patients mildly disabled, in the t-PA treated group. On the other hand, both age and severity are associated with increased risk of hemorrhage *(2)*. Therefore, given this patient, physician judgment should be exercised, and a decision to use t-PA discussed with the patient and family.

The role of diffusion weighted MRI is unclear at present. In this case, a large area of altered water diffusion suggested to the clinician that there may be a large area of brain that could not be salvaged. Although this is a reasonable hypothesis, in fact no data yet exist to prove this contention. Therefore, we do not advise that patients undergo acute MRI scanning. Research may eventually confirm the utility of MRI scanning in this setting, but until such confirmation exists, MRI should be viewed as experimental.

Case kindly provided by Dr. Philip Ente, MD.

REFERENCES

1. NINDS TPA Stroke Study Group. Generalized Efficacy of t-PA for Acute Stroke. *Stroke* 1997; **28:** 2119–2125.
2. NINDS TPA Stroke Study Group. Intracerebral Hemorrhage After Intravenous t-Pa Therapy for Ischemic Stroke. *Stroke* 1997; **28:** 2109–2118.

Case 6

This patient is a 15-yr-old white male, who developed a stroke-like syndrome one morning. His stepmother stated that he got up as usual and was in his room with the door shut. He yelled out suddenly at approx 6:50 AM and was found lying on the floor. He estimates that he was on the floor for perhaps ten minutes before he was found. There was no loss of consciousness, incontinence, or evidence of seizure. Thus the onset of the stroke was at approx 6:40 AM. The patient was transported to the hospital immediately. He was noted to have a dense left hemiplegia and a left facial droop. He was referred for a CT scan of the brain. The patient never had problems like this previously. He had no known risk factors for stroke. He admits that he was smoking marijuana the previous night, but denied any other drug use. He apparently had migraine headaches in the past, however, these were not problematic for him recently. Otherwise he is very healthy (Fig. 6A).

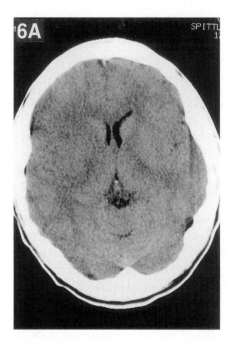

From: *Thrombolytic Therapy for Stroke*
Edited by: P. D. Lyden © Humana Press Inc., Totowa, NJ

At this point you consider the following options:

1. Abort the Code because the patient is too young,
2. Abort because the CT scan shows excessive edema,
3. Continue.

Upon examination, the blood pressure was 115/58, temperature 98.6, pulse 80 and regular, respiratory rate 16. Auscultation of the heart revealed a regular rate and rhythm without murmurs. There was visual extinction on the left and a gaze preference toward to the right. There was a pronounced left facial asymmetry. Motor testing of the upper and lower limbs reveals that the patient could not lift his left arm at all. In the leg, the patient was barely able to lift the leg off the bed: it drifted to the bed within 2 s. Reflexes were slightly brisker in the left hemibody than on the right. Plantar responses were down-going on the right, and up-going on the left. The patient was anesthetic on his left side to all modalities. Laboratory work-up was unremarkable; his platelet count was 172,000. Prothrombin time and partial thromboplastin time were normal. Urine drug screen was positive for cannabinoids, negative for barbiturates, benzodiazepines, opiates, amphetamines, and cocaine. A 12-lead electrocardiogram appeared normal.

At this point you consider these options:

1. Cancel the Code Stroke because there is no obvious cause for the stroke,
2. Cancel because this might be arterial dissection, and thrombolysis might worsen the dissection,
3. Hold the thrombolysis pending an angiogram to evaluate for dissection,
4. Continue with thrombolysis.

The situation was discussed at length with the parents, who requested that thrombolytic therapy be used. The patient was treated with the adult dose (*see* Chapter 17). Within 2 h his left-sided weakness improved dramatically. At long-term follow-up he exhibited only minimal deficits.

An extensive search for causes of stroke was undertaken. Erythrocyte sedimentation rate was 5 mm/h. PT and PTT were normal. A circulating lupus anti-coagulant was negative. Angiotensin-converting enzyme level was normal at 44 U/L. Antithrombin 3 level and anticardiolipin antibody profile was normal. Serum homocysteine level was 5 (normal). Serum immunoelectrophoresis was normal. Protein C was 97% and protein S total was 121%. These were both normal results. SSA and SSB antibody titers were negative.

A CT scan of the brain performed without contrast 24 h after thrombolysis revealed subtle abnormalities involving the right cerebral hemisphere, suggesting an acute right MCA infarct involving about one-third of the middle cerebral artery territory. An MRI of the brain performed with and without contrast on revealed multi-focal cortical edema, consistent with a known acute right middle cerebral artery distribution infarction (Fig. 6B). Abnormal flow was also noted in the right internal carotid artery.

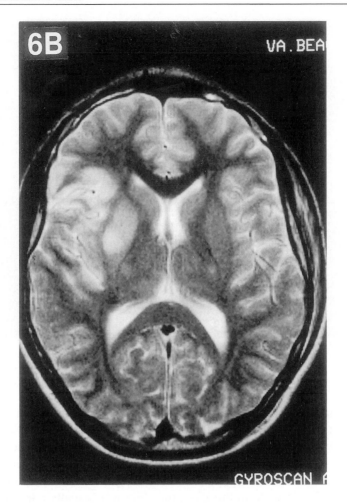

A neck magnetic resonance angiogram revealed a high-grade apparent long-segment stenosis of the cervical internal carotid artery on the right (*see* Fig. 6C; arrows mark the narrowed internal carotid). The abnormalities were most consistent with a carotid artery dissection without occlusion. A four-vessel cerebral angiogram confirmed dissection of the right internal carotid artery from the petrous portion to a point several centimeters above the carotid bifurcation.

Upon re-review of the history with the patient and family, it was learned that he had been involved in a game of tackle football the afternoon prior to the stroke. A surgeon felt that the carotid lesion could require repair, but he did not favor a surgical approach to the problem currently. The patient was heparinized and then converted to Coumadin therapy. The patient was discharged home on Coumadin, 2.5 mg daily and one aspirin.

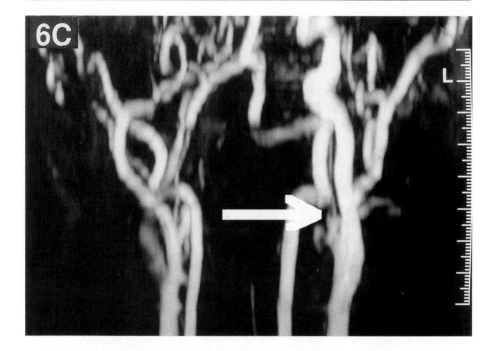

COMMENT

Most clinical stroke trials are conducted in adults (age older than 18 yr) so the utility of stroke therapy in children is unknown. There is almost no experience available with thrombolytics in children, although the authors are aware of several cases. Based on anecdotal experience, it seems that children tend to exhibit dramatic recoveries, but then the natural history of stroke in children is quite favorable to begin with. In this case, the child was actually a teenager, closer physiologically to an adult.

Whether to use thrombolytic therapy in patients with carotid dissection is not resolved. In the NINDS study, many dissection patients were included (*see* Chapter 8). The probable pathophysiology of dissection involves the formation of blood clot on the intimal flap, from which an embolus arises, lodging in the intracerebral circulation. For this reason, anticoagulation is now favored for dissection, although once it was viewed with considerable trepidation. At this time, we suggest that anticoagulation should be strongly considered for dissections, but should not preclude thrombolytic therapy for acute embolic stroke.

The presence of early ischemic changes on CT scan did not constitute a contraindication to thrombolytic therapy (*see* Chapters 15 and 17). Subtle findings such as blurring of the gray/white matter border or loss of the insular ribbon are valuable markers, but do not indicate propensity to hemorrhage. Such findings, however, should prompt a careful review of the time of onset, as was done in this case, to assure that less than 3 h have elapsed. In contrast, large areas of hypodensity, representing frank edema, should prompt considerable caution, and may represent a relative contraindication to thrombolysis, especially if the edema subsumes greater than one-third of the MCA territory.

This case was kindly provided by Dr. Sidney Mallenbaum, MD.

REFERENCES

1. Biousse V, D'Anglejan-Chatillon J, Touboul P-J, Amarenco P, Bousser M-G. Time Course of Symptoms in Extracranial Carotid Artery Dissections: A Series of 80 Patients. *Stroke* 1995; **26:** 235–239.
2. Biller J, Hingtgen WL, Adams HP, Smoker WRK, Godersky JC, Toffol GJ. Cervicocephalic Arterial Dissections: A Ten Year Experience. *Arch Neurology. Dec.* 1986; **43:** 1234–1238
3. Mokri B, Sundt TM, Houser OW, Piepgras DG. Spontaneous Dissection of the Cervical Internal Carotid Artery. *Ann Neurol.* 1986; **19:** 126–138.

Case 7

The emergency department calls you at about 11 PM for a 67-yr-old woman brought in with sudden left-sided weakness at 10:30 PM. She has no prior past medical history that anyone is aware of. EMS reported a blood pressure of 134/86. Finger stick blood glucose is 110.

After hearing the history do you:

1. Cancel the Code Stroke since it is late in the evening,
2. Continue the Code Stroke by ordering a STAT head CT scan and labs,
3. Do nothing until the emergency room physician has time to evaluate the patient.

You arrive at the CT suite as the CT scans are being reconstructed and projected onto the video screen. You interpret the images off of the screen and wait for the hard copy films, which are shown in the figure, to confirm your impression. The patient is transported back to the emergency room. It is now 11:42 PM.

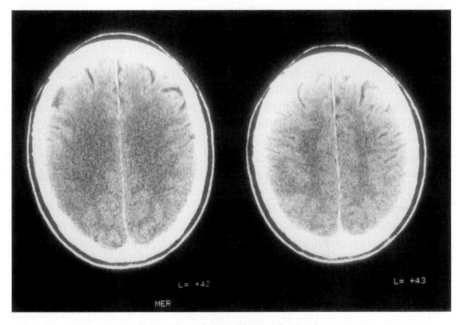

From: *Thrombolytic Therapy for Stroke*
Edited by: P. D. Lyden © Humana Press Inc., Totowa, NJ

After reviewing the images, you note a dense middle cerebral artery on lower cuts. Do you:

1. Abort because of the dense middle cerebral artery sign,
2. Abort because there is minimal effacement of the sulci,
3. Continue.

The husband arrives to report that the patient had been in the kitchen when she suddenly said her left arm felt funny. She then fell to the floor unable to move the left side of her body within 5 min of the arm complaint. He immediately called 911. From the emergency room records and EMS run sheet, you determine that the call to 911 occurred at 10:05 PM. You therefore set stroke onset at 9:55 PM. It is now midnight.

She is alert and oriented. There is slight dysarthria and a dense left homonymous hemianopia, and gaze deviation to the left. There is left facial weakness and the left arm and leg are plegic. There is no response to pinprick, temperature, and touch on the left. Severe left-sided neglect is present. Reflexes are depressed on the left-side. Blood pressure is 148/90. Pulse is 78 and regular and there are no other pertinent general exam findings.

You now present the issue of acute management to the husband. It is now 12:20 AM. you recommend:

1. Not to use t-PA because the stroke is too severe,
2. Not to use t-PA because the CT scan is abnormal,
3. Try t-PA realizing that it most likely will not help but could hurt.

After discussion of the issues, the husband agrees. You explain the situation to the patient as she is alert and oriented although not necessarily legally able to give valid consent. She also wishes to proceed. She receives the standard dose of t-PA, using the standard protocol.

At mid-afternoon following treatment, strength in the left arm and leg was almost normal. The visual field defect was not detectable. There was mild left facial weakness. Pinprick and light touch were normal but she extinguished on the left side to either sensory or visual stimuli.

A 24-h posttreatment head CT scan revealed a small, deep parietal infarct. No obvious cause of the stroke was found. One week later, she was home with minimal facial asymmetry and occasional left-sided extinction that did not interfere with her activities of daily living.

COMMENT

This case illustrates two very important points. First, Code Stroke can occur at any time of day, although most events do cluster in the early morning *(1)*. A well-managed Stroke Team, therefore, will have systems in place to ensure that late night patients are handled efficiently and rapidly. In most hospitals, this means that CT technicians must be on-call, and the Code Team physicians should be readily available. Such a Team may be implemented differently in different communities *(2,3)*. The second point concerns the presence of the dense middle artery sign *(4)*. The prognostic implications of this sign are presented in Chapter 15. There appears to be considerable misunderstanding about this sign. Whereas it is true that the dense MCA sign carries a poor prognosis, thrombolysis can be effective in some cases, such as this one and the one presented as Case 14. Therefore, it is reasonable to present the options to the family and the patient, alerting them that although the prognosis is very poor, there is a chance that the treatment may help. Obviously this is also an opportunity to consider intra-arterial therapy (*see* Chapter 10).

REFERENCES

1. Zweifler RM, Drinkard R, Cunningham S, Brody ML, Rothrock JF. Implementation of a stroke code system in Mobile, Alabama. Diagnostic and therapeutic yield. *Stroke* 1997; **28:** 981–983.
2. Lyden PD, Rapp K, Babcock T, Rothrock J. Ultra-rapid identification, triage, and enrollment of stroke patients into clinical trials. *J. Stroke Cerebrovasc. Dis.* 1994; **4:** 106–113.
3. The National Institute of Neurological Disorders and Stroke rt-PA Stroke Study Group. A system approach to immediate evaluation and management of hyperacute stroke. Experience at eight centers and implications for community practice and patient care. *Stroke* 1997; **28:** 1530–1540.
4. Tomsick TA, Brott TG, Chambers AA, Fox AJ, Gaskill MF, Lukin RR, Pleatman CW, Wiot JG, Bourekas E. Hyperdense middle cerebral artery sign on CT: Efficacy in detecting middle cerebral artery thrombosis. *Am. J. Neur. R.* 1990; **11:** 473–477.

Case 8

At 1:40 PM on a Saturday afternoon a 70-yr-old man presented unable to speak and not following commands since about noon. Blood pressure was 160/92 and his pulse was irregularly irregular.

As soon as the patient is removed from the CT scanner, an NIH stroke scale is performed: a total score = 7. CBC, platelet count, PT, PTT, and glucose were normal. EKG showed atrial fibrillation without acute ischemic changes. Work-up was complete by 2:25 PM.

The neighbor said the patient was speaking fine at 11:45 AM and then suddenly stopped speaking and appeared confused. The emergency room physician spoke with the patient's internist who said the atrial fibrillation is new and that he had had a "TIA" 6 mo ago without a cause found. He was on Mevacor for elevated cholesterol. No other t-PA exclusions were identified.

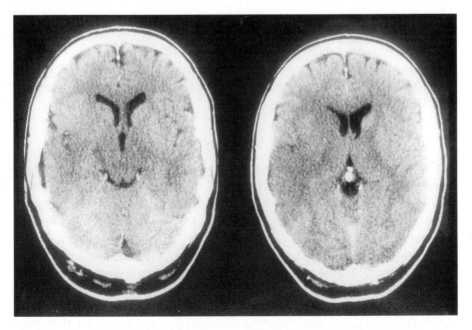

From: *Thrombolytic Therapy for Stroke*
Edited by: P. D. Lyden © Humana Press Inc., Totowa, NJ

After reviewing the brain CT scan, you decide to:

1. Give t-PA per protocol assuming the patient would agree,
2. Try to contact next of kin for consent,
3. Estimate patient weight and order pharmacy to mix drug STAT,
4. Not treat if next of kin cannot be contacted.

The head CT shows no intracranial hemorrhage. There is some blurring of the left insular ribbon and loss of clarity of the basal ganglia margins. Also, there is loss of the distinction of the grey-white matter border in the temporal and parietal lobes. The patient's son was contacted at 2:40 PM and had concerns about treatment because of the risk of bleeding.

At this point, consider whether:

1. To cancel the Code Stroke given the son's concerns,
2. Cancel because the signs of early edema constitute more than one-third the territory of the MCA,
3. Proceed with treatment.

The son consented for treatment, which was given via the protocol, with the bolus started at 2:44 PM. There was no significant language improvement at 24 h and head CT showed an infarct in the insular cortex and lateral basal ganglia. No hemorrhage was present. Echocardiography did not show a thrombus. He was anticoagulated with heparin and Coumadin and was seen by speech therapy. At 3 mo post-stroke, he followed simple commands and was able to speak in short sentences although fluency and comprehension was moderately impaired: NIHSS score = 5.

COMMENT

The original report of the ECASS study suggested that hemorrhage might be more common in patients with early ischemic change in a zone comprising more than one-third the territory of the MCA (1). In subsequent studies, this relationship has been very difficult to confirm. Also, there is poor agreement between experienced examiners looking at test scans as to whether the changes are present (2). There is little question, however, that if the first CT scan shows much early ischemic change then the prognosis for a favorable outcome is poor, compared to patients without such findings. The prudent clinician presented with such a scan should first go back to the bedside and reestablish the onset time: early edema may indicate that the stroke has been present for longer than first suspected. If the onset time is shown less than 3 h, thrombolysis may still be offered, but the patient should be advised that the odds for excellent recovery are lessened.

This case was kindly provided by Dr. Steven Levine, MD.

REFERENCES

1. Kaste M, Hacke W, Fieschi C, ECASS Study Group. Results of the European Cooperative Acute Stroke Study (ECASS). *Cerebrovasc. Dis.* 1995; **5:** 225–273.(Abstract)
2. Grotta J, Chiu D, Lu M, Patel S, Levine S, Tilley B, Brott T, Haley EC, Jr., Lyden P, Kothari R, Frankel M, Lewandowski C, Libman R, Kwiatkowski TG, Broderick J, Marler J, Corrigan FM, Huff S, Mitsias P, Talati S, Tanne D. Agreement and variability in the interpretation of early CT changes in stroke patients qualifying for intravenous rtPA therapy. *Stroke* 1999; **30:** 1528–1233.

Case 9

You are paged by an internist colleague for a patient in the hospital who had been improving after treatment for congestive heart failure. The nurses gave the patient his usual medication at 7 AM and he was fine. At 7:10 AM, the patient's roommate called a nurse in because the patient fell on the way to the bathroom and was unable to get up. The nurse noted decreased movement on the right side, slurred speech, and a blood pressure of 195/110. She paged the Internist.

The Internist reviews with you by telephone the inclusion and exclusion criteria: There is no exclusion. The patient was in the process of being transported to CT and the necessary blood work was drawn by 7:30 AM.

His blood pressure was 190/108. His NIHSS score = 11. At 7:45 AM the blood pressure was 195/105. The laboratory results were normal. The patient wished to be treated after detailed discussion of the risks and benefits by 7:55 AM.

You decide to:

1. Call pharmacy to mix drug and then treat,
2. Call pharmacy for two 10 mg syringes of IV labetolol,
3. Cancel the t-PA treatment protocol,
4. Wait 30 min and retake blood pressure.

Pharmacy delivered two 10-mg syringes of labetolol at CT scan. The blood pressure was 198/106. 5 mg of labetolol iv (one-half of one syringe) were given. The CT scan was completed and shown. In the emergency room, at 8:15 AM, the blood pressure was 190/96.

After reviewing the CT scan, you decide to:

1. Administer t-PA 86.4 mg and give 8.6 mg as a bolus over 1 min,
2. Wait 15 min to see if the blood pressure remains above the exclusion criteria,
3. Cancel the t-PA treatment because you treated the blood pressure,
4. Place an arterial line in to monitor blood pressure.

A recheck of the blood pressure was 180/95. His dysarthia and weakness were unchanged. t-PA was given and the patient moved to an intensive care unit for monitoring as per the t-PA protocol. Four hours later (about 12:30 PM) the

From: *Thrombolytic Therapy for Stroke*
Edited by: P. D. Lyden © Humana Press Inc., Totowa, NJ

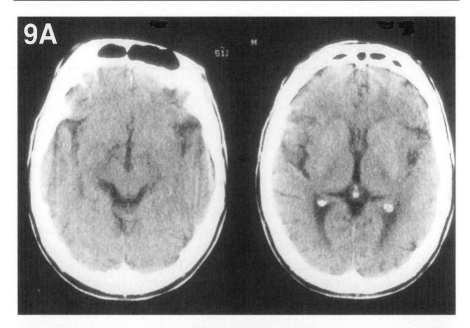

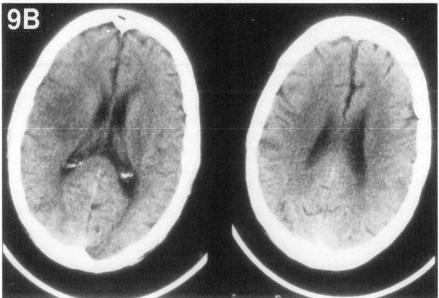

ICU nurse called because the patient became less attentive and arousable. His blood pressure was 180/95.

The patient underwent a STAT head CT scan without contrast, which demonstrated a small parenchymal hemorrhage in the left lateral basal ganglia. There

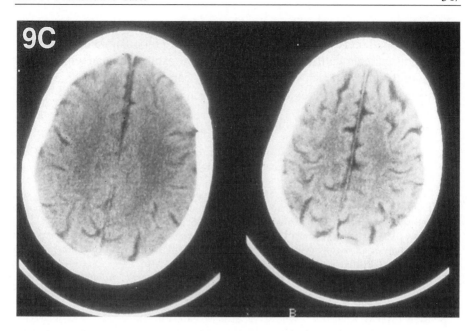

was minimal mass effect. The PT, PTT and platelets were normal and the fibrinogen was 130. Blood pressure is 185/110.

A neurosurgeon recommended nonsurgical management with careful attention to blood pressure and frequent neuro assessments in the ICU for at least 24 h. The patient slowly improved to the point of regaining an alert level of consciousness. At 3 mo post-stroke after rehabilitation, he was hypophonic, mildly dysarthric, with moderately severe right hemiparesis and mild right hemisensory loss.

COMMENT

There is now considerable evidence that hypertension during thrombolysis predisposes to hemorrhage (1–4). The protocol (Chapter 17) mentions that patients with blood pressure greater than 185/110 should not receive thrombolysis, unless the blood pressure comes down with gentle treatment such as the single dose of labetolol used in this case. After thrombolytics are given, the blood pressure must be kept below the limit 185/105 using all possible measures. Such doses of antihypertensives were not associated with any deleterious effects in a large group of stroke patients (5). More worrisome in this case is the obvious hypodensity in the basal ganglia on the baseline scan (see Fig. 9B). This amount of hypodensity exceeds the characteristics of "subtle early ischemic change" as defined in Chapter 15 and illustrated in Case 8. Such a finding strongly suggests that the onset time has been reported incorrectly, or for some other reason, this patient is suffering an atypical degree of blood brain barrier breakdown. This patient qualified for treatment, but the astute clinician will consider the use of thrombolytics in such a patient very carefully.

This case was kindly provided by Dr. Steven Levine, MD.

REFERENCES

1. Hårdemark H-G, Wesslén N, Persson L. Influence of Clinical factors, CT Findings and Early management on Outcome in Supratentorial Intracerebral Hemorrhage. *Cerebrovasc Dis.* 1999; **9**: 10–21.
2. Levy DE, Brott TG, Haley EC, Jr., Marler JR, Sheppard GP, Barsan W, Broderick JP. Factors related to intracranial hematoma formation in patients receiving tissue-type plasminogen activator for acute ischemic stroke. *Stroke* 1994 ;**25**: 291–297.
3. Bowes MP, Zivin JA, Thomas GR, Thibodeaux H, Fagan SC. Acute hypertension, but not thrombolysis, increases the incidence and severity of hemorrhagic transformation following experimental stroke in rabbits. *Exp. Neurol.* 1996; **141**: 40–46.
4. Fagan SC, Bowes MP, Lyden PD, Zivin JA. Acute hypertension promotes hemorrhagic transformation in a rabbit embolic stroke model: Effect of labetalol. *Exp. Neurol.* 1998; **150**: 153–158.
5. Brott T, Lu M, Kothari R, Fagan SC, Frankel M, Grotta JC, Broderick J, Kwiatkowski T, Lewandowski C, Haley EC, Marler JR, Tilley BC. Hypertension and its treatment in the NINDS rt-PA stroke trial. *Stroke* 1998; **29**: 1504–1509.

Case 10

A 58-yr-old African-American woman with a history of poorly controlled hypertension, diabetes, and hyperlipidemia is noted stumbling and slurring her words at work. She complains of blurry vision and a headache. She is unsure exactly when the symptoms started. A coworker noted that the woman was fine and talking clearly at 3:00 PM. It is now 4:50 PM when her employer calls 911.

Her current medications include an ACE inhibitor, clonidine, aspirin, glucophage, and pravastatin. You are told that the EKG shows left ventricular hypertrophy, a first degree AV block, and nonspecific T wave changes. There is no prior history of stroke, seizures, or recent head trauma. Her fingerstick glucose is 200. Her blood pressure is 180/96. It is now 5:20 PM.

What is the time of onset of this stroke:

1. When she awoke that morning?
2. When she went to bed the night before?
3. 3:00 PM?
4. 4:50 PM?

You meet the patient in the CT scanner room as she is being placed onto the CT table. Immediately after the CT is complete, you perform an examination which reveals mild lethargy, bilateral ataxia of all four limbs, left greater than right, a left superior homonymous quadrantanopia, moderate dysarthria and coarse horizontal gaze nystagmus. The CT is shown below (Fig. 10A).

From: *Thrombolytic Therapy for Stroke*
Edited by: P. D. Lyden © Humana Press Inc., Totowa, NJ

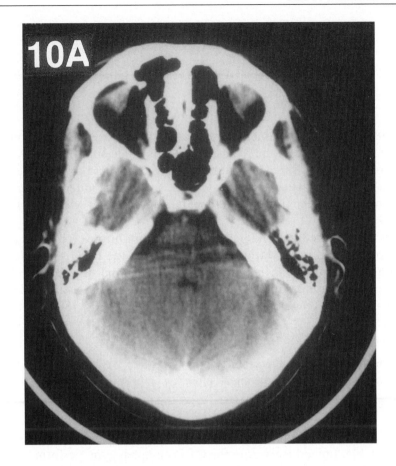

At this point, you consider whether to:

1. Abort because of the density in the basilar artery,
2. Abort because basilar thrombosis is progressive and requires heparin,
3. Continue.

CBC shows a mild anemia and platelet count is normal. Serum glucose is 245 and blood pressure is 182/96. The CT (Fig. 10A) shows a dense basilar artery sign at the level of the midbrain without evidence of acute ischemic changes or hemorrhage. There is an old lacune in the left caudate nucleus and mild periventricular leukomalacia. It is now 5:40 PM.

Pharmacy brings the t-PA. As the patient weighs about 200 lbs., she is dosed for 91 kg. = 81.9 mg. The bolus is to be 8.2 mg over 1 min and then 73.7 mg over the next hour. It is now 5:48 PM. You have 12 min to discuss risks and benefits and decide to treat. The patient wants to discuss the risks and benefits with her daughter and gives you her telephone number.

After reviewing the CT brain scan you:

1. Call the daughter, explain the risks and benefits, suggesting that treatment would be better than doing nothing even when taking the risk of bleeding into account and that you have only minutes left to treat and you therefore need a quick decision.
2. Tell the patient that there is not enough time to both call her daughter and treat her. Therefore she should just be treated.
3. Decide not to treat because you can't reach the daughter in time.
4. Try to convince the patient to be treated because her daughter is not home.

Fortunately the daughter is home and agrees to have you treat her mother. You treat her per protocol at 5:59 PM. By the next morning the patient is less dysarthric and her ataxia is not as pronounced. She still has the same visual field deficit and nystagmus. She has improved 3 points on the NIHSS. A transcranial Doppler suggests basilar artery stenosis. She undergoes a CT scan 24-h post-stroke onset which shows small bilateral cerebellar infarcts and a right inferior temporal infarct.

COMMENT

Basilar thrombosis can be a challenging entity; the response to thrombolysis can be dramatic, but if no response occurs, the patient is likely to die. Progressing basilar stenosis is considered an indication for heparin, to try to halt the formation of further basilar occlusion (1,2). On the other hand, no clear documentation of the efficacy has been published, and the t-PA protocol prohibits heparinization for 24 h. To complicate matters further, in the authors' experience, basilar cases tend to recanalize with thrombolysis, only to re-occlude again. One seasoned Neurologist has given heparin and t-PA together for a series of basilar cases, claiming excellent results (Personal communication from Clarke Millikan, MD, 1999). No clear recommendations can be given based on evidence, and a clinician can do no wrong if the protocol is followed. Nevertheless, basilar patients do recanalize very nicely, and are prone to reocclusion. Therefore, providing heparin to such patients after thrombolysis, despite the protocol restrictions, seems reasonable.

The CT hyperdensity in the basilar artery could have indicated calcification, or a intra-luminal thrombus. The MRI confirmed that there was luminal narrowing due to thrombus, with a small flow void remaining (Fig. 10B).

The onset time in this case was problematic. There is the coworker report that the patient appeared to be at baseline around 3:00 PM. The astute clinician should telephone the coworker, and personally verify that the timing of that conversation was accurate and reliable. If so, that time can be taken as the onset time. Otherwise, the time must be set back to the last time that the patient was known to be normal.

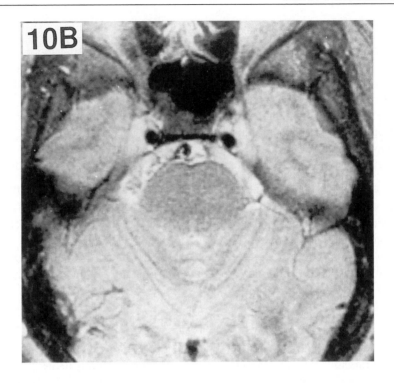

This case was kindly provided by Dr. Steven Levine, MD.

REFERENCES

1. Adams HP, Jr., Brott TG, Furlan AJ, Gomez CR, Grotta J, Helgason CM, et al. Guidelines for thrombolytic therapy for acute stroke: A supplement to the guidelines for the management of patients with acute ischemic stroke. *Circulation* 1996; **94:** 1167–1174.
2. Rothrock JF, Hart RG. Antithrombotic therapy in cerebrovascular disease. *Ann. Intern. Med.* 1991; **115:** 885–895.

Case 11

This 74-yr-old patient was brought into the Emergency Room at roughly 1:30 PM after being involved in a single-vehicle motor vehicle accident at 1:00 PM. Upon arrival in the Emergency Room, she was noted to have a right facial droop and some problems with verbal expression and comprehension. At roughly 3:30 PM the Neurologist was called by the Emergency Room Physician because the patient's expressive-comprehensive problems had worsened. On initial evaluation there was a central type right facial paresis, no weakness of any of the extremities, no reflex asymmetry. There was a moderate global aphasia. Past history included a diagnosis of diabetes mellitus Type II, hypertension, paroxysmal atrial fibrillation, aortic sclerosis, sleep apnea, and vitamin B12 deficiency. She has had multiple surgeries in the past including partial gastrectomy with a vagotomy, multiple surgeries of the right lower extremity for osteomyelitis, a hysterectomy, and cataract surgery.

Baseline CT of the brain is shown.

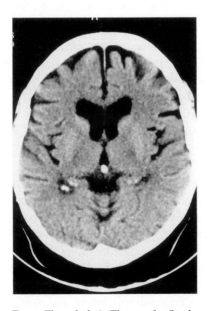

From: *Thrombolytic Therapy for Stroke*
Edited by: P. D. Lyden © Humana Press Inc., Totowa, NJ

At this point you consider these options:

1. Cancel the Code Stroke because of the delay in summoning the Neurologist,
2. Cancel because of the extensive co-morbidities,
3. Cancel because the deficit is too mild (no motor findings),
4. Continue.

After explaining risks and benefits with family members and after further discussions with the patient's primary care doctor over the phone, it was decided to administer t-PA. The standard 10% bolus of t-PA was given and roughly 5 min later there was a dramatic improvement in both comprehensive and expressive aphasia. There was then a partial loss of improvement.

She had lab work done: B12 level was 815, TSH 2.23, creatinine 1.1, BUN 25, sodium 139, potassium 5, chloride 104, bicarb 23, hemoglobin 12.5, hematocrit 36.8 with a history that she had been running an anemia in the low 11 range prior to the B12. Speech therapy, physical therapy, and occupational therapy were consulted. Initially she could only speak single words. However, facial asymmetry resolved. By the second day of admission she was speaking multiple word sentences with pauses and her strength and movement in her right upper and lower extremity were improving. By discharge she had no detectable motor weakness, she could write but she continued to have trouble finding words. Her speech would be in the maximum of 1–3-word sentences. She struggled finding the right word.

By one week after hospital discharge, there was further improvement in language and reading/writing abilities. The patient showed apparently normal levels of comprehension, but there was a slight nonfluency of speech owing to pauses for word finding. Writing had returned to normal. Reading was nearly recovered but the patient reported difficulties with registration of the significance of what she read. She was, however, able to follow written commands. Her previous right facial paresis resolved.

COMMENT

This patient presented with a mild but disabling stroke consisting of severe aphasia. Whether to treat such deficits with thrombolytic therapy is open to considerable physician judgment, including careful consideration of the patient's lifestyle and wishes. In this case, the patient and family felt that lifelong aphasia would impair her quality of life considerably. Certainly, the same could be said for any patient in whom language plays an essential role in the occupation, such as lawyer, teacher, broadcaster, or preacher. Fortunately, with milder strokes, the risk of hemorrhage is correspondingly lower, and considerable data analysis has shown that the benefit/risk ratio is favorable even for mild strokes (*see* Chapter 9). On the other hand, if the NIHSS is less than 5, there is a higher likelihood of spontaneous resolution. In this case, the patient was improving within 5 min of the bolus, which almost certainly reflects spontaneous, and not drug-related, response. It cannot be predicted in any individual case if the improvement would continue absent the therapy. Group data suggest that therapy is beneficial in mild cases.

The presence of comorbidities, especially diabetes, certainly impacts prognosis adversely. No data suggest, however, that any comorbidity should preclude therapy (*see* Chapter 9). That is, although the overall prognosis is worse, there is still a significant likelihood that thrombolytic therapy will benefit the patient. Physician judgment is needed, though, in cases where comorbidity has significantly diminished the quality of life; stroke may be an end-of-life event that is consistent with the wishes of a severely disabled patient.

The delay in summoning the Neurologist represents a common situation. Until Emergency Department protocols are in place, and practiced, such delays will continue (*see* Chapters 14 and 16). This patient was still treated within 3 h of symptom onset, despite the delay. In any hospital with repeated delays activating the Stroke Team, a rigorous training program, including mock drills, should be considered. The Neurologist who is called late should consider proceeding with the therapy, since there remains a chance for benefit, and might use the occasion to educate the Emergency Department staff.

This case was provided by Dr. Philip Ente, MD.

Case 12

A 49-yr-old right-handed male presented with a history of cerebrovascular accident affecting the right frontal cortical region approx 10 yr ago. At that time, the patient had a full neurologic evaluation which included an angiogram, transthoracic echocardiogram, transesaphogal echocardiogram and some labs for hypercoagulable state, all of which were negative. The patient subsequently had a single generalized seizure and he was placed on Dilantin, which was discontinued after approx 3 yr without a seizure. The patient was in his usual state of good health until approx 7:00 PM when he noted some slurring of speech. This was followed shortly by gait instability and weakness of the left side. The patient noted some diaphoresis but denied any vertigo, nausea, chest pain, or chest palpitations. The patient was improving upon arrival in the emergency room, going from flaccid left hemiparises to some movement. He denies any history of hypertension, diabetes mellitus, cardiac arrhythmia, smoking or drug abuse. The patient is a medical doctor.

At this point consider whether to:

1. Abort the Code Stroke because the patient is improving,
2. Abort because he is a physician, and more complications occur in doctors and nurses,
3. Continue.

On examination, there was a normal left-right differentiation and the patient was able to follow multi-step commands without difficulty. Graphesthesia, stereognosis, and proprioception were all absent in the left upper extremity. Cranial nerve examination demonstrated a left upper motor neuron type seventh nerve paresis. Motor examination demonstrated a mild hemiparesis over the left side of his body, face equal to arm, greater than leg. Left-sided coordination was not tested given the patient's weakness. The patient had significant ataxia upon ambulation.

CT scan revealed an old infarct in the distribution of right middle cerebral artery, without acute changes (Fig. 12A). CT scan later in the evening revealed no definite change. Carotid Doppler studies were negative. Chest X-ray revealed borderline cardiomegaly but otherwise within normal limits.

From: *Thrombolytic Therapy for Stroke*
Edited by: P. D. Lyden © Humana Press Inc., Totowa, NJ

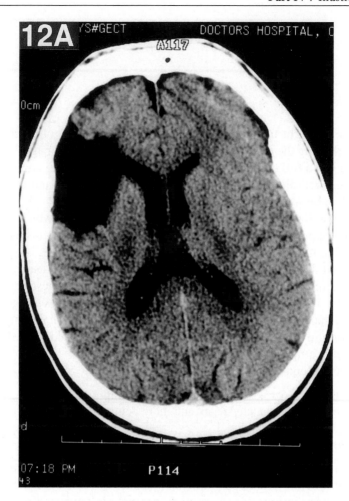

At this point consider whether it is appropriate to:
1. Cancel Code Stroke due to previous stroke,
2. Cancel because of minimal symptoms,
3. Continue.

The patient was admitted for observation, but continued to rapidly improve, so no thrombolysis was offered. He was admitted to CCU, given aspirin and monitored. Myocardial infarction was ruled out. He continued to improve over the first few hours but about 6 h after admission (at about 3:00 AM) he suffered a relapse with flaccid left hemiparesis and dense anesthesia. A repeat CT scan was obtained (Fig. 12B1).

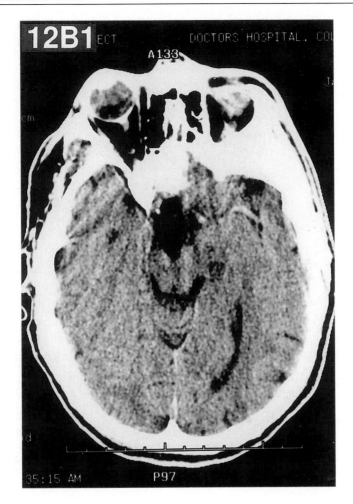

At this point you consider whether to:

1. Give thrombolysis since the admitting event was likely a TIA,
2. Do not give thrombolysis, since he may have been ischemic for many hours,
3. Consult with Radiology about obtaining an angiogram,
4. Start heparin.

Repeat CT scan revealed a new hyperdense middle cerebral artery (Fig. 12B1). Higher cuts revealed early ischemic changes (Fig. 12B2). After thorough explanation of the risks and benefits, the patient requested intravenous t-PA, which was administered per protocol. He had gradual clearing of his deficit to a point where he had just some mild incoordination of the left upper extremity with

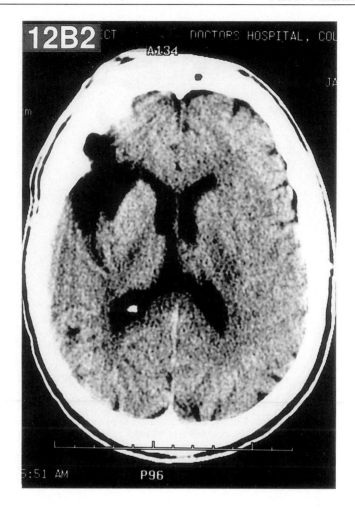

normal strength. Thorough work-up failed to yield a cause of stroke, but the trans-esophageal echocardiagram showed a small region of hypokinesis in the apex of the left ventricle. The patient completed rehabilitation on aspirin and ticlopidine, and returned to work with minimal disability.

COMMENT

This dramatic case, fortunately, represents an atypical situation. The sudden deterioration after admission could have signaled a second embolic event, perhaps from the heart. This idea is supported by the fact that both events were sudden in onset, and followed by improvement. Also, since there was an event many years prior, one is led to suspect an embolic source. On the other hand, the patient could also have had an *in situ* thrombosis; the waxing and waning clinical symptoms could have reflected changes in collateral perfusion. The second CT scan clearly shows a dense MCA sign, a poor prognostic indicator (Fig. 12B1) *(1)*. This may not have been present after the first embolus, or it may have been missed by the first CT scan. The decision to use t-PA after the second event was made easier by the fact that the patient was a physician who could rationally participate in decision making. Nevertheless, a clinician would be justified in withholding treatment in this case, given the uncertainties about the first event. The decision to treat proved the right one.

An angiogram may not have helped in this case, since the CT scan clearly shows the thrombus (Fig. 12B1). Also, it is unlikely that the Angiography Team could have been assembled rapidly, given the time of the night. On the other hand, intra-arterial delivery of thrombolytics may produce greater success, especially with large, proximal MCA occlusions (*see* Chapter 10).

This case was kindly provided by Dr. Jonathan Liss, MD.

REFERENCE

1. Tomsick TA, Brott TG, Chambers AA, Fox AJ, Gaskill MF, Lukin RR, et al. Hyperdense middle cerebral artery sign on CT: Efficacy in detecting middle cerebral artery thrombosis. *Am. J. Neur. R.* 1990; **11:** 473–477.

Case 13

An 85-yr-old white female, left-hand dominant, was brought in by paramedics complaining of left facial droop, slurred and incoherent speech beginning at approx 1:00 PM on the day of admission. The patient was her usual self at 10:00 PM the day prior to admission when her daughter spoke to her on the phone. At approx 12:30 PM, the patient's daughter phoned the patient without a response. Approximately 15 min later, the patient's daughter received a phone call from the patient and at that time noted the slurred speech. At approx 1:00 PM, the patient's daughter found the patient in front of the dining room table with a half-eaten sandwich. At that time, her daughter noted that the patient had a left facial droop, slurred and incoherent speech. The patient was occasionally following commands, was able to walk to the bathroom and urinate appropriately by herself. The patient denied dizziness, nausea, vomiting, fevers, chills, chest pain or shortness of breath. The patient arrived in the emergency department at approx 1:45 PM.

She had a history of migraine headaches for 1 1/2 yr. She had suffered five spells characterized as TIA, the last being approx 4 yr ago with symptoms of mild slurred speech, facial droop, visual changes lasting 15 to 20 min. On all occasions, the symptoms resolved completely. Carotid ultrasound approx 1 yr ago was normal. The patient was divorced, with one daughter, and lived alone in her home approximately two blocks away from the daughter. Upon examination, she was awake, alert and oriented to self only on arrival to the Emergency Department; she was aphasic. The patient had a left facial droop; otherwise cranial nerves II-XII were intact. Strength was 4/5 in the left upper extremity otherwise 5/5 in all other extremities. Rapid alternating movement in left arm was decreased. Reflexes were 3+ in the left biceps otherwise 2+ in all other areas. Toes were equivocal on the left and downgoing on the right. The patient had astereognosis but no graphesthesia or visual neglect. Her brain CT scan showed mild leukoariosis and no signs of acute stroke (Fig. 13A).

At this point, would you consider it appropriate to:

1. Stop the Code Stroke because of the patient's age,
2. Stop the Code because the onset time is uncertain,
3. Proceed with the evaluation.

From: *Thrombolytic Therapy for Stroke*
Edited by: P. D. Lyden © Humana Press Inc., Totowa, NJ

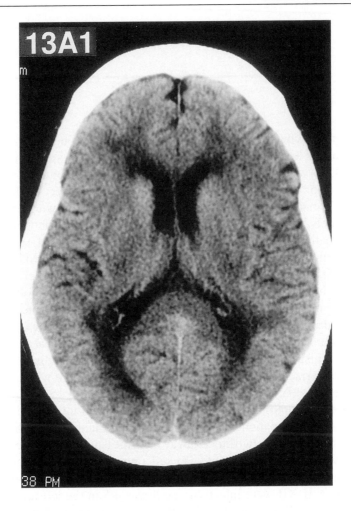

Initially, she was able to speak coherently although she was intermittently aphasic and only oriented to self. At approx 2:45 PM en route to the CT scanner, the patient became more incoherent and mumbling, unable to recognize her daughter. The patient's neurological condition waxed and waned over the next hour. Because of concern of her mother's neurological condition, the patient's daughter gave her ASA 325 mg in the Emergency Department without telling anyone. After a lengthy and extensive discussion of the risks and benefits of thrombolytic therapy at this time, after strong urging from the patient's daughter, t-PA was administered. After the bolus, the patient was transferred to the IMU. A few minutes after arrival, the patient complained of a severe headache in the frontal area and at this time the t-PA was stopped. Approximately 50% of the t-PA infusion had been given. The patient soon experienced nausea and vomit-

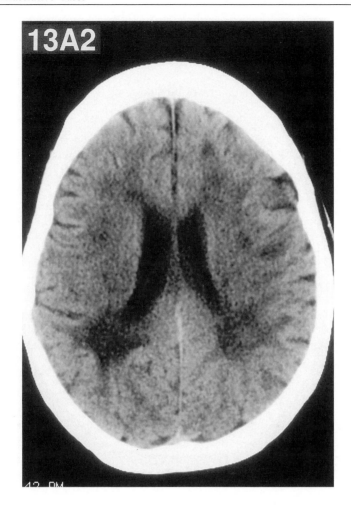

ing. Emergent CT scan was obtained at this time, which showed a left occipital lobe hemorrhage close to the midline with slight edema in the left hemisphere (Fig. 13B1). A small right occipital bleed was also noted.

The patient was transferred to the SICU for a closer cardiovascular and neurological monitoring. A neurosurgery consult was also obtained at this time. Approximately 1 h later, the patient's blood pressure increased for which labetalol iv was given. Her heart rhythm went into atrial fibrillation with an initial rapid ventricular response for which digoxin was given. The neurological examination at this time revealed decreased mental alertness, lethargic with no pupillary response and poor corneal/gag reflexes. The patient started to have labored breathing with respiratory distress and she was therefore intubated for airway protection and possible hyperventilation.

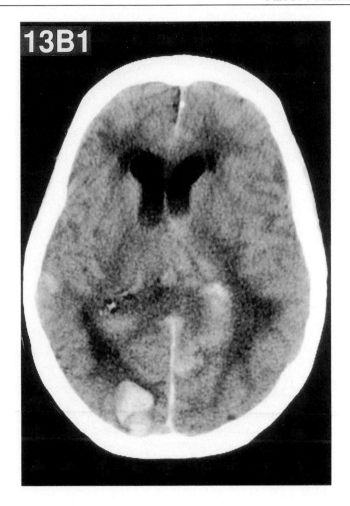

A third head CT scan was obtained at this time, which revealed enlargement of left occipital bleed with multiple area of bleeding in right occipital lobe and blood in the fourth ventricle (*see* Fig. 13B2). Neurosurgery had discussed options of evacuation versus ventriculostomy with the patient's daughter at this time. The patient's daughter considered that with the patient's current status and prognosis, she would like her mother to be NO-CODE, COMFORT-CARE. The patient expired within 24 h.

COMMENT

This tragic case illustrates many of the pitfalls associated with the use of thrombolytic agents. First and foremost, there was no clear onset time. The

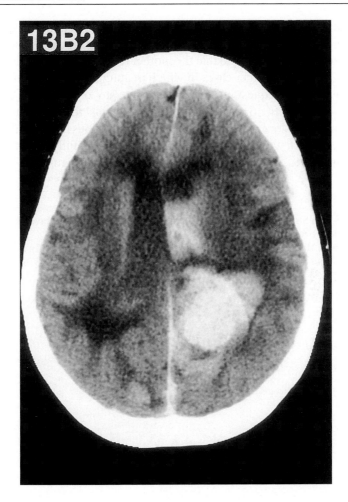

patient's daughter, an experienced Registered Nurse, argued forcefully in the Emergency Department that the patient must have been intact during the morning hours, since she had prepared a sandwich around her typical lunch time. However, patients with moderate deficits of cortical function may complete some tasks, especially if motor function is spared. The treating team did not have independent confirmation of the patient's status, and could have used the time that she was last known to be normal, the prior night's telephone call, as the onset time. The patient's age and the presence of leukoariaosis also may predispose the patient to hemorrhage *(1)*. The daughter's surreptitious administration of aspirin to the patient may or may not have contributed to the hemorrhage. In the clinical trials, aspirin has not been associated with increased risk of hemorrhage, although some limited preclinical data suggested aspirin could be a risk *(2)*.

To illustrate the absurdity of the modern American healthcare system, note that the daughter filed a lawsuit alleging that the physicians caring for this patient erred in agreeing to her demand that the mother receive thrombolysis. The editor is aware of at least two other cases in which treating physicians, acting in accordance with a patient request, used t-PA for acute stroke outside of the accepted protocol boundaries. In no case has a jury found against the physician. Nevertheless, treatment decisions involving a potentially hazardous drug should always be made in accordance with accepted medical guidelines. Family and patient wishes must be considered, but should not overrule physician judgment.

REFERENCES

1. NINDS TPA Stroke Study Group. Intracerebral Hemorrhage After Intravenous t-Pa Therapy for Ischemic Stroke. *Stroke* 1997; **28:** 2109–2118.
2. Clark WM, Madden KP, Lyden PD, Zivin JA. Cerebral hemorrhagic risk of aspirin or heparin therapy with thrombolytic treatment in rabbits. *Stroke* 1991; **22:** 872–876.

Case 14

You receive a call from your Emergency Department at 9:30 PM regarding a 64-yr-old man with the sudden onset of left sided weakness about 9:00 PM tonight. There is no prior medical history that anyone is aware of. The blood pressure in the ambulance is reported as 130/82 and the finger stick blood sugar is 120. Upon your arrival in the Department, you learn that the patient has gone to CT scan. You arrive in the control room as the scans are being reconstructed and projected onto the video display screen. You wait for the hardcopy films to print and confirm your impression of the scan. The patient is transported back to the Department while you finish up in CT. It is now 10:12 PM. The films reveal a dense artery sign and some effacement of the temporal sulci (Fig. 14A).

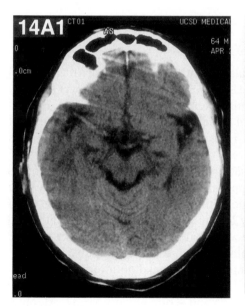 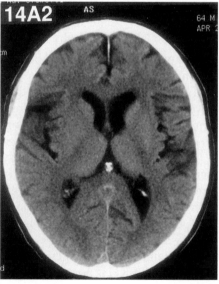

From: *Thrombolytic Therapy for Stroke*
Edited by: P. D. Lyden © Humana Press Inc., Totowa, NJ

At this point consider whether you would:

1. Cancel the Code Stroke because the dense middle cerebral artery is associated with poor outcome after stroke,
2. Cancel because there is minimal effacement of the sulci over the right temporal parietal cortex,
3. Cancel since it is late in the evening,
4. Do nothing until the ED physician has time to evaluate the patient,
5. Continue.

When you return to the Emergency Department you find that the wife has arrived by private car. Upon your direct questioning you learn that the wife observed the onset of the stroke. She states that the patient was working at the computer when he suddenly stated that his arm felt numb. He stood up and walked into the kitchen. Suddenly, he stated that his arm felt weak, then he fell to the floor unable to move the left side, all within 5 or 10 min of his first complaint of numbness. She immediately called 911. From the records available in the Emergency Department you determine that the call to 911 was placed at 9:15 PM. You therefore set the time of onset as 9:05 PM. It is now 10:30 PM.

Would you like to:

1. Learn more history,
2. Perform an examination,
3. Obtain laboratory results.

The patient has been in excellent health recently, but underwent a three-vessel coronary artery bypass graft 15 yr ago. He exercises regularly, has never smoked, and although he drank while in the military, has abstained for 20 yr. He was severely wounded in Korea, with loss of muscle mass, but not function, of the left arm and calf. He takes no medications. He is retired from the military and works as a computer consultant.

He is alert, oriented, and slightly dysarthric. There is a dense left homonymous hemianopsia, left facial weakness (upper motor neuron type), and a left gaze preference. The arm and leg are plegic with no observable proximal or distal movements. There is a dense sensory loss to pin, temperature, and touch and profound neglect of the left hemispace with moderate anosognosia. Reflexes are diminished throughout. At this time blood pressure is 142/88, pulse is regular, and the remainder of the general examination is normal or unremarkable.

A 12-lead EKG is normal. INR = 1.13 and the partial thromboplastin time is 23.3 (control of 25.1). Platelet count is 165 and serum glucose is 237. All other routine chemistries and hematology studies are normal.

At this point you present the issue to the wife. It is now 10:44 PM. Consider whether you would recommend to her:

1. Not to use t-PA because the stroke is too severe,
2. Not to use t-PA because the CT scan is abnormal,
3. To try t-PA realizing that it most likely will not help, and could hurt.

After discussion of the issues, the wife agrees to the therapy. You explain the situation to the patient as well, for even though he may not be able to give consent, he is alert, oriented, and able to verbalize his desires. He too wishes to proceed.

After treatment in the ED, the patient is transferred to the Intensive Care Unit for overnight monitoring. The next morning the patient is able to move his left arm and leg with normal strength; there is a mild pronator drift. The homonymous hemianopsia is completely resolved. He still manifests a left facial weakness and although sensation is intact to pin, touch, and temperature, he extinguished to double simultaneous presentation of visual or tactile stimuli. A CT scan is obtained (Fig. 14B). Despite a detailed work-up, no obvious cause is found for his stroke. One week later he is at his pre-morbid activities, including his work with the computer.

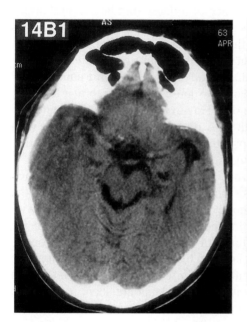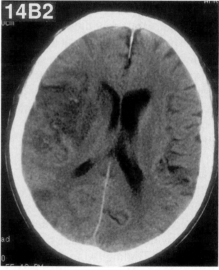

COMMENT

Most Code Strokes occur in the early morning, or late afternoon *(1)*. Invariably they occur at inopportune times; it is important when setting up a stroke call schedule that this phenomenon be considered, and that there be a sufficient number of individuals in the schedule. For most groups the min. safe number is four persons.

It is highly appropriate to order a CT scan STAT without first examining the patient. Every minute counts and needless delays must be avoided. In this case, the history obtained by telephone indicated that the patient had suffered a major neurologic event, so no matter what diagnosis might be suggested by further history, a CT scan will likely be needed. In some centers where Stroke Codes are frequent, a standing order is written for STAT brain CT on appropriate patients *(2,3)*. Although it is true that the ED Physician may obtain history to exclude the patient from further consideration for thrombolysis, it is also true that the sooner you are in motion toward the hospital, the sooner treatment can begin. Although it is permitted to treat up to 3 h after symptom onset, better results are obtained with quicker treatment. While driving in to the hospital, further information can be obtained by telephone. If you learn of a reason to cancel the Code, you can turn around and return to home or office. On the other hand, if you wait, and the patient is a good candidate, nothing can then be done to make up for the lost time and wasted brain.

The CT scan indeed reveals the presence of a dense middle cerebral artery sign. The frequency of this finding in acute stroke patients depends on scanning technique, especially the thickness of the CT slices (*see* Chapter 15). This sign can be overdiagnosed and it is important to note the finding only when one artery is clearly more dense than the surrounding brain *(4)*. It is best if the contralateral artery can be seen to be less dense. When a true dense middle cerebral artery sign is present, it indicates a very poor prognosis. However, even though the outcome is generally poor, patients treated with t-PA do better than those treated with placebo. Therefore, it is prudent to inform the patient and family of the finding, that the prognosis is poor, but that t-PA should be considered.

Very early after large ischemic stroke there may be mild swelling which manifests as effacement of the sulci over the involved cortex (Chapter 15). In the NINDS t-PA study, this finding was not exclusionary and many patients with early signs of edema were successfully treated. Early subtle signs of ischemia are not a contraindication to treatment within 3 h of stroke. However, in the European trial, in which patients were treated as late as 6 h after stroke with a higher dose of t-PA, CT findings were correlated with a higher risk of disabling or fatal brain hemorrhage. Therefore, when CT signs of early edema are seen, it is best to question the family/witnesses again about the time of onset. If it can be established with certainty that the stroke began within the past 3 h, it is probably best to proceed with thrombolysis.

The National Institutes of Health Stroke Scale score for this patient was about 17, above the average for acute stroke patients, but not the most severe. Importantly, he was wide awake with no evidence of encephalopathy. Based on the examination, he was an ideal candidate for thrombolysis.

REFERENCES

1. Zweifler RM, Drinkard R, Cunningham S, Brody ML, Rothrock JF. Implementation of a stroke code system in Mobile, Alabama. Diagnostic and therapeutic yield. *Stroke 1997*; **28:** 981–983.
2. Tilley BC, Lyden PD, Brott TG, Lu M, Levine SR, Welch KMA. Total quality improvement method for reduction of delays between emergency department admisison and treatment of acute ischemic stroke. *Arch. Neurol.* 1997; **54:** 1466–1474.
3. Lyden PD, Rapp K, Babcock T, Rothrock J. Ultra-rapid identification, triage, and enrollment of stroke patients into clinical trials. *J. Stroke Cerebrovasc. Dis.* 1994; **4:** 106–113.
4. Tomsick TA, Brott TG, Chambers AA, Fox AJ, Gaskill MF, Lukin RR, Pleatman CW, Wiot JG, Bourekas E. Hyperdense middle cerebral artery sign on CT: Efficacy in detecting middle cerebral artery thrombosis. *Am. J. Neur. R.* 1990; **11:** 473–477.

Case 15

An 84-yr-old male presented to the Emergency Department at 8:30 AM with a complaint of right arm numbness and weakness for 1 h. The patient was at a hotel to attend a conference where he was to be the keynote speaker. While practicing his speech, he suddenly stopped talking and could not move his right side. A friend who was present when the patient's symptoms began brought him to the Emergency Room. The friend noted the time to be approx 7:00 AM in the morning.

The patient had a history of hypertension, diabetes, gout, but no history of TIA or heart attack. He regularly took medications for the above, including aspirin 81 mg/d. On neurological examination, the patient had mild aphasia with features consistent with both receptive and expressive deficits. There was a right upper motor neuron facial weakness and no visual field cut. The arm was weak on the right with near complete paralysis of the hand. The right leg was mildly weak. The patient did not appreciate pain or light touch over the right arm or leg.

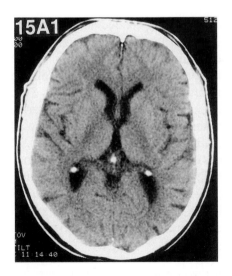 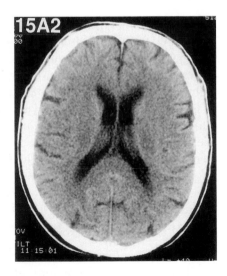

From: *Thrombolytic Therapy for Stroke*
Edited by: P. D. Lyden © Humana Press Inc., Totowa, NJ

The initial EKG revealed first-degree heart block and a right frontal branch block, prompting a troponin and CPK to be sent. Noncontrast brain CT was normal for age (Fig. 15A).

At this point, consider whether you would:

1. Cancel the Code Stroke, as the EKG does not permit you to rule out a myocardial infarction,
2. Cancel the Code Stroke because the patient is too old,
3. Continue the Code Stroke.

After the CT scan showed no evidence of hemorrhage (Fig. 15A) the patient returned to the Emergency Department and preparations were made for the administration of t-PA. The wife was contacted out of state and by long distance, she gave consent for administration of t-PA. Initial laboratory studies revealed an INR of 1.1, a platelet count of 328,000.

At the completion of your examination, you are informed that the troponin is less than 0.2, which is considered normal in your laboratory.

At this point, consider whether you might:

1. Cancel the Code Stroke since it is too early for the troponins to reliably indicate micro ischemia.
2. Cancel the Code Stroke because the patient's wife cannot physically sign the consent form.
3. Cancel the Code Stroke because the patient's deficits are too mild.
4. Continue the Code Stroke.

With the concurrence of the patient and the family the decision was made to proceed with the treatment at 9:48 AM, 2 1/2 h after the onset of symptoms. The patient was treated with t-PA according to protocol. At 5:00 PM on the same evening the patient was examined and found to have cleared his aphasia completely. However, his repeat troponin returned elevated at 2.7. His CPK was slightly elevated at 227 with a MB isoenzyme fraction at 5.6%. Cardiology determined that the patient in fact had suffered a mild inferior wall ischemic injury. He underwent coronary catheterization and no acute vessel occlusion was found. However diffuse areas of narrowing were found including a 60–70% distal left anterior descending artery lesion, and a 50–60% stenosis of the mid-right coronary artery. The patient continued to suffer additional coronary events, despite maximum medical therapy, and expired owing to congestive heart failure, pneumonia, and sepsis 10 d after the stroke.

COMMENT

This case illustrates several nuances of thrombolytic therapy. In general, patients who are suffering myocardial infarction and stroke simultaneously should not be treated if one or the other process is more than 6 h old. The typical scenario is represented by a patient with myocardial infarction who does not seek medical attention because of an atypical presentation. Between 1 to 4 d later, the patient presents with a cardioembolic event owing to an akinetic wall segment with adherent mural thrombus. In patients admitted to coronary care units for heart attack, as many as 5% were noted to have simultaneous acute stroke symptoms, whereas in stroke unit admissions, the incidence of myocardial ischemia may be as high as 30% (1–3). During a Code Stroke, it may not be clear whether EKG changes reflect new myocardial damage or not. The editor has seen several such cases and in none was it prudent to treat with t-PA. A recent stroke contra-indicates thrombolytic therapy for heart attack due to the possibility of transforming a late stroke into a hemorrhage. Likewise if a patient has suffered a myocardial event recently, acute treatment for stroke might cause pericardial wall rupture and tamponade. The present example illustrates the truly exceptional situation: it was clear that this stroke was less than 3 h old. If a myocardial infarction were happening, it was certainly not old or recent because the troponins were negative. Therefore, a case was made to proceed with thrombolytic therapy. The next question was to select a dose: the myocardial dose or the calculated cerebral dose. Although experience in this setting is quite limited, most clinicians prefer to use the lower of the two doses, that is the cerebral dose of 0.9 mg/kg. Intra-arterial therapy might also be a reasonable alternative, especially if the myocardial ischemia is more than 24 h in duration, to reduce the chance of pericardial rupture.

The patient was elderly at 84 yr, but there is no upper age limit in the protocol. Patients over the age of 80 have been treated successfully with t-PA although responsiveness declines with increasing age. It is not clear whether there is an increased risk of hemorrhage owing to increasing age although this point is being studied (4,5).

Since t-PA for acute stroke is approved by the FDA, no consent form is required. However, many practitioners choose to use the consent form to document that all issues have been thoroughly discussed with the family and patient prior to using t-PA. Whether telephonic consent is permissible is decided individually in different localities by either state or local government regulations or by the human subjects protection committee. In some settings, medical staff bylaws will address this issue.

The question of severity is one that requires physician judgement in individual circumstances. Patients with a mild aphasia may be severely disabled if their occupation depends on communication skills. In this particular case, the patient was a frequent lecturer and guest speaker; he decided that he would rather proceed with therapy because of his need for a return of his communication function.

REFERENCES

1. Komrad MS, Coffey CE, Coffey KS, McKinnis R, Massey EW, Califf RM. Myocardial infarction and stroke. *Neurology* 1984; **34:** 1403–1409.
2. Dimant J, Grob D. Electrocardiographic changes and myocardial damage in patients with acute cerebrovascular accidents. *Stroke* 1977; **4:** 448–455.
3. Myers MG, Norris JW, Hachinski VC, Weingert ME, Sole MJ. Cardiac sequelae of acute stroke. *Stroke* 1982; **13:** 838–842.
4. Tanne D, Verro P, Mansbach H, Levine S. Overview and Summary of Phase IV Data on Use of t-PA for Acute Ischemic Stroke. *Stroke Interventionalist* 1998; **1:** 3–5.
5. NINDS TPA Stroke Study Group. Intracerebral Hemorrhage After Intravenous t-Pa Therapy for Ischemic Stroke. *Stroke* 1997; **28:** 2109–2118.

Case 16

This 50-yr-old male presented to the Emergency Department with the sudden onset of right arm weakness and inability to speak. According to witnesses, he sat down for lunch with his coworkers at 11:30 AM, then at approx 12:12 PM they noticed that his speech was incomprehensible and his right arm would not move normally. The coworkers saw him suddenly droop to the right and in 5 min they called 911. The patient arrived at the Emergency Department at 12:56 PM. A CT scan was performed at 1:36 PM, which showed no evidence of intracranial bleed (Fig. 16).

The patient was diagnosed with hypertension about 2 yr ago and was given hydrochlorothiazide; he stopped taking the medication shortly after. The patient denies tobacco. He drinks approximately three glasses of red wine per week. He is a computer engineer.

At this point consider whether you would:

1. Cancel the Code Stroke because he has no vascular risk factors, is young, and is likely to have a rare or unusual cause of stroke,
2. Cancel the Code Stroke because the symptoms are too mild,
3. Continue.

On examination, the patient was alert but had difficulty with comprehension, following only one-step commands. His speech was aphasic: he was able to say only "okay," "yes," and "no." There was a right facial droop in an upper motor neuron pattern. The patient had a pronator drift on the right but strength was otherwise normal. Sensory system testing revealed the patient had a right-sided neglect, but was intact to pin prick and light touch. His total NIH Stroke Scale Score was 6. All laboratory studies and the EKG returned within normal limits.

From: *Thrombolytic Therapy for Stroke*
Edited by: P. D. Lyden © Humana Press Inc., Totowa, NJ

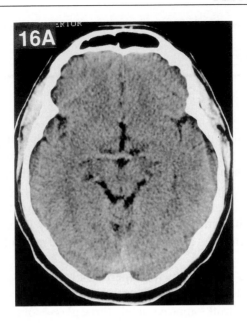

At this time would you:

1. Cancel the Code Stroke since the examination confirms the mild deficit,
2. Consider an MRI to try to determine the size of the lesion,
3. Offer thrombolysis.

After a full discussion of the risks and benefits, the patient received t-PA according to the standard protocol at 2:03 PM ,1 h and 45 min after the onset of the symptoms. Over the next day the patient had dramatic improvement. His severe aphasia and right-sided neglect improved the next day to a transcortical motor aphasia. By hospital day 3 the patient's aphasia was essentially resolved with just mild slowing on repetition. The patient was given aspirin and a carotid duplex showed no significant stenosis. A transthoracic echocardiogram with Valsalva and bubble studies showed no evidence of clot and no evidence of patent foramen ovale. Extensive search for other rare causes of stroke yielded no diagnosis.

Three months after treatment the patient was back at work full time with no observable deficits. He reported occasional word finding difficulty, especially under stress, but could detect no deterioration in his job performance.

COMMENT

The protocol admonishes the clinician to avoid thrombolysis in the setting of mild symptoms (*see* Chapter 17). In practice, this means that patients with purely

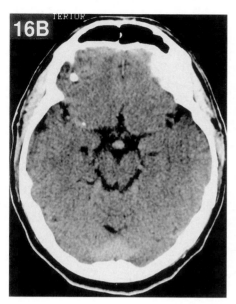
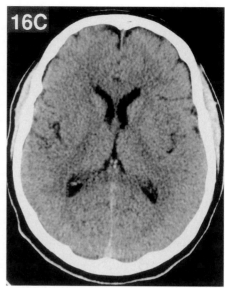

sensory symptoms, or isolated ataxia, could be excluded from therapy. Some authorities have suggested that patients with an NIH Stroke Scale score of less than 5 or 6 should be excluded. However, the use of a specific value of the NIH Stroke Scale to select patients could be hazardous, as this case illustrates. Since the patient's occupation required language, his initially mild deficit would actually have proven quite disabling. Even if the aphasia had been his only symptom, most experienced stroke Neurologists would strongly consider treating such a young, employed patient.

Young patients do exhibit a higher incidence of unusual causes of stroke. Most of these rare entities are likely to occlude arteries through a thrombotic mechanism, however. There is no reason, *a priori*, to assume that thrombolysis would offer such patients no benefit. An MRI scan would not have clarified the situation, since it would likely have shown early abnormalities that indicate ischemia, but not specific pathologic diagnosis. Similarly, it is difficult to imagine any findings on angiography that would dissuade the clinician from using thrombolysis.

REFERENCES

1. Adams H, Kappelle J, Biller J, Gordon D, Love B, Gomez F, Heffner M: Ischemic Stroke in Young Adults. *Arch. Neurol.* 1995; **52:** 491–495.
2. Bevan H, Sharma K, Bradely W: Stroke in Young Adults. *Stroke* 1990; **21:** 382–386.

Case 17

This patient, a 73-yr-old white female, was brought in by Paramedics at approx 1:30 PM. Paramedics were called when witnesses observed the patient drive her car at low speed into a roadside barrier. Witnesses immediately attended to her and found that she was slumped over and not moving her right side. No seizure activity was noted. She was wide-awake with her eyes open, and although she attempted to speak she was not able to make any coherent sounds. There was no evidence of trauma at the scene and there was no damage to the car other than scratched paint. During the paramedic evaluation, the patient was noted to be normotensive with a finger stick blood sugar of 136. Cardiac rhythm was normal.

Upon arrival in the Emergency Department, the patient was stable with eyes open and no verbal response. Her right side was not moving, but her left moved normally. Initial Code Stroke laboratory bloods were drawn and sent and the patient was prepared to go to CT scan. The initial CT scan is shown (Fig. 17A).

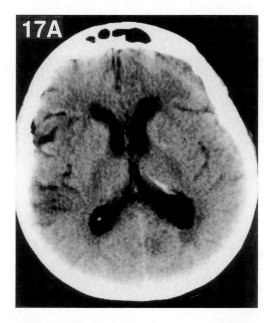

From: *Thrombolytic Therapy for Stroke*
Edited by: P. D. Lyden © Humana Press Inc., Totowa, NJ

At this point you decide to:

1. Cancel the Code Stroke because the patient may have suffered trauma,
2. Cancel the Code Stroke because there is no witnessed onset time,
3. Cancel the Code Stroke because the patient cannot give consent,
4. Continue Code Stroke.

At 2:45 PM the CT scan was completed and the patient's daughter arrived in the Emergency Department. The daughter was informed of the situation and agreed to continue with evaluation for possible t-PA therapy. At 2:55 PM while returning from CT scan the patient suffered a grand mal seizure. She was transferred expeditiously back to the emergency room and loaded with Dilantin. The seizure cleared and the patient was left with an alert mental status, continued unresponsiveness, and right-sided weakness. Formal neurological exam revealed that she had a global aphasia and was mute. There was a right homonymous hemianopsia and a right upper motor neuron type facial weakness of the face. Her right arm and leg were totally paralyzed and her sensory exam revealed that she did not withdraw from painful stimulus on the right but did from the left. Her platelet count returned at 390,000, coagulation studies were normal and a 12-lead EKG showed normal sinus rhythm. During the Dilantin load the patient suffered one more tonic clonic seizure which was easily managed with airway protection and oxygenation. After the seizure was completed, the patient returned to the above examination. Repeat CT Scan was done and is shown below (Fig. 17B).

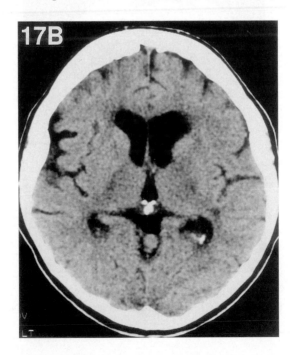

At this point you decide to:

1. Cancel the Code Stroke because of seizures,
2. Cancel the Code Stroke because the patient's CT scan is abnormal,
3. Cancel the Code Stroke because the patient is too severe,
4. Continue the stoke evaluation.

After a discussion of all the potential risks and benefits, the patient's daughter consented to t-PA therapy, which was administered. Since the patient weighed 125 lbs. A total of 51 mg was delivered as a 5-mg bolus with the remainder diffused over 1 h. The bolus was given at 3:29 PM, which was about 2 h and 15 min after the presumed onset.

Examination the next morning the patient was markedly improved with normal language, no hemiparasis, no sensory deficit, and normal coordination. No further seizures occurred but an EEG did reveal left temporal parietal slowing. The patient was discharged home 3 d later. Follow-up carotid ultrasound revealed no stenosis and cardiac work revealed wall motion abnormalities at the apex. She was treated with long-term antiplatelet therapy and after 3 yr follow-up has suffered no further spells.

COMMENT

This patient was driving her car when her stroke presumably occurred. A conference was held with Paramedics in the Emergency Room to locate a witness, but unfortunately witnesses could not be reached by telephone. However, witnesses did tell Paramedics that the patient had been driving normally then suddenly she veered to one side and ended up striking the barrier. Witnesses called 911 immediately and that call was recorded as being received at 1:30 PM. Therefore, the onset time is reasonably established to be shortly before 1:30 PM and for practical purposes this was set at 1:15 PM. There were no external signs of trauma at the scene or when the patient was examined thoroughly in the hosptial. The CT scan clearly showed absence of any extracranial soft tissue injury; there was no intracranial contusion or hemorrhage. The impact was witnessed to occur at low speed and in fact there was no damage to the car and the airbag did not deploy. Therefore it is reasonable to conclude that the patient did not suffer serious head or back trauma. The astute clinician should note that the patient was at risk for a carotid dissection and that an ultrasound should be done urgently, but not to delay therapy.

The patient suffered two generalized seizures. The package insert states that t-PA is contraindicated if seizure occurs at the onset of stroke. The purpose for this exclusion criterion is to avoid treating post-ictal paralysis, which may mimic stroke. In this case the patient had a clear-cut history of stroke initially and in fact her initial event was witnessed to lack any seizure activity. Rarely, a patient will suffer seizures immediately following a large cortical stroke, as happened in this case. As Dr. Caplan has pointed out (*see* Chapter 13) thrombolytic therapy should be reserved for patients in whom vascular occlusions are proven. In this case, Dr. Caplan's approach would be ideal in that if we would obtain vascular imaging promptly we could know whether the patient had an appropriate vascular occlusion to support our theory that the convulsions followed the stroke. However, this type of imaging was not available at the time this patient presented (1994) and therefore a decision had to be made without the benefit of vascular imaging. The patient was severely affected, with an NIH stroke scale score >20. As we have discussed in previous chapters (especially Chapters 8 and 9), this is not a contraindication to thrombolytic therapy. However, elevated stroke scale score may be associated with risk of hemorrhage. In this case, the family was informed that although there was a potential for benefit there was also an increased likelihood of hemorrhage. The patient's response was gratifying, but does not prove whether her event was stroke or seizure. The observation that no further seizures occurred, in the absence of anticonvulsant therapy, supports the diagnosis of stroke.

Case 18

Paramedics were called to see a 56-yr-old female patient for 1 h of right-sided weakness and unresponsiveness. The family noted that she had been complaining of headache for approx 3-5 d. Although she does not have a history of migraine she had suffered some vomiting and had not been eating. The patient has a history of diabetes. During the Paramedics' initial evaluation, she was noted to be unresponsive but did open her eyes to name-calling. She followed no commands and did not appear to recognize her family. According to the medics, her right face was markedly paralyzed and her right arm and leg did not move at all; her left arm and leg moved in response to painful stimulation. The Code Stroke was called from the field and the above history was given by the nurse on duty in the Emergency Department radio room.

At this point, consider whether you would:

1. Cancel the Code Stroke since you cannot personally examine the patient,
2. Cancel the Code Stroke since this is probably migranous stroke,
3. Cancel the Code Stroke because this could be hypoglycemia,
4. Continue the Code Stroke.

Medics began to transport the patient as a potential Code Stroke. About 10 min later, the medics radioed to report that the patient's finger stick glucose was 26 mg/dl. They administered two ampules of 50% Dextrose and continued an intravenous of 50 mL/h 5% Dextrose in water. When the patient arrived in the Emergency Room she was wide-awake and conversing normally. She was found to have a persistent right facial droop but the right arm and leg were moving normally. There was a right pronator drift. Sensory testing and reflexes were entirely normal. Over the ensuing 20 min of observation, all deficits, including the facial weakness, cleared up and the patient regained a completely normal neurological examination. The Code Stroke was canceled and no brain CT was performed.

COMMENT

It is appropriate to notify the stroke team from the field: very often paramedics can be asked by radio to conduct a maneuver in the field that may illuminate a

From: *Thrombolytic Therapy for Stroke*
Edited by: P. D. Lyden © Humana Press Inc., Totowa, NJ

diagnosis other than stroke. In this particular case, migraine would be a possibility, but would not necessarily exclude the patient from thrombolysis.

This case illustrates the under-appreciated incidence of focal findings with hypoglycemia. The history of diabetes and reduced oral intake suggested the possibility of hypoglycemia, confirmed by the finger stick glucose in the field. In patients with severe hypoglycemia, focal findings were noted in about 2% of patients (1–3). In our experience there is usually some change of mental status, as was noted in this patient, but this can often be mistaken for aphasia. It is therefore an essential part of the Code Stroke that a finger stick glucose be drawn and tested. In this particular case it resulted in the proper therapy being applied and no thrombolytic therapy was needed.

REFERENCES

1. Shanmugam V, Zimnowodzki S, Curtin J, Gorelick PB. Hypoglycemic hemiplegia: insulinoma masquerading as stroke. *Journal of Stroke and Cerebrovascular Diseases* 1997; **6**: 368–369.
2. Malouf R, Brust JCM. Hypoglycemia: Causes, Neurological manifestations, and outcome. *Ann. Neurol.* 1985; **17**: 421–430.
3. Rother J, Schreiner A, Wentz KU, Hennerici M. Hypoglycemia presenting as basilar artery thrombosis. *Stroke* 1992; **23**: 112–113.

Case 19

While trying to open a can of soda, a 51-yr-old right handed physician was noted by his family to suddenly become aphasic with right sided hemiparesis and right facial droop at about 1:45 PM. The patient was a physician visiting family because of his father's recent death. Since the witnesses were also physicians and nurses, a call to 911 was made immediately; the patient was brought to the Emergency Department within 30 min. After Code Stroke laboratory studies were drawn and sent, the patient was examined and found to be awake, but globally aphasic with no intelligible output and following no commands. There was an upper motor neuron like facial weakness, but the visual fields could not be accurately assessed. The right arm and leg were weak but moving. He did not withdraw to sensory stimulation on either side. The patient was taken urgently to the CT scanner, where a normal CT scan was obtained.

At this point, you decide to:

1. Cancel the Code Stroke because the patient is a physician and would not be appropriate for potentially hazardous treatment.,
2. Cancel the Code Stroke because the symptoms are too severe,
3. Continue the Code Stroke.

Further history was obtained from the wife after the CT Scan. She noted that he had been complaining for 2 mo of episodes of difficulty with speech, balance, dizziness, nausea, vomiting, and restlessness. About 2 wk prior to the present admission, the patient had an episode where he was unable to dial a number on a touch tone telephone and he was unable to add the restaurant bill. He continued working until the day prior to the stroke, however, and was able to dictate radiographic reports without a problem. He had obviously been under considerable stress recently due to the death of his father.

At this point consider whether you would:

1. Cancel the Code Stroke resulting from the history of multiple TIA-like episodes,
2. Cancel the Code Stroke since the episode could be a conversion reaction,
3. Send the patient for a brain MRI scan to see if any of the prior events left any residual damage,
4. Offer thrombolysis.

From: *Thrombolytic Therapy for Stroke*
Edited by: P. D. Lyden © Humana Press Inc., Totowa, NJ

In consultation with the patient's brother, also a physician, and the wife, the decision was made to treat with t-PA. The prothrombin time returned back normal and the platelet count was 192,000. The patient was treated with t-PA according to protocol.

By the next morning the patient's neurologic symptoms had cleared to a gratifying extent. He continued to exhibit episodes of aphasia, but his motor, sensory, and other cranial nerve functions returned to normal. However, within another 24 hours the patient worsened with quite clear deterioration in mental status. An extensive evaluation was conducted over the ensuing 2 mo, which included lumbar puncture, angiography, EEG, and extensive cultures of blood and cerebrospinal fluid. He was treated with Acyclovir against the possibility of herpes encephalitis, but all tests for this were negative. Eventually the diagnosis of granulomatous angiitis was entertained: a biopsy of the meningies was consistent with this diagnosis. Over the ensuing 3 yr the patient was treated with imunosuppression. On multiple occasions, an attempt was made to wean him from therapy and on each occasion his symptoms returned. Eventually after 5 yr it was possible to taper the imunosuppressent and the patient remained symptom free.

COMMENT

In retrospect, the patient's stroke-like presentation is consistent with the known spectrum of presentation of granulomatous, or isolated, angiitis of the nervous system. The key to the diagnosis was the history of the waxing and waning symptoms, including restlessness, over the 2 mo prior to presentation. Stroke or TIA syndromes are rarely the initial manifestation of isolated angiitis.

It is not clear whether a thrombosis was present in a cerebral artery at onset, since vascular imaging was not possible. It could have been coincidental that the patient's focal symptoms resolved after the t-PA. Nevertheless, it was appropriate to consider the patient for thrombolytic therapy, since the clinical picture was initially consistent with stroke. In this patient, the usual differential diagnosis of stroke in the young was considered, with particular emphasis in ruling out migraine, dissection, drug abuse, vasculitis, cardiac disease, and coagulopathy. Any of these conditions could cause stroke by a mechanism that would be expected to respond to thrombolytic therapy.

REFERENCES

1. Moore PM: Central Nervous System Vasculitis. *Current Opinions in Neurology* 1998; **11:** 241–246.
2. Alhalabi M, Moore PM: Serial angiography in isolated angiitis of the central nervous system. *Neurology* 1994; **44:** 1221–1226.
3. Lie JT: Primary (Granulomatous) Angiitis of the Central Nervous System: A Clinicopathologic Analysis of 15 New Cases and a Review of the Literature. *Human Pathology* 1992; **23:** 1640–1671.

Case 20

This 62-yr-old, right-handed, white female with no history of previous stroke or TIA, was taking aspirin for chronic atrial fibrillation first diagnosed in 1989. While out shopping with her husband, she suffered the sudden onset of left-sided weakness at 5:35 PM. The husband noted the time on his watch, because he had recently seen a public television show about warning signs of stroke and the need for accurate timing of the onset. Paramedics were called to the shopping center, and the patient was transported to the Emergency Department. On Coumadin, the patient had difficulty maintaining a therapeutic prothrombin time and was taking aspirin instead. A brief examination prior to CT scanning showed a left hemiparesis, hemi-sensory loss, profound neglect, and a left homonomous hemianopsia. The patient exhibited classic atopagnosia and denial of her deficit. She denied that she was having any problem at all. An admission electrocardiogram showed atrial fibrillation, but no acute ischemic changes. Admission coagulation parameters were within normal limits. A CT brain scan was done without contrast (Fig. 20A).

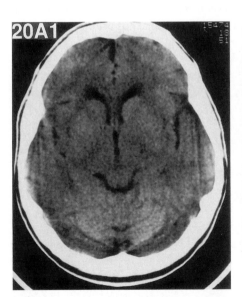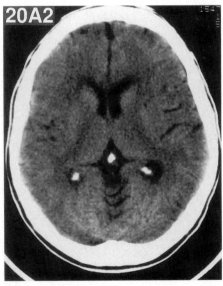

From: *Thrombolytic Therapy for Stroke*
Edited by: P. D. Lyden © Humana Press Inc., Totowa, NJ

At this point, consider whether you would:

1. Discontinue the Code Stroke because she was taking aspirin,
2. Start heparin to prevent recurrent cardioembolic stroke and avoid thrombolysis,
3. Discontinue the Code and use neither heparin or thrombolysis because the CT scan shows sulcal effacement in the right parietal area,
4. Continue the Code, proceeding to an examination and history.

After full discussion of risks and benefits with the the husband, and complete description of the same to the patient, the husband decided to authorize thrombolytic treatment. At 85 minutes after stroke onset she received a bolus of t-PA, followed by the remainder of her infusion over 60 min, for a total dose of 0.9 m/ kg. Her symptoms resolved quite remarkably by 2 h following the bolus. Her residual deficit 24 h after stroke onset included some decreased sensory function in the left lower and upper extremities, but no extinction, or anosognosia. The motor system examination revealed normal strength in all muscles and there was no evidence of visual field deficit. The patient was re-started on Coumadin prior to discharge to home, in consultation with her cardiologist.

A follow-up CT of the head 24 h after the onset of symptoms showed a lucency in the right middle cerebral artery distribution, especially at the right caudate nucleus with some mass effect on the right frontal horn of the ventricle. One week later, only a lucency in the head of the caudate nucleus could be seen (Fig. 20B). There was no hemorrhagic transformation seen at that time. A carotid duplex was negative for significant stenosis of the right internal carotid artery.

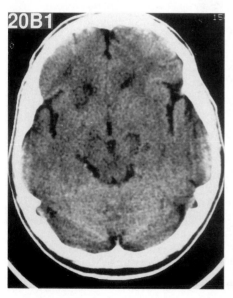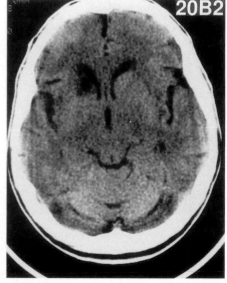

COMMENT

Use of aspirin prior to the stroke was not a contraindication to thrombolysis, although the protocol prohibits use of aspirin AFTER thrombolytic therapy for 24 h. In the original NINDS trial, about one-third of patients had taken aspirin prior to the stroke; no harmful interaction with t-PA was noted. Nevertheless, the protocol used in that study prohibited aspirin use for 24 h for safety reasons. When t-PA was approved for use by the US Food and Drug Administration, the study protocol was adopted intact, and the 24-h limit against aspirin was included. Thus, although prior use of aspirin is not a contraindication, it probably should not be used for 24 h.

The use of heparin after cardioembolic stroke is more problematic. The risk of early recurrent embolization after such stroke is much lower than traditionally taught. The TOAST study *(1)* and the International Stroke Study *(2)* both contain data to suggest that after cardioembolic stroke, there is a 3 to 5% risk of recurrence over the first 2 wk. Anticoagulation did not appear to alter this. Thus, there is probably no compelling reason to start heparin in the first 24 h. For the safety reasons outlined above, heparin was prohibited for 24 h after thrombolysis in the original t-PA study. Heparin use after stroke remains highly controversial, and open to physician judgement, but no data support its use in the acute setting after stroke, whereas considerable data supports the use of thrombolysis.

The role of the sulcal effacement in selecting patients has been discussed previously (*see* Chapter 15). The only contraindication to thrombolytic therapy on CT scan is hemorrhage. Large areas of edema suggest that the onset time may be incorrect. Cortical effacement and other subtle signs of early ischemia may in fact predict a patient that has the best chance of a good response to t-PA.

REFERENCES

1. The Publications Committee for the Trial of ORG 10172 in Acute Stroke Treatment (TOAST) Investigators. Low Molecular Weight Heparinoid ORG 10172 (Danaparoid), and Outcome After Acute Ischemic Stroke: A Randomized Controlled Trial. *JAMA* 1998; **279:** 1265–1272.
2. International Stroke Trial Collaborative Group. The international stroke trial (IST): a randomised trial of aspirin, subcutaneous heparin, both, or neither among 19435 patients with acute ischaemic stroke. Lancet 1997; **349:** 1569–1581.

Case 21

The patient was a 77-yr-old, right-handed male in good health, who had just finished a book at 12:38 AM. He attempted to place the book back on a shelf, but was unable. He then realized he could not speak, even though five minutes prior to this he was speaking and functioning normally per his family. At 12:39 AM the family called 911. The Paramedics found him completely aphasic, with no seizure activity and purposeless movements of his right hand. The EMTs also noted him to improve during transit, with one to two words and increased purposeful movements of his right arm. His past medical history included hypertension, a nosebleed requiring cautery 3 to 4 wk ago, and tooth extraction 1 wk ago.

At this point, consider whether you would:

1. Cancel the Code Stroke since he is improving,
2. Cancel because of the nosebleeds and tooth extraction,
3. Continue the Code for the time being.

Upon arrival in the Emergency Department, you find that the patient was awake and alert, aphasic, with minimal speech: "yeah," "I don't know," "God damn it," "no." He had some receptive aphasia, as well. Cranial nerve examination was unremarkable. Motor power was 5/5 in all extremities at the time of examination, but there was increased tone diffusely. Sensory function and coordination appeared to be intact but were difficult owing to the patient's inability to cooperate. Reflexes in the triceps, biceps, and brachio-radialis were 2+ on the right, 3+ on the left. The lower extremities were 1+ bilaterally and symmetric. Toes were downgoing. The noncontrast CT brain scan is shown in Fig. 20A.

From: *Thrombolytic Therapy for Stroke*
Edited by: P. D. Lyden © Humana Press Inc., Totowa, NJ

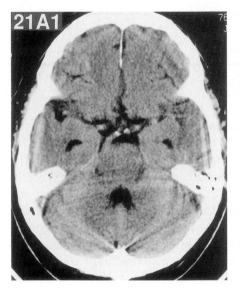 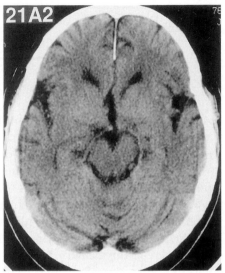

At this point, consider whether you would:

1. Offer thromboblysis since the CT scan shows no hemorrhage,
2. Obtain an ENT consult to evaluate a source of potential bleeding,
3. Cancel the Code Stroke.

The patient initially had a negative head CT and was improving in terms of his language: he was able to utter monosyllables in the ED. Therefore, he was not considered a t-PA candidate. After admission, his initial clinical symptoms did not change significantly. He continued to exhibit receptive and expressive aphasia. He showed excellent motor strength, however.

The patient underwent MRI of the brain, which showed two large lesions, anterior and posterior, left middle cerebral artery distribution, sparing his motor cortex (Fig. 21B). He had carotid ultrasounds that were negative. He had a cardiac echo that showed an intra-atrioseptal aneurysm with a positive bubble study and bi-atrial enlargement. Magnetic resonance angiography showed a paucity of vessels in the left hemisphere, consistent with emboli (Fig. 21C). He had lower extremity ultrasounds, which were negative for deep venous thrombosis. After 3 mo, the wife reported that "physically" her husband was doing fine. However, she reports that it was a rare occasion when he could get a word out. He remained blind to his right side and unable to read which she stated, "is devastating to him." "There is only so much TV one can watch."

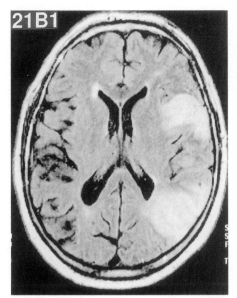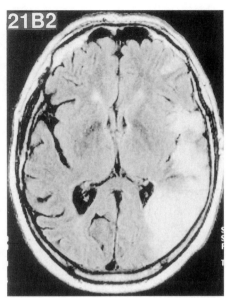

COMMENT

The protocol specifies that t-PA should not be given if a patient exhibits mild symptoms or is rapidly improving (*see* Chapters 14 and 17). It can be a very difficult judgement to decide when a patient is improving. The clinician should keep in mind that during the first 90 to 180 min after stroke, symptoms can oscillate, sometimes considerably. Oscillating symptoms rarely improve, however. In this case, the patient improved from mutism to global aphasia with a few monosyllables output. After a period of observation, no more than 20 min or so, if the patient is not improved, one could consider proceeding with thrombolysis. The vast majority of transient ischemic attacks resolve within 60 min (*1*), so if considerable improvement is not seen by then, the odds are high that the patient is suffering a stroke, not a TIA.

It is also difficult to decide what symptoms are too mild to treat. The visual field cut must have been present on admission, but was missed. The patient was also globally aphasic. Either deficit alone could have justified use of t-PA in certain patients: Homononmous hemianopsia can be disabling if the occupation involves driving or reading. In this case, the patient's avocation included reading, which may or may not justify the use of thrombolysis. Similarly, aphasia could be career-ending for some professions, and could justify use of thrombolysis for minimal symptoms. The MRI (Fig. 20B) shows the large amount of brain that was actually involved in this presentation.

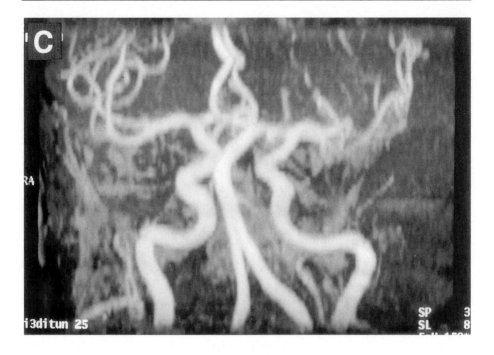

The history of nose bleeding is problematic. If the cauterization worked, presumably the site is stable enough to allow thrombolysis. However, such bleeding can be notoriously difficult to control. An ENT surgeon should be available to see the patient, should bleeding commence. The history of the tooth extraction is not a contraindication, since bleeding at such a site can be controlled with local pressure.

REFERENCE

1. Levy DE. How transient are transient ischemic attacks? *Neurology* 1988; **38:** 674–677.

INDEX

A

Abciximab, intra-arterial thrombolysis adjunctive therapy, 181

Alteplase, *see* Recombinant tissue plasminogen activator

γ-Aminobutyric acid (GABA) receptor,
agonists in neuroprotection, 50
modulators, 51
subtypes, 50

Ancrod, phase 2 clinical trials of intravenous therapy for acute ischemic stroke, 136, 137, 218

Anisoylated plasminogen streptokinase activator complex (APSAC),
activity, 14
exogenous plasminogen activation, 6, 10

α_2-Antiplasmin, fibrinolysis regulation, 16

Apoptosis,
features, 51, 52
therapeutic targets for inhibition, 52

APSAC, *see* Anisoylated plasminogen streptokinase activator complex

Arterial dissection, thrombus formation and sites, 37, 38

Aspirin, case study of thrombolytic therapy, 391–393

Atherosclerosis, large arteries, 36, 37

B

Benefits, thrombolytic therapy,
agent diversity, 217, 218
cost-effectiveness, 212
imaging independence, 215, 216
long-term results, 214, 215
subgroup selection independence, 216, 217
summary, 218, 219
variety of therapeutic medical centers, 212–214

Blood pressure,
case studies of thrombolytic therapy, 323, 324, 328, 345–348
hypertension as contraindication to thrombolytic therapy, 292, 293, 301, 345–348
monitoring following stroke, 246, 247, 302

N-tert-Butyl-α-phenylnitrone (PBN), reperfusion injury
neuroprotection, 80
therapeutic window, 77

C

Calcium flux,
calmodulin binding effects, 77
ischemic cascade role, 49

Cardioembolic stroke, *see* Embolism

Cardiopulmonary resuscitation (CPR), importance of rapid initiation, 238

Carotid dissection, case study of thrombolytic therapy, 331–335

CD18, antibody combination therapy with recombinant tissue plasminogen activator, 87

Cerebral hemorrhage, *see* Intracranial hemorrhage

Cerebral venous/sinus thrombosis, thrombolytic therapy trials, 111–114

Cincinnati Prehospital Stroke Screen (CPSS), 285, 286

Citicholine, neuroprotection, 310

Clomethiazole, recombinant tissue plasminogen activator combination therapy trials, 88

Code Stroke,
  airway management, 244, 245
  blood pressure monitoring, 246, 247, 292, 293
  box for tools and supplies, 288, 292
  breathing evaluation, 245
  case study of readiness, 337–339
  Cincinnati Prehospital Stroke Screen, 285, 286
  circulation evaluation, 245, 246
  coagulation assessment, 293
  computed tomography, 289, 290, 292, 300, 369–372
  differential diagnosis, 249, 288, 289, 297
  emergency medical services,
    first responders, 285, 286
    911 system, 285
  triage in emergency department, 286, 287
  intravenous access, 246, 247
  obstacle identification and tracking improvement, 294, 295
  pretreatment clinical pathway for thrombolytic therapy, 288, 290
  public awareness of stroke treatment urgency, 283, 284
  standing orders, 288, 289
Stroke Chain of Survival and Recovery,
  data, 247, 249
  decision, 250
  delivery, 244
  detection, 243
  dispatch, 244
  door, 244–247
  drug, 250, 251
Stroke Team,
  definition, 240
  duties, 240
  evolution, 243
  members, 239, 240
  stroke severity assessment, 247–249, 288
  system development,
    documentation, 242
    education, 242, 243
    flow charting, 240, 241
    information gathering, 241
    patient evaluation, 241
  therapy initiation time goals, 293, 294
  time of day of stroke onset, 371
  time of stroke onset determination, 287, 288, 299, 300
Computed tomography (CT),
  angiography, 265

artifacts, 316
attenuation of X-rays, 256–258
calcification of basal ganglia, 264
case studies of thrombolytic
    therapy,
    dense basilar artery sign, 349–351
    dense middle cerebral artery,
        357–361, 369, 371, 372,
        391, 392
    hypodensity in basal ganglia,
        345–347
    initiation after time limit, 313,
        316–319
    intracranial hemorrhage following
        treatment, 365, 366
    ischemic changes, 341, 342
    normal scans, 375, 376, 379,
        383, 384, 389, 395, 396
    older patients, 327, 375, 376
    parietal infarct, 337, 338
    young patients, 331, 332, 334, 381
cerebral artery occlusion, 257, 258
Code Stroke, 289, 290, 292, 300,
    369–372
consequences for thrombolytic
    therapy, 272, 275, 280
findings within first 6 h of stroke
    onset,
    incidence of findings among
        studies, 267–270
    negative findings and
        sensitivity, 265, 267
    third hour and beyond, 267
goals, 255, 256
Hounsfield Unit scale, 256, 257
intra-arterial thrombolysis patient
    selection, 176
intracranial hemorrhage, 261, 262

ischemic edema and vasodilation,
    261, 280
parenchymal hypodensity, 258–261
pathologic findings in acute
    stroke, overview, 257
perfusion imaging, 265
technique for acute stroke, 265
thrombolytic therapy requirement
    studies, 215, 216, 231–233
voxels, 256
CPR, *see* Cardiopulmonary
    resuscitation
CPSS, *see* Cincinnati Prehospital
    Stroke Screen
CT, *see* Computed tomography
Cyclohexamide, reperfusion injury
    neuroprotection, 80

D

DCLHb, *see* Diaspirin crosslinked
    hemoglobin
Desmodus salivary plasminogen
    activator (DSPA), features, 15
Diabetes, case studies of
    thrombolytic therapy, 353–
    355, 387, 388
Diaspirin crosslinked hemoglobin
    (DCLHb), middle ceerbral
    artery occlusion in animal
    models, 82, 83
DSPA, *see* Desmodus salivary
    plasminogen activator
Duteplase, *see* Recombinant tissue
    plasminogen activator

E

ECASS, *see* European Cooperative
    Acute Stroke Study
EKG, *see* Electrocardiography

Electrocardiography (EKG),
    changes in stroke, 245, 246
    myocardial infarction diagnosis
        with stroke, 300, 375–377
Embolism,
    cardiac risk factors, 31–33
    case study of onset following
        hospital admission, 357–361
    definition, 29
    donor sites for embolic material,
        30, 31
    materials of embolism, 31, 32, 34
    recipient sites and infarct patterns,
        anterior cerebral artery, 33, 34
        basilar artery, 35
        carotid arteries, 32, 33
        intracranial vertebral arteries,
            34, 35
        middle cerebral artery, 33, 34
        posterior cerebral arteries, 35
        posterior inferior cerebellar
            artery, 35
Emergency management, *see* Code
    Stroke
European Cooperative Acute Stroke
    Study (ECASS),
    computed tomography findings,
        268–272, 276–280
    ECASS-II outcomes, 147, 218
    outcomes, 143, 146, 217, 218
    patient selection, 145, 146
    therapeutic window, 145

F

Fibrin, proteolytic digestion, 3, 4
    crosslinking, 5
Fibrinogen, fragments, 10
Fibrinolysin, pre-computed
        tomography era studies, 94

Fibrinolysis,
    endogenous system,
        overview, 5, 7
        regulation, 16, 17
    plasminogen,
        activators, 6, 8
        inhibitors, 7
    thrombus dissolution, 10
Fibromuscular dysplasia (FMD),
    arterial lesions, 38
    embolism association, 30, 31
FMD, *see* Fibromuscular dysplasia

G

GABA receptor, *see* γ-Aminobutyric
    acid receptor
Glutamate, neurotoxicity, 48, 49
Granulocyte,
    antibody inhibition in
        neuroprotection therapy, 54
    neurotoxic effects, 53, 54
    no-reflow phenomenon mediation, 53
Granulomatous angiitis, case study of
    thrombolytic therapy, 389, 390

H

Hematoma,
    definition, 55
    etiology, 55, 56
    management, 56
Heparin, intra-arterial thrombolysis
    adjunctive therapy, 180, 199, 216
Hypercoagulable states, diseases,
    38, 39
Hypertension, *see* Blood pressure
Hyperthermia, minimization in
    stroke management, 305, 309

I

ICAM-1, *see* Intercellular adhesion
    molecule-1

ICH, *see* Intracranial hemorrhage
Intercellular adhesion molecule-
1 (ICAM-1), antibody in
neuroprotection therapy,
54, 55, 86, 87
Intra-arterial thrombolysis,
adjunctive therapy,
abciximab, 181
heparin, 180, 199, 216
agents, 180
case series,
carotid artery territory
occlusions, 181–183
vertebrobasilar artery territory
occlusions, 183, 186, 187
combination intravenous
thrombolysis with
recombinant tissue
plasminogen activator,
cardiology experience, 205, 206
Emergency Management of
Stroke Trial, 201–203, 206
Interventional Management of
Stroke Study, 206
prospects, 207
rationale, 201
University of Cincinnati
experience, 203–205
differential response of lesions,
226–228
indications, 190, 191
intracerebral hemorrhage risks, 188,
189
intravenous thrombosis comparison,
189
limitations, 190
patient selection, 176, 191, 192
Prolyse in Acute Cerebral
Thromboembolism trials,

PROACT I, 187, 199
PROACT II, 187, 188, 199,
200, 216
rationale, 181
technique,
catheter design, 179
diagnostic catheter, 177
recanalization, 179, 180
thrombolysis, 179
transfemoral approach, 176, 177
treatment algorithm, 190
Intracranial hemorrhage (ICH),
causes and locations, 272
computed tomography, 261, 262,
365, 366
hematoma versus hemorrhagic
infarction, 55
prevalence, 55
thrombolytic therapy complications,
clinical studies, 104, 106, 107
intra-arterial thrombolysis
risks, 188, 189
myocardial infarction
thrombolytic therapy,
dose response, 105
onset of stroke, 104
streptokinase, 104, 105,
108–110
tissue plasminogen activator,
104, 105, 108–110
prevalence, 304, 305
Ischemic cascade, overview, 47–51
Ischemic penumbra,
apoptosis versus necrosis in cell
death, 51, 52
definition, 44
duration of neuron survival, 44–46
granulocyte role, 53, 54
imaging studies, 45

neuroprotection,
  anti-intercellular adhesion
      molecule-1 antibody, 54
  combinatorial neuroprotection,
      54, 55, 79
  excitotoxicity inhibition, 47–51
  neurosteroids, 51
  rationale, 46, 47
  overview, 43, 44
  zones, 45, 46

L

Lacune, *see* Penetrating artery
    disease
Limitations, thrombolytic therapy,
  differential response of lesions,
      intra-arterial thrombolysis,
        226–228
      intravenous thrombolysis, 228, 229
  ethical considerations, 232
  patient selection criteria inclusion of
      nonvascular or nonresponsive
      conditions, 228, 230, 231, 232
  protocol, 224
  unanswered questions,
      adjunctive therapies, 225
      administration routes, 225
      agent selection and dose, 224, 225
      comparison with other
        therapies, 225
      hematological-coagulation
        factor roles, 224
Lubeluzole,
  recombinant tissue plasminogen
      activator combination therapy
      trials, 88
  reperfusion injury neuroprotection,
      80, 83

M

Magnetic resonance imaging (MRI),
  case studies of thrombolytic therapy,
      319, 328, 332, 333, 351, 380,
      381, 396, 397
  goals, 255, 256
  thrombolytic therapy requirement
      studies, 215, 216, 231–233
N-Methyl-D-aspartate (NMDA)
    receptor,
  antagonists in neuroprotection, 49
  ischemic cascade role, 48, 49
MI, *see* Myocardial infarction
Migraine, arterial vasoconstriction, 38
MK-801,
  neuroprotection in combination
      therapy, 54, 55, 82, 86
  therapeutic window, 77
MRI, *see* Magnetic resonance
    imaging
Myocardial infarction (MI),
  case study of stroke thrombolytic
      therapy, 375–378
  electrocardiographic diagnosis
      with stroke, 300, 375–377
  emergency management, 238, 239
  intra-arterial combination intravenous
      thrombolysis, 205, 206
  thrombolytic therapy, intracranial
      hemorrhagic complications,
      dose response, 105
      onset of stroke, 104
      streptokinase, 104, 105, 108–110
      tissue plasminogen activator,
        104, 105, 108–110

N

National Institute of Neurologic
    Disorders and Stroke recombinant

tissue plasminogen activator
(NINDS rt-PA) Stroke Study,
cost effectiveness analysis,
assumptions, 154–156
disability status, 156, 157
disposition results, 156, 157
implications for clinicians,
159, 160, 212
methods, 154–156
sensitivity analysis, 156–159
long-term outcome analysis,
implications for clinicians,
172, 173, 214, 215
methods, 168
multivariate analysis, 171, 172
rationale, 166, 167
recurrent stroke, 170, 171
6 month outcome, 168
survival, 170, 171
12 month outcome, 168–170
outcomes, 143–145, 198, 199
parts, 142
patient selection, 142, 143, 292, 293
prospective analysis,
necessity, 153
summary of results, 173
protocol recommendations, *see*
Recombinant tissue
plasminogen activator
stroke severity assessment,
247–249
sub-group analysis,
age effects, 161, 164
baseline covariate relationship
to outcome, 161–163
implications for clinicians,
164–166
methods, 160, 161
rationale, 160

stroke severity effects, 161
stroke subtype effects, 161
summary of results, 161, 164,
167, 216, 217
therapeutic window, 142
Necrosis,
injury triggers, 51, 52
overview, 51
Neuroprotection-thrombolytic
combination therapy,
animal model studies, 80, 82, 83,
85–87
clinical trals, 88
end points, 77, 78
neuroprotectant monotherapy
failure, 76–79
reperfusion therapy, 80
study design, 76–78
Nimodipine, neuroprotection with
MK-801, 54, 82
NINDS rt-PA Stroke Study, *see*
National Institute of Neurologic
Disorders and Stroke
recombinant tissue plasminogen
activator Stroke Study
NMDA receptor, *see* N-Methyl-D-
aspartate receptor
Nosebleed, case study of
thrombolytic therapy, 395–398

P

PAI-1, *see* Plasminogen activator
inhibitor-1
PAI-2, *see* Plasminogen activator
inhibitor-2
PAI-3, *see* Plasminogen activator
inhibitor-3
PBN, *see* N-*tert*-Butyl-α-
phenylnitrone

Penetrating artery disease, overview, 39
Plasmin,
    animal model studies of
        thrombolysis, 66, 67
    formation, 8
    function, 8
    pre-computed tomography era
        studies, 94, 96
    protein complexes, 16
Plasminogen, *see also specific*
        activators and inhibitors,
    activation, 6, 8–10
    consequences of therapeutic
        activation, 17
    forms, 8
    inhibitors, 7
    proteases, 6, 10, 11
Plasminogen activator inhibitor-1
        (PAI-1),
    induction, 16
    specificity of inhibition, 16
Plasminogen activator inhibitor-2
        (PAI-2), features, 17
Plasminogen activator inhibitor-3
        (PAI-3), features, 17
PROACT, *see* Prolyse in Acute
        Cerebral Thromboembolism
        trials
Prolyse in Acute Cerebral
        Thromboembolism trials
        (PROACT),
    PROACT I, 187, 199
    PROACT II, 187, 188, 199, 200, 216
Public awareness, stroke treatment
        urgency, 283, 284, 298, 299

R

Recombinant tissue plasminogen
        activator (rt-PA),

animal model studies of cerebral
        ischemia, 19
animal model studies of thrombolysis,
    analog analysis, 71
    baboon, 69
    clinical prediction, 77, 78
    overview, 66, 68
    rabbit, 66, 69, 70, 83, 85, 86
    rat, 87
anti-CD18 antibody combination
        therapy, 87
anti-intercellular adhesion molecule-1
        antibody combination therapy,
        55, 86, 87
case studies, 313–398
contraindications, 18
cost effectiveness analysis, *see*
        National Institute of Neurologic
        Disorders and Stroke
        recombinant tissue plasminogen
        activator Stroke Study
differential response of lesions,
        228, 229
end points in clinical trials, 77, 78
intra-arterial thrombolysis,
    carotid artery occlusions, 182,
        183, 200
    combination with intravenous
        thrombosis,
    cardiology experience, 205,
        206
    Emergency Management of
        Stroke Trial, 201–203,
        206
    Interventional Management
        of Stroke Study, 206
    prospects, 207
    rationale, 201

University of Cincinnati
experience, 203–205
intracranial hemorrhage risks, 56,
101, 198, 304, 305
ischemic complications, 110, 111
limitations, 198, 199
MK-801 combination therapy, 54, 86
mutants, 15, 16, 71
National Institute of Neurologic
Disorders and Stroke protocol
recommendations,
development, 298
dosage, 293, 302
laboratory tests, 300–303
medical history, 300
nonspecific therapy, 305
patient selection criteria, 301,
302, 304
prospects, 305, 306
rationale, 298
time of onsert determination,
299, 300
Web sites, 298, 299
neuroprotection combination
therapy clinical studies, 88
phase 2 clinical trials of intravenous
therapy for acute ischemic
stroke,
controlled trials,
alteplase, 136, 137
duteplase, 135, 136
historical perspective, 129, 130
open-label trials,
alteplase, 131–135
dose escalation studies, 133
duteplase, 130–132
summary of results, 137, 138
platelet function effects, 17

posttreatment monitoring, 251,
302, 303
randomized clinical trials, *see also*
European Cooperative Acute
Stroke Study; National Institute
of Neurologic Disorders and
Stroke recombinant tissue
plasminogen activator Stroke
Study,
Alantis study, 145
historical perspective, 141, 142
therapeutic window, 3, 72, 92, 148,
151, 198
Reperfusion injury, neuroprotection
studies, 80
Riluzole, neuroprotection, 47
rt-PA, *see* Recombinant tissue
plasminogen activator

S

scu-PA, *see* Single-chain urokinase
plasminogen activator
Seizure, case study of thrombolytic
therapy, 383–386
Single-chain urokinase plasminogen
activator (scu-PA),
conversion of proenzyme, 12
endogenous plasminogen activation,
6, 10
SK, *see* Streptokinase
Staphylokinase (STK),
exogenous plasminogen activation,
6, 10
protein complexes, 14, 15
STK, *see* Staphylokinase
Streptokinase (SK),
animal model studies of
thrombolysis, 66, 67
elimination kinetics, 14

exogenous plasminogen activation,
        6, 10, 14
intra-arterial thrombolysis,
        carotid artery territory
                occlusions, 181, 182
        vertebrobasilar artery territory
                occlusions, 186
ischemic complications, 110
myocardial infarction thrombolytic
        therapy and intracranial
        hemorrhagic complications,
        104, 105, 108–110
post-computed tomography era,
        early studies, 97, 99, 100, 102
pre-computed tomography era
        studies, 96
protein complexes, 14
randomized clinical trials,
        Australian Streptokinase Trial,
                148
        Multicenter Acute Stroke
                Trial–Europe, 148, 150
        Multicenter Acute Stroke
                Trial–Italy, 150
        summary of results, 149, 150
therapeutic window, 148, 151
Stroke Chain of Survival and
        Recovery, *see* Code Stroke
Stroke Team, *see* Code Stroke

T

Thrombin, function, 4, 5
Thrombolysin, pre-computed
        tomography era studies, 94, 96
Thrombolytic therapy, *see also*
        specific agents,
        benefits, *see* Benefits,
                thrombolytic therapy
        case studies, 313–398

cerebral venous/sinus thrombosis
        trials, 111–114
hemorrhagic cerebrovascular
        disease treatment, early
        studies,
        intracerebral hemorrhage, 115
        intraventricular hemorrhage, 116
        subarachnoid hemorrhage, 115,
                116
imaging requirement studies, 215,
        216, 231–233
intra-arterial thrombolysis, *see*
        Intra-arterial thrombolysis
        intracranial hemorrhagic
        complications,
        clinical studies, 104, 106, 107
myocardial infarction
        thrombolytic therapy,
        dose response, 105
        onset of stroke, 104
        streptokinase, 104, 105, 108–110
        tissue plasminogen activator,
                104, 105, 108–110
ischemic complications, 110, 111
legal cases, 368
limitations, *see* Limitations,
        thrombolytic therapy
neuroprotectant combination
        therapy, *see* Neuroprotection-
        thrombolytic combination
        therapy
post-computed tomography era,
        early studies,
        overview, 98
        small series and case reports,
                102–104
        streptokinase, 97, 99, 100, 102
        tissue plasminogen activator,
                100–102

urokinase, 97, 99, 100, 102
pre-computed tomography era
    studies,
    fibrinolysin, 94
    limitations of studies, 92, 93
    plasmin, 94, 96
    streptokinase, 96
    thrombolysin, 94, 96
    urokinase, 96, 97
prospects, 309, 310
successful outcome factors, 117
therapeutic window, 92, 233
training and community experiences,
    212–214, 232, 233
Thrombus,
    arterial dissection, 37, 38
    atherosclerosis of large arteries, 36,
        37
    dissolution, *see* Fibrinolysis
        formation,
        fibrin crosslinking, 5
        overview, 4, 5
Time of onset, determination for stroke,
    287, 288, 299, 300, 366, 367
Tissue plasminogen activator, *see also*
    Recombinant tissue plasminogen
    activator,
    cell types in expression, 12
    cerebral tissue activity, 18, 19
    domains, 11
    endogenous plasminogen activation,
        6, 10
    forms, 12
    myocardial infarction thrombolytic
        therapy and intracranial
        hemorrhagic complications,
        104, 105, 108–110
    post-computed tomography era,
        early studies, 100–102

stimulation of release, 5, 12
Trauma,
    field resuscitation, 238
    rapid response teams, 237, 238
    time window for major trauma, 238
Triage, *see* Code Stroke

U

u-PA, *see* Urokinase plasminogen
    activator
Urokinase,
    animal model studies,
        global ischemia, 72
        thrombolysis, 66, 67
    intra-arterial thrombolysis,
        carotid artery territory
            occlusions, 181–183
        Prolyse in Acute Cerebral
            Thromboembolism trials,
            187, 188, 199, 200
        rationale, 180
        recombinant prourokinase,
            180, 187, 188
        vertebrobasilar artery territory
            occlusions, 186
    limitations of intravenous
        therapy, 200
    post-computed tomography era,
        early studies, 97, 99, 100, 102
    pre-computed tomography era
        studies, 96, 97
Urokinase plasminogen a
    ctivator (u-PA),
    cerebral tissue activity, 18
    domains, 13
    endogenous plasminogen
        activation, 6, 10
    exogenous plasminogen
        activation, 13

forms, 13
processing, 12

V

Vampire bat salivary plasminogen
    activator (Bat-PA), features, 15